The Personal Computer for Speech, Language, and Hearing Professionals

The Personal Computer for Speech, Language, and Hearing Professionals

Edited by

Jerry L. Northern, Ph.D.

Professor of Otolaryngology,
University of Colorado School of Medicine;
Head, Audiology Division,
University of Colorado Health Sciences Center,
Denver

Little, Brown and Company
Boston/Toronto

First Edition

Library of Congress Catalog Card No. 85-82262

ISBN 0-316-611972

Printed in the United States of America

DON

Contents

Preface

A new generation of electronics is upon us, and we find ourselves in an age of computers that invade our lives and manage nearly every aspect of our existence. Ten years ago, we could not have predicted that the personal computer would be so highly developed and readily available at low cost for use in our homes and our offices, offering untapped potential for speech-language-hearing applications. The incredible usefulness of the personal computer, and the ease with which it can be adapted to a wide variety of daily tasks, makes knowledge of small-computer technology a necessity for all communication-disorders specialists.

For the most part, speech-language practitioners and audiologists have been hesitant to utilize computer technology. Our reactions perhaps are based on the fact that the wave of computer information struck following completion of our graduate coursework, and, after all . . . "computers are so complex and expensive" . . . "I just don't have a computer mind" . . . "we have never had a computer, so why do we need one now?" The purpose of this book is to address these common excuses, and at the same time provide a basic introduction to the fascinating world of microcomputers.

The Personal Computer for Speech, Language, and Hearing Professionals was developed for those working in speech-language pathology and audiology who have a real interest to include computers in their daily professional lives. It is also aimed at the rest (including students) who know little or nothing about personal computers, except that everybody seems to be talking in "computerese." Or perhaps there is a small computer in the clinic that is not used very often—and what can be done with it? Many must have a general curiosity about how personal computers are used in various areas of the communication-disorders field. My most optimistic hope is that if we have a textbook available on microcomputer applications in speech and hearing, specialized courses for students will be included in university curricula.

The text has been written specifically for the nontechnical background of most speech-language pathologists and audiologists. Although literally hundreds of "how to" computer books are available at your local neighborhood bookstore, this text has been written by experts who are actively involved in speech, language, and hearing applications with personal computers. The intent is to provide a readable, useful textbook. Because of the variety of employment settings, chapters have been included that will interest clinicians and researchers, the private practitioner, the university-oriented instructor, and the undergraduate and graduate student majoring in speech, language, special education, or audiology.

The chapters deal with various aspects of personal computing and speech-language pathology and audiology professional issues. Following my introductory chapter, Michael Seilo of Western Washington University and William Yost of Loyola University have written chapters dealing with selection of the basic components of personal computers and the basic operation of microcomputers. Chapter 4, prepared by Gary E. Rushakoff, Director of the Microcomputer Laboratory at New Mexico State University, discusses computer-based client-record management. Jackson Roush and Yoshiyuki Horii present an outstanding description in Chapter 5 of how microcomputers may be used for a wide variety of tasks within the university speech and hearing program.

The next six chapters deal with various patient-oriented uses of personal computers including the use of personal computers in speech disorders programs (R. Ann Howard), applications in aphasia and head trauma (Russell Mills), microcomputers in language assessment, intervention and enhancement (Mary Wilson and Bernard Fox), applications in the area of audiology and hearing measurement (Brad Stach and James Jerger), computer technology in school and industrial mass hearing screening programs (David Lipscomb and Russell Fankhouser) and an excellent discussion of computer-assisted instruction for hearing-impaired students by Donald Sims and E. William Clymer of the National Technical Institute for the Deaf in Rochester, New York.

The last sections of this book deal with more technical aspects of personal computer utilization. Conrad LaRiviere and John Sherblom discuss the rapidly developing area of speech synthesis and speech recognition. James Curran and David Preves cover the comprehensive area of computer intervention in various aspects of hearing aid design, manufacture, assessment, fitting and management. James Murphy, a biometrics statistician, discusses elementary computer application in research design and analysis. In the final chapter, Larry Ball, Charlie D. Anderson, and Christopher Schweitzer present a useful summary of the use of microcomputers in office management procedures.

Fred D. Minifie, past-president of the American Speech and Hearing Association (ASHA), summarized our current professional status with personal computers in a speech delivered in Las Vegas in 1984 (*Asha*, 26:6, 1984). Dr. Minifie stated, "From the perspective of speech-language pathology and audiology, we must recognize that personal computers are simply one tool which can be used to enhance the quality of services provided by our profession. With the heady swirl of the rapid expansion of personal computers it is easy to stand back and admire the new products and fail to get on with the important business of *using* the computer technologies to our advantage."

This book is in no way intended to be comprehensive on the topic of personal computers, but rather our purpose is to stimulate thought and action by speech-language-hearing professionals who work with the communicatively disabled. On behalf of all the contributing authors, I hope that the interested reader will have a difficult time holding back enthusiasm for hands-on practice with a personal computer. And then it is just a small step to think about the many possible microcomputer applications that can enhance our professional activities.

J. L. N.

Contributing Authors

Charlie D. Anderson, M.S.E.E.
President, And/Or Corp., Golden, Colorado

Larry L. Ball, Ph.D.
President, American Cyber Med, Ltd., Atherton, California

E. William Clymer, M.S., M.B.A.
Assistant Professor and Instructional Developer, Department of Communication Research, National Institute for the Deaf, Rochester Institute of Technology, Rochester, New York

James Curran, M.S.
Research Audiologist, Starkey Laboratories, Inc., Eden Prairie, Minnesota

Russell J. Fankhouser, M.S.
Edatauga Hearing Conservation, Inc., Johnson City, Tennessee

Bernard J. Fox, B.S.
Vice President, Laureate Learning Systems, Inc., Burlington, Vermont

Yoshiyuki Horii, Ph.D.
Professor, Department of Communication Disorders and Speech Science, University of Colorado, Boulder, Colorado

R. Ann Howard, M.A.
Vice President, MAXXAM Dataware, and Speech-Language Pathologist, Lakewood, Colorado

James F. Jerger, Ph.D.
Professor of Audiology, Baylor College of Medicine, Houston, Texas

Conrad LaRiviere, Ph.D.
Associate Professor, Department of Audiology, University of Maine at Orono, Orono, Maine

David M. Lipscomb, Ph.D.
Professor of Audiology and Speech Pathology, University of Tennessee, Knoxville, Tennessee

Russell H. Mills, Ph.D.
Director, Brain-Link Software; Senior Speech Pathologist, Audiology and Speech Pathology Service, Veterans Administration Medical Center, Ann Arbor, Michigan

James R. Murphy, Ph.D.
Associate Professor, Department of Preventive Medicine and Biometrics, University of Colorado School of Medicine, Denver

Jerry L. Northern, Ph.D.
Professor of Otolaryngology, University of Colorado School of Medicine; Head Audiology Division, University of Colorado Health Sciences Center, Denver

David Preves, Ph.D.
Starkey Laboratories, Inc., Eden Prairie, Minnesota

Jackson Roush, Ph.D.
Assistant Professor, Department of Communication Disorders and Speech Science, University of Colorado, Boulder, Colorado

Gary E. Rushakoff, Ph.D.
Assistant Professor, Division of Communication Disorders, New Mexico State University, Las Cruces, New Mexico

Christopher Schweitzer, Ph.D.
Vice President, And/Or Corp., Golden, Colorado

Michael T. Seilo, Ph.D.
Chair, Department of Speech Pathology/Audiology, Western Washington University, Bellingham, Washington

John Sherblom, M.A.
Programmer/Analyst, Computing Center, University of Maine at Orono, Orono, Maine

Donald G. Sims, Ph.D.
Associate Professor, Rochester Institute of Technology; Research Associate, Department of Communication Research, National Technical Institute for the Deaf, Rochester Institute of Technology, Rochester, New York

Brad A. Stach, M.A.
Director of Clinical Services, Audiology Service, The Methodist Hospital, Houston, Texas

Mary Sweig Wilson, Ph.D.
Professor of Communication Science and Disorders, University of Vermont; President, Laureate Learning Systems, Inc., Burlington, Vermont

William A. Yost, Ph.D.
Director, Parmly Hearing Institute, and Professor of Psychology and Otolaryngology, Loyola University of Chicago, Chicago, Illinois

The Personal Computer for Speech, Language, and Hearing Professionals

1

The Personal Computer as a Professional Tool

Jerry L. Northern

Let there be no doubt, we are in the Computer Age. Our society is almost totally controlled by computers. The personal computer is the tool of the 1980s, and if you are not already working with your own computer, you will be soon. The personal computer is a fantastic asset, and not a fad, passing fancy, or short-term whim. And the good news is that you do not have to be a "nerd" to learn how to incorporate personal computers into your daily professional life. You just need an open and inquisitive mind and a commitment to set aside time to ingest this innovation.

There is a difference between *using a computer* and *personally computing*. Personal computing is the interaction between a desk-top computer and an individual. The personal computer is entirely under the control of the individual who turns it on, decides what operations to work on, and shuts it off when the day's task is completed. Personal computing is like an individual fitness program—you get as much out of it as you are willing to put into it. Personal computing is similar to learning a new sport—it is fun even for a beginner, and it gets better as your skills increase.

The personal computer is only a tool, and it will never replace the professional. Nearly every profession these days depends on computers in some fashion: business, banking, insurance, law, travel, engineering, publishing, art, medicine, communications, etc. Nevertheless, speech-language-hearing professionals, those individuals who specialize in the identification and management of communication disorders, have been slow to accept and develop computer programs to assist them in their daily duties.

Personal computing can quickly improve your outlook on life. You do not *have* to know about bytes and bits, but the more you know, the more you will be able to derive from your computer. Professionals do not necessarily do more work with their computers, but they tend to do better work, more efficiently, with ample time for review and revision. The personal computer will help you do tasks that you already do, while leaving time for you to conduct new projects. Chances are, at this time you do not know all the applications you will be able to achieve with your personal computer. New users often admit, "I had no idea this could be done with a computer!"

The personal computer is a master at managing tedious and routine tasks without error. It "crunches" number problems with ease and presents facts and figures with speed and accuracy previously unimagined. The benefits of having a personal computer on your desk include easy completion of all writing tasks, incredible accuracy and precision in record keeping, standardization of tasks and data collection, and increased availability of patient records in a format that lends itself to easy data collection, retrieval, and storage. You will have more facts and figures at hand to help you extrapolate, evaluate, and make better decisions than ever before.

But some cautionary statements are in order. The personal computer is so useful that you might find yourself wallowing in an overabundance of irrelevant information and data. It is easy to be swept up in a consumer's frenzy to buy at least one of every piece of hardware—some of which you may never use—leaving you financially strapped when you want to purchase the software you need to accomplish the tasks for which you bought the computer. Most important, you must have a commitment to interact with the computer *yourself*. Too often the system is purchased by the professional and then dropped in the lap of a secretary or assistant without instruction. Computer manuals are notoriously poor when you get stuck in the middle of a software program, or the screen freezes in "gridlock," or when a keystroke is forgotten, the wrong command is inadvertently struck, and you find you cannot get back to the proper place in the program without losing all the data entered.

An important but intangible cost of the computer is professional time. You can lose hours of work in an instant with a single incorrect keystroke. One of the most important assets of the personal computer as a professional tool is that it conducts mundane tasks in a new light. Working with your computer can be fun, and your efforts will unconsciously stimulate new outlooks and approaches to daily tasks (Fig. 1-1). The personal computer has been called an imagination machine, and it truly is limited only by the user's creativity. There are always new frontiers to be tamed with your computer; you will be able to reach new heights and accomplish tasks with ease that you never thought possible.

The personal computer is not a panacea for your problems, but you surely will understand why your professional friends who use a computer say, "I wonder how I ever got along without it." Professionals tend to use their computers in five different areas: (1) managing information files and numbers, (2) writing, (3) education, (4) converting figures into easily understood graphics, and (5) communicating with other computers and other professionals. Following a general discussion about how to get started in personal computing, this chapter will present information about each of these applications.

GETTING STARTED IN PERSONAL COMPUTING

According to some authors, the personal computer is "the most important invention since fire," or "the most significant event since man climbed down from the trees." It is truly incredible that the first personal computers arrived on the scene in 1977. It is estimated that 15% of the American population now has a personal computer at work or at home, and some three million units were sold in 1984. The *Complete Sourcebook of Personal Computing* (Bowker, 1984) indicates that there are now at least 400 computer manufacturers and 1000 peripheral hardware items such as disk drives, printers, and cathode-ray tube (CRT) screens.

The typical professional person attacks new problems by reaching for something to read. In the field of personal computing, it is easy to in-

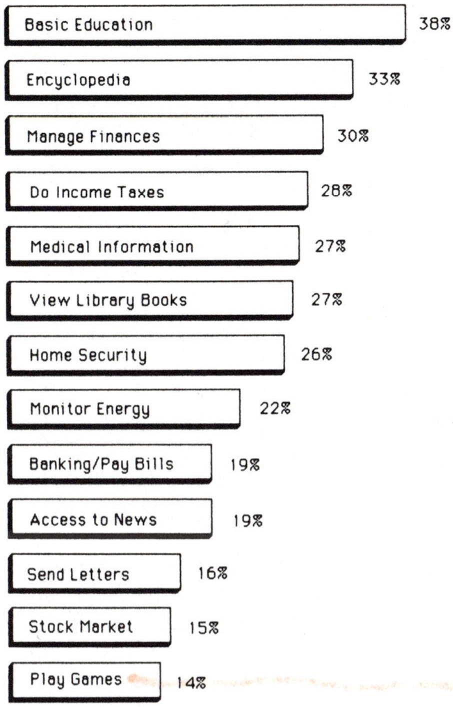

Fig. 1-1. *Results of a survey conducted by* USA Today *concerning the services people are "very interested" in having computers provide.*

undate yourself with reading material. There are at least 3000 books on personal computers at the time of this writing (make that 3001 with the publication of this book), and magazine racks are about to collapse under the weight of the growing number of computer magazines. *Popular Computing* and *Personal Computing* are good introductory general magazines, whereas *Creative Computing* offers more technically oriented articles. Specialized magazines devoted to particular personal computers are also good reading and include *Macworld, Applesoft, Softalk,* and *Incider* for the Apple Computer family, and *Peanut* and *PC World* for the IBM systems. Other excellent sources of computer information are the users' groups located in most cities; more than 1100 clubs have been organized across the nation.

It is important to decide what you want to use a computer for before you buy one. Otherwise, the computer is likely to be just a dust collector. Although first-time buyers can hesitate too long, being too meticulous and careful, you must thoroughly consider exactly what problems the new computer will help resolve. Never buy a computer as an instant answer to a problem. Buy the computer during a slack period, before the emergency of a pressing problem, so you will have time to orient yourself to the basic operation of the unit. It bears repeating that there are no shortcuts to learning about personal computers. You must be prepared to set aside nights and weekends to read the manuals and work on the basic operational procedures. No one else can learn it for you, and there is absolutely no substitute for hands-on experience.

It is no longer acceptable to believe that computer users must be, first and foremost, computer programmers. In the early days, everyone had to develop and write his or her own programs. And it is still a deterrent to people who enroll in basic computer courses that the instructors initially teach computer programming. There is no doubt that it is useful to understand the logic of programming, but the large majority of today's professionals use computers with commercially available software and little or no knowledge of programming.

Software is the vital link to successful computing. Without software, the computer is just a hunk of plastic, metal, and silicon. At least 1000 companies manufacture software, and it is estimated that there exist nearly 40,000 software packages, including some 1300 public data bases available to anyone who wishes to subscribe to or pay for them. According to *Newsweek* magazine, software sales in 1984 were expected to exceed $1.5 billion. Computer magazines publish monthly best-seller lists of software in categories such as games, home use, education, business, and word processing. New applications for your personal computer usually are accomplished with new software, not new hardware.

Experts indicate that today's hardware is at an evolutionary peak, and that we are unlikely to see any significant hardware advances in the immediate future. Today's emphasis in computer advancement lies in the development of software. A new generation of software, known as integrated software, combines many routine applications such as a data-base program, a word-processing program, and a graphics program into one piece. Integrated software eliminates the need to change programs and retype information when you want to include data from a spread sheet into a written report or letter. With integrated software, when you change a number in the spread sheet, the corresponding figures in related word-processing and graphic documents automatically change also.

A clever essay by Quinn (1983) divided potential computer users into two groups, *R-people* and *S-people*. He described R-people as persons who are comfortable with syntactic reasoning and symbolic conclusions that are devoid of "meaning." R-people are happier dealing with models of reality than with reality itself, and they often deal in generalizations and abstractions. R-people probably already own computer equipment and are involved in writing their own programs. The other group, S-people, think in terms of meaning rather than symbols and regard themselves as "practical-minded." These people are more interested in the outcome than in the process. S-people are goal-directed and productive. Quinn thinks these qualities orient S-people toward well-designed "friendly" computer systems with practical analysis and writing capabilities.

As a final word on getting started in personal computing, take the time to review the chapters in this textbook to gain appreciation of the wide variety of possible applications for professionals working in the area of communication disorders. Beware of hidden costs such as training time, additional software, extra hardware, and input/output circuit boards, and give careful consideration to the ergonomics of computer use—a comfortable chair, table, lights, expendable supplies, a power-surge protector, dirt and dust protectors, etc.—and stop procrastinating and making excuses for not getting started with your own personal computer.

INFORMATION MANAGEMENT

To many professionals the most useful application of a personal computer is as an information management tool. The term *information management* refers to a centralized collection of stored data that an individual can call up—in its entirety or in part—for display on a screen or in hardcopy format. In data-base programs, this information can be handled in a variety of ways, including searching and index identification, arithmetical manipulation, reporting capabilities, data-sequencing alternatives, matching-merging or updating two or more separate collections of information (data files), hierarchical or relational file structures, table look-up capability, etc. Is it any wonder that data-base management programs are among the most widely used computer software?

The electronic spread sheet is often a key portion of an information management system. Using the computer keyboard, you fill out rows and columns with data numbers. You can instruct the computer to manage the cells created by the crossing of a row and a column to be added, subtracted, multiplied, or divided with any other cell value. In addition, you can calculate percentages and averages wherever you need them. When you want to evaluate the "bottom line" after changing the figure in one cell, the computer can perform all the necessary calculations to keep the spread sheet balanced. As a forecasting tool, the electronic spread sheet has no equal, since you can manipulate all the figures until you find the best combination of facts to help you reach your goal.

One aspect of an efficient information management system is that it can reduce the amount of paper you deal with on a daily basis. It has been said that the vast majority of all paper you place in the traditional file folder is never used again—because it cannot be found easily, or because the contents become dated or forgotten. The data base created for personal use can provide base line or reference data from which you can derive statistical information and group or individual performance trends, which can then be applied to the assessment of future needs.

There are at least 6000 data bases maintained by colleges for their researchers, by trade organizations for their members, and by companies that provide information services for their customers. Many data bases supply abstracts or summaries of published materials. A tremendous resource is the availability of topical bibliographies that can be searched by subject area, author, journal or book title, year, etc. Most computer data bases are also cross-indexed so a searcher can arrange the printout of a bibliography in alphabetical order of the author's last name or in chronological order by date of publication. These software systems have progressed so far that some programs even "read" every word in an abstract or summary (or even the entire article, if it is on file) and identify all the items that contain the key words in which you are interested.

Related forms of information management software are programs that let you create your own bibliographies. With a little diligent attention to keeping such bibliographies up to date, you can cross-index an incredible collection of journal articles for use by students and colleagues, or in your next research proposal. With careful planning and consistent data entry, your computer video screen can become your own personal reference librarian.

Anything you do that generates lists or written records can be done better with an information management program. To be sure, this application has been carried out *ad nauseam*, with software to help you with Christmas card lists, telephone numbers, recipe and food-shopping information—most of which really can be done with less trouble by pencil, paper, and index cards. On the other hand, many people use their personal computers effectively for such lists. Inventory and operational schedules often are monitored through computerized information database systems.

A properly used information management system can help you generate profiles, perform analyses, and organize reference materials that would be prohibitively time-consuming if done manually. Be warned, however, the price of such an information-access system is a lot of keyboarding by someone to make the initial transfer of data from paper to computer, as well as the time and cost required to update the computer entries.

WORD PROCESSING

Every professional working in speech, language, and hearing has volumes of writing to face every day. Our writing requires all kinds of formats including general correspondence, patient progress notes, memorandums to colleagues, hospital-chart reports, news items, journal articles, and maybe even chapters or entire books. Anyone who uses a pencil and can type—no matter how slowly—will benefit immediately from the use of word-processing software and a printer for his or her personal computer. Word processing with a computer is probably the single best way to simplify your writing chores.

Typically, a word processor stores your first draft on a disk, while you review your words on the computer screen. You may choose to print your draft out on paper to be corrected by hand, or you may choose to correct it by manipulating the word-processing program in the edit mode. In the edit mode, you move a cursor through the material, correcting spelling, rearranging words and paragraphs, and deleting or moving sentences as necessary. In fact, you can reorder entire pages of text if you wish. The advantage to making corrections on material stored in the computer is that the entire manuscript does not have to be retyped to include the corrections and changes. The word processor's printing program usually lets you decide the margins, spacing, line justification, placement of titles and page numbers, etc., so the final printed manuscript looks neat and professional. Since the corrections are done in the computer, your documents and letters will no longer include erasure scars and globs of correction fluid.

Word processing is the most common application of personal computers, and it is not too much to say that the technique has revolutionized writing, according to Fluegelman and Hewes (1983) in their excellent book, *Writing in the Computer Age*. Word processing does not really help you write better, but it does make the task of setting down the words considerably easier. A word-processing program is a stimulating boost, a new kind of tool that permits you to outline, draft ideas, arrange your thoughts, fill in the gaps, correct technical errors, check your writing style, fix errors in spelling and punctuation, and then print out a perfect version.

A number of valuable related programs are easily added to the word-processing procedure. These programs include spelling "dictionaries" that scan each word in your document and highlight words that are spelled incorrectly. A proofreading program scans your document in seconds, and correction of a single error in the manuscript causes the computer to correct the error automatically throughout the document. Programs are also available to check grammar and punctuation. Other special programs include a thesaurus to help you find synonyms and a mail-list merger. The mail-list merger can take a list of names and addresses from a separate program and merge them with a letter. With such a program you can avoid retyping the same document over and over (perhaps changing only the names of the people addressed), and you have your own mass-mailing system. With a quick change from computer paper to mailing labels, your mail-merge program can run a list of addresses by alphabetical order of names or numerical order of zip codes for easy bulk bundling, or the mail-merge can be instructed to scan the entire mailing list to cull out mailing labels for certain groups that you identified previously, such as speech-language pathologists, physicians, or certain agencies.

All creative writing is improved by review and revision. The word processor makes laborious corrections fun and easy. The personal computer cannot evaluate the content of your writing, but it can produce a clean manuscript in minimal time with minimal pain and effort (Bates, 1984). Furthermore, it is a simple matter to create a standard format for referral letters, or to fill in a form letter to describe the results of a hearing evaluation and hearing-aid fitting, or the results of a language evaluation in a 4-year-old youngster.

TELECOMMUNICATION APPLICATION

Telecommunication innovations not only are altering the ways in which computer users communicate with colleagues, acquire information, shop, and bank, but also are providing a system for working at home. All that is needed is (1) a personal computer, (2) a tone telephone, (3) a special serial card that converts the information in the computer to units that can be relayed on the telephone, (4) a communications software package, and (5) a modem.

The modem (a short name for modulate-demodulate) cradles the telephone receiver and translates the computer's binary language into tones that a telephone can understand (modulation) and reconverts incoming tones into binary language that the receiving computer can understand (demodulation). Modems operate at different speeds, typically 300 baud or 1200 baud (300 bits per second or 1200 bits per second). Most modems used in business are 1200 baud and cost \$300 to \$600; the 300-baud units cost less, \$80 to \$250. It is useful to have a software system that includes automatic dial and answering programs.

Telecommunication offers a speedy way to disseminate information through an open communications system. Also known as electronic mail, the system is not exactly like written mail, nor is it exactly like communicating through the telephone. It offers an entirely new form of communication that speech-language-hearing clinicians have been slow to accept and use.

Utilization of the electronic communications network requires careful management and planning, but such a system could tie together a group of professionals who wish to share data or debate some clinical problem.

Electronic mail saves time in communication and is, in fact, cheaper than other means of speedy mail including overnight carrier or Express Mail. Such a system provides for completeness of thought and understanding, and works as quickly as you can type the information onto your computer screen. Telecommunication sends the message directly from your personal computer to various electronic storage receptacles, where the message waits to be retrieved, read, and, if necessary, responded to at the receiver's convenience.

The idea of two computers communicating with each other does sound a bit bizarre, but the opportunity for teleconferences is wide open. Everything can be written and waiting in files, including assignments and discussions, and any member of the conference can review a manuscript, make changes, or contribute comments as appropriate. A number of electronic mail services are available, offering subscribers information such as updated stock market quotations or even airline schedules.

The modem input/output device makes it possible for professionals to work at home with a computer and send material directly to the office computer, where it will be waiting in the morning for the office staff. It is an interesting comment on office business that whenever any of us has a really important project to complete, we stay at home to do it! Many businesses now permit staff members to work at home with their computers, since studies show that nearly half of the time spent in the office is devoted to nonbusiness activities.

EDUCATIONAL APPLICATIONS

The outlook for the use of personal computers in education is absolutely phenomenal. The number of personal and desk-top computers in elementary, middle, and high schools is growing by leaps and bounds. Youngsters have a definite advantage over adults by being born into the Computer Age and accepting computers in their daily activities without apprehension. Today's students seem to have an innate aptitude for sitting down at a computer keyboard and getting right into the task at hand. The students understand simple programming and simple graphics. The home computer has put a whole new slant on the age-old problems related to homework.

Education through computer instruction is easy in the familiar environment of home, school, or office. Suddenly there is a thin line between education and entertainment. Surveys show that nearly 50% of home computers are used entirely for entertainment, in spite of the attempt to install the computer in the home as an educational tool. The computer is a patient, consistent tutor that can innovatively present new material. Repetitive drill work is now a video game, and many of the exercises are enhanced with brilliant splashes of color and clever graphics.

Educational software packages are overwhelming in number and cover fields from aeronautics to zoology. Packages are available to help students prepare for all types of standardized examinations, from the Scholastic Aptitude Test (SAT) to pre–law and pre–medical school examinations, as well as the Graduate Record Examination (GRE). Foreign-language programs abound and are outnumbered only by business-oriented educational courses such as finance and accounting. You can even learn to type with a computer program that reports your speed per minute, identifies keys that need additional practice, and presents practice work in ever-changing random sequences.

Of course, much of the clinical activity related to speech, language, and hearing therapy is, in fact, educational in nature. A mistake that clinicians may make is thinking that placing a client in front of a personal computer will automatically resolve all problems. There is no question that educational software is far more effective when the clinician and the client (child or adult) work at the computer together, even if only for a short time during the therapy session. In fact, a lack of proper supervision and commitment may make the computer worthless as a therapy aid.

Knowledge of computer-assisted educational techniques should be of incredible value to the practicing communication-disorders specialist. The computer's ability to interact with the client can provide hours of innovative therapy with repetitive drill practice. We are on the forefront of a whole new world of computer-assisted therapy. Suffice it to say that most of the clinically oriented chapters in this book deal with educational and therapeutic applications of personal computers.

GRAPHIC APPLICATIONS

Graphics programs let you convert numbers to charts and graphs, often in the colors of your choice. Today's graphics software is incredibly simple to use on a personal computer. Anyone who needs charts and graphs for documents and presentations can create them as easily as answering questions on the screen about the data to be charted. The personal computer automatically sizes and scales your numbers to fit the chart you select. You will see on the screen a preview of the information in several graphic formats (bar graphs, pie charts, etc.) before you commit the graph to hard copy with your printer. Current printers are capable of printing in color—assuming you can afford a color printer.

Graphics programs can help you make sense of rows and columns of data. As you change the data, the charts change automatically. Graphic software will let you quickly show data in relation to other data, or pre- and post-treatment analyses. Even the simplest graphics programs will display data in a wide variety of formats including basic bar graphs, stacked bar graphs, multiple bar graphs, line graphs (with a variety of line configurations), area graphs, pie charts, or any combination thereof, such as a combination line chart and bar graph. Some software programs include a graphics illustrator feature that lets the user start from scratch and draw images on the screen to fit any particular need.

Modeling-type programs are used to predict trends. Perhaps the most common type of model is the architectural type that shows in scaled format what a final construction will look like. Manipulation of the model is also possible with a personal computer. Mass storage and data manipulation techniques are quite well developed for the desk-top computer and are constantly being improved. A number of three-dimensional graphics packages are available that enable you to draw three-dimensional objects on the two-dimensional screen. The object drawn can be nested, rotated on any axis, put into motion, or moved around the screen while your viewing perspective is moved independently. Of course, all these functions can be stored on disks or printed out as hard copy.

Graphics are presented in either low-resolution or high-resolution format. The low-resolution format is so simple to program that school-aged children can learn to create pictures on a personal computer in very little time. Naturally, the pictures are considerably rougher than graphics drawn to high resolution where every dot on the screen is programmed. High-resolution graphics are often associated with advanced software programs, while low-resolution graphics may be sufficient for certain therapeutic activities or simple video games.

A final use of graphics for the professional is the creation of color charts that can be photographed with a standard 35-mm camera to produce slides for oral presentations. High-quality slides are easily made with such a system, although some experimentation is required to identify the proper settings for the camera.

REFERENCES

Bates, P. How to turn your writing into communication. *Personal Computing* 8:60–67, 1984.

Bowker's Complete Sourcebook of Personal Computing. New York: Bowker, 1984.

Fluegelman, A., and Hewes, J. J. *Writing in the Computer Age: Word Processing Skills & Style for Every Writer.* New York: Doubleday, 1983.

Quinn, F. B., Jr. What to do about computers. *Arch. Otolaryngol.* 109: 243–244, 1983.

2

Considerations in Selecting a Microcomputer System

Michael T. Seilo

The future is now with respect to microcomputer use in the pathology and audiology of speech and language. Perhaps no single past event had the potential to influence the development of the field of communication disorders as the computer has. The practical applications of the microcomputer to the administrative, clinical, educational, and research components of the speech and hearing profession are seemingly limitless. Massive amounts of patient data and other clinical information can be stored and later retrieved with relative ease. Programmed learning units can assist professors by helping them introduce and reinforce important academic and clinical concepts. Newly developed special-purpose instrumentation reduces diagnostic test time, thereby allowing more testing to be performed in the same time frame. The incorporation of microprocessors into therapy techniques with nonvocal individuals, for example, greatly enhances patient-clinician interaction, among other things. The contributions of the microcomputer to research, in terms of controlling design sequences and storage of data, to name but two applications, is unlimited.

The current preoccupation of our culture with computers places a certain amount of pressure on everyone to become a computer user. For some, the decision to buy a microcomputer is based totally on a life-long fascination with gadgets rather than on a bona fide need. The temptation to purchase a microcomputer just to have another toy should be avoided. Instead, one should determine what jobs could be performed better with a computer than by the old method. An analysis should also be done to identify activities that could be carried out by a computer that could not be accomplished without one. Only if it can be said honestly that the computer would noticeably increase, improve, enhance, streamline, or otherwise extend one's capabilities should a microcomputer be considered.

Purchasing a microcomputer system is somewhat similar to buying a new car. That is, the final decision usually is based on some combination of personal preference, individual needs, advice from others, and, to a considerable extent, one's budget.

THE BASIC COMPONENTS OF A MICROCOMPUTER SYSTEM

The configuration of the microcomputer system is often depicted in terms of devices that put information into the computer, devices that allow input information to be displayed in some manner, and devices that can either input or output information (Fig. 2-1).

Microcomputers that are self-contained are sometimes referred to as *appliance* computers. Some computers purchased for home use that are

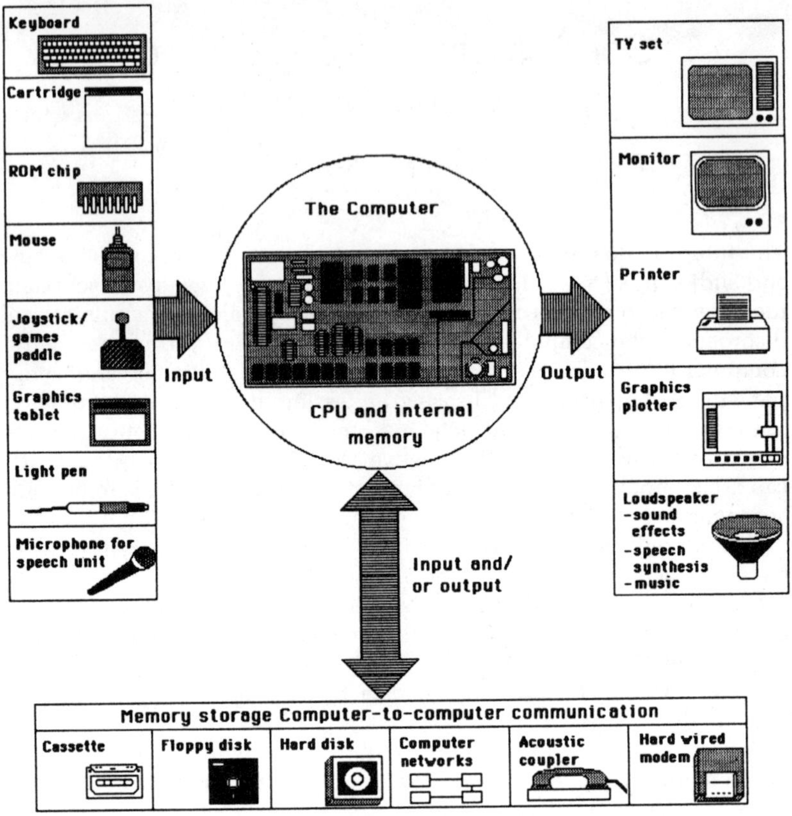

Fig. 2-1. Input and/or output devices available for use with many microcomputers.

simply taken from the box, connected to a television set, and plugged in ready for use belong in this category.

It is best to think of a microcomputer as a *system* rather than a single unit, however. As shown in Figure 2-2, a typical microcomputer system consists of several different components connected together, each performing a different function. Intended uses and available finances, among other things, will determine which and how many components are included in the system.

Central Processing Unit

Despite some variability in the configuration of different systems, each contains a microprocessor, which is nothing more than an integrated circuit etched onto a wafer-thin silicon chip and soldered into a small plastic case. This central chip circuit, called the central processing unit, or simply the CPU, controls and directs the flow of millions of pieces of information each second. In some systems the CPU is a separate component; in others it is part of the keyboard console. Essentially, the CPU is the brains of the system where all the computing occurs. All calcula-

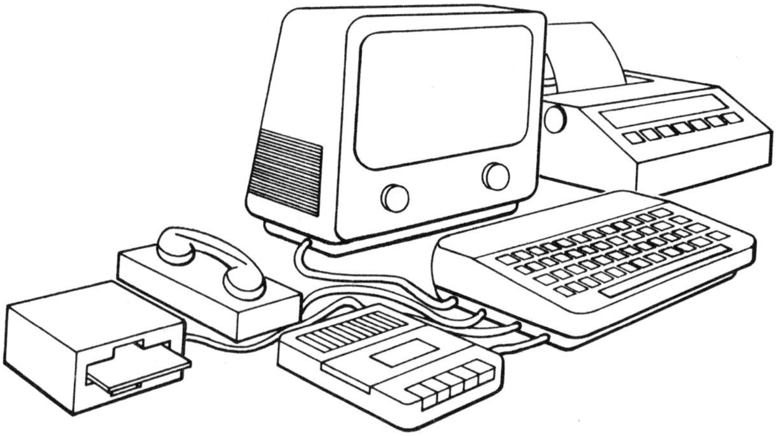

Fig. 2-2. A functional microcomputer system. (Appreciation is expressed to the University of Tennessee, Agricultural Extension Service, for granting use of the figure. Publication No. 1080, Home Computers, *author LaVerne Farmer, artist, Gary Dagnan.)*

tions, memory functions, and movement of information are controlled by the CPU.

The CPU and memory circuits of a microcomputer can be interfaced (connected) to an assortment of other devices. For instance, most microcomputer systems contain a keyboard, viewing screen, and storage system. Other systems may incorporate special-purpose devices for graphics work, speech input and output, or the synthesis of music. Also, if communication with other computers is desired, it can be accomplished either by some sort of networking arrangement wherein two or more computers are linked together by wire, or by telephone transmission through a coupling device called a modem.

Keyboard

A staple of any microcomputer system is the keyboard, which allows the operator to input various kinds of information that is subsequently acted on in some way by the CPU. Although computer keyboards have not been standardized, most include a space bar and fifty or so keys that represent the letters of the alphabet, special symbols such as $ and #, brackets, arithmetic symbols, punctuation and quotation marks, and several special-function keys that allow the operator to do things like *delete* text, *return* the cursor to a new line, and *escape* from one mode of operation to another. Also, a *control* key struck simultaneously with an alphabet key changes the meaning of that key. For example, the *control* key hit in unison with the G key might delete an unwanted letter from a misspelled word.

Although most microcomputer keyboards are patterned after a typical typewriter, a few manufacturers feature membrane-type keyboards. A membrane keyboard has a clear plastic covering over touch-sensitive keys for greater durability and protection against dust and other debris. Because users have found conventional typing to be difficult on a membrane surface that provides no sensation of movement when keys are touched, the membrane keyboard has not been popular in professional office environments.

Mass Storage Devices

If there is information to be stored, or stored information to be used, one or more disk-drive units or a cassette tape recorder must be added to the system. These input/output devices allow for the storage of information placed in the microcomputer either in response to an existing software program or as independently generated material. Although the cassette tape recorder provides adequate storage for most basic computer activities, the disk drive is preferred because of the increased storage capacity of the diskette and speed of access to previously stored information.

To avoid accidental loss of information already stored on a diskette, it is strongly recommended that a backup copy always be made. Usually, a single disk drive is sufficient when only an occasional backup copy is needed. When circumstances dictate the need for frequent backup copies, however, two disk drives are highly recommended because copies can be produced more easily and rapidly this way.

Video Display

A viewing screen of some sort (i.e., a television or a special video monitor) is useful because it exhibits the information as it is being entered into the microcomputer. It is recommended that the video display unit purchased for use with the microcomputer be dedicated to that activity alone instead of serving a number of other functions. Switching back and forth among functions is time-consuming, frequently inconvenient, and can become a source of friction among those competing for its use.

In most cases, a monitor is preferable to a television set for displaying the video output because it has superior resolution. Furthermore, the fact that a less expensive monochrome monitor produces sharper images than a color monitor makes it the video screen of choice, except when color games or graphics are important.

If a monochrome monitor is selected for the video display, the text will appear in a single color (e.g., white, green, or amber) and typically will be embedded in a black background. The fact that an amber screen is easier on the eyes when viewed for extended periods may be important, especially if the microcomputer system is to be used in the treatment of communicatively handicapped individuals, and particularly if they possess visual deficits also.

Increasingly, educational and therapy-oriented software programs incorporate color because it makes the information more interesting for the viewer. Therefore, a color video display unit would be useful if graphics, animation, or both are employed in any of the following ways: (1) in programs designed for use in the rehabilitation of the communicatively handicapped, (2) in computer-assisted instruction (CAI) in the classroom, or (3) in programs providing information about the prevention of communication disorders. In rare instances, where precision color graphics are required routinely, an RGB (or red-green-blue) monitor supplying a superior high-resolution picture will be required (Goodman, 1983).

A word of caution is in order regarding the use of video display devices, whether monochrome or color. Because the images on the screen are created by electrons hitting a phosphorescent surface, radiation is emitted. Moreover, the amount of radiation emitted can be up to five times as great for a color video than for a monochrome unit (McWilliams, 1982). Nevertheless, a 1983 study by the National Research Council indicated that video display terminals give off very low amounts of radiation and should not be a cause of concern to users.

Although it is difficult to determine exactly how much radiation reaches the operator, how much can be tolerated safely, and what the long-term effects might be, one thing is known for sure—the amount of radiation decreases considerably as the user's distance from the screen increases. Therefore, an operator seated a few feet from the video screen is exposed to significantly less radiation than someone who is situated just a few inches away (McWilliams, 1982). For some people this might be motivation enough to purchase a system in which the keyboard and the video display device are separate pieces so that the distance between them can be controlled.

Finally, video display devices that can handle only 40 characters across the screen for any given line are not sufficient for word processing or accounting and should be avoided in favor of an 80-column screen.

Printer

Although the printer is categorized routinely as a peripheral device that is expendable, or at least deferrable, in a home or personal microcomputer system, it is essential in most professional settings where printed material is needed on a continual basis. Available printers are of two basic types: *daisywheel* (letter quality), and *dot matrix*. The former utilizes any of several impact-printing techniques to produce letter-quality print. The consequences of obtaining letter-quality printouts are reduced speed (approximately 10 to 45 characters per second) and increased equipment cost.

Thermal printers burn characters onto special heat-treated paper. Although quieter than their impact-printing counterparts, thermal machines print more slowly, and the paper is more expensive. A relative newcomer to the market is the ink-jet printer, which generates characters by firing minute drops of ink at the paper. Also, the laser printer, although not yet practical for conventional use, holds promise for the future.

In cases where print quality is not a factor, dot-matrix printers can provide a less expensive alternative. Essentially, a dot-matrix printer creates a mosaic of dots on paper. Although speeds of 50 to 150 characters per second can be reached by this print method, character resolution is sacrificed, resulting in printed text that is difficult to read for long periods of time. However, some dot-matrix units now produce pseudo-letter-quality print that is hard to distinguish from the daisywheel type.

Interesting graphics can be produced with the addition of a peripheral package such as a graphics printer, plotter, or graphics tablet of some sort. A plotter is the best graphics peripheral for high-quality work, but the creation of complex designs and shapes requires tedious programming. An alternative is a graphics tablet that allows the user to draw free-hand designs on the tablet itself with a special pen. The microcomputer tracks and digitizes the emerging design and stores it in memory or on a disk for subsequent use with a printer or plotter. The best way to determine which peripheral is most appropriate for the user's needs is to try them out individually.

SPECIAL-PURPOSE PERIPHERAL DEVICES

A growing assortment of accessories is available to the computer user with unique needs. For example, graphic designs can be produced on paper by a specialized printer called a *plotter*. When properly connected to the microcomputer, the plotter draws charts, graphs, and other designs, often in a variety of colors. Frequently, lettering can be done in different styles and sizes.

Another device sometimes employed with a microcomputer system is the *modem*. When properly employed between the computer and a telephone, modems allow computers to talk to each other by converting electronic signals into audible tones that can be passed back and forth over telephone lines. Also, a modem can connect a microcomputer to a centralized storage bank or network, providing access to potentially useful information on a variety of topics.

The ability of the microcomputer to generate synthetic speech, music, or both is a requirement for some buyers. Although this function is not available as a standard item on many current systems, it can be purchased as an optional feature. At this point, most microcomputer-produced synthetic speech is of limited quantity and quality. As research continues, however, increasingly sophisticated speech synthesis chips and software will be developed that will produce amazingly humanlike speech (see Chapter 12).

FACTORS INFLUENCING THE PURCHASE OF A MICROCOMPUTER SYSTEM

If one anticipates that a microcomputer could facilitate the operation of a clinical practice, the matter of its purchase should be examined carefully. In settings with a large number of employees, a group of existing and potential computer users can be formed to assist in assessing the need for a microcomputer system. The things such a group can provide to improve and expedite the process include (1) an analysis of current procedures and needs, (2) an evaluation of employee interest in microcomputers, (3) an investigation of suitable microprocessing systems, (4) a determination of specific hardware and software needs related to employee requests for microcomputers, (5) a prioritization of microcomputer requests, (6) identification of sources of financial support, (7) development of procedures for employee training and supervision, (8) establishment of policies for access and usage, and (9) setting up an implementation timetable. Even if the purchasing decision is an individual matter, adherence to these guidelines should result in a much more informed choice.

Software

It is often mentioned that software should be the number-one consideration in the selection of a microcomputer system (Rodwell, 1983; Staples, 1983). Once the tasks have been identified, an assessment should be made of the software available to accomplish these tasks. By joining an organization like CUSH (Computer Users in Speech and Hearing), one can gain immediate access to a wide variety of potentially useful software programs. Once suitable software has been found for the desired applications, the choice of hardware becomes easier. In some cases it may narrow the choice down to a single make and model. For instance, much of the desired educational, diagnostic, and rehabilitative software may be compatible with only one brand of computer. Business-related functions, on the other hand, might be handled best on another system because of its strong orientation in that direction.

Ease of Operation

For the majority of computer users a system that is simple to operate is the preferred choice. The best way to determine the ease of operation is actually to try out various systems. Often, a short trial period will uncover personal likes and dislikes regarding a particular microcomputer. If anything in the operation of the system generates concern or doubt, chances are the system will not be acceptable if purchased. This can be true of even a seemingly small matter, such as the feel of the keys on the keyboard.

Also, the software selected for use with the system should be easy to work with, or "user friendly." A program that displays the instructions for its use on the screen is easier to use than one that requires continual reference to a manual. Furthermore, built-in safeguards should make it virtually impossible to erase information from within the system.

Cost

Price reductions in computer hardware have been precipitated to a large degree by competition among manufacturers. It is not certain, however, exactly how long this bonanza will continue, so it is not necessarily helpful to delay buying a microcomputer system solely for reasons of price.

The capabilities and speed of the microcomputer will, to a considerable extent, determine its ultimate cost. In general, if the microcomputer is intended strictly for home use, where its functions are limited and simple, then the price could be as low as a few hundred dollars. However, the variety and complexity of computer uses in an institutional or private practice setting would be greater. Furthermore, many of the functions best performed in these environments by a microcomputer are repetitive in nature, such as producing forms, letters, invoices, and mailings.

In many clinical settings, word processing would account for a sizeable amount of computer time each day, in which case a letter-quality printer would become essential. A microcomputer system that included such a printer in addition to two disk drives would undoubtedly cost several thousand dollars.

If finances are limited, there is a growing market in used computers. Many of these can be found listed in the classified sections of newspapers.

System Expansion

If expansion of the original microcomputer system is probable, this fact should be taken into account prior to the initial purchase of any system. The expansion capabilities of a microcomputer have been largely predetermined by its manufacturer. Of preference to most users are machines that allow a peripheral such as a graphics plotter to be plugged directly into the main unit, rather than those that require the use of an interface device, usually at considerable extra cost.

Another factor is whether the proposed microcomputer can accept peripherals from other manufacturers. In some cases the choice of peripheral devices is limited to those made by the manufacturer of the microcomputer itself. This limitation can greatly reduce the expansion options and also increase the overall price.

Service

Although most machines operate flawlessly, breakdowns do occur and can create serious problems because the number of service centers for the repair of microcomputers has not kept pace with the industry. Another source of concern is the fact that the type, amount, and cost of service can vary substantially.

Two basic types of repair service are available, *mail-in* service and *on-call* service. The first requires packing up the malfunctioning component and shipping it back to the manufacturer or some repair center by mail. For many, this is time-consuming and inefficient and can be surprisingly expensive when insurance costs are included in the total. Also, damage during shipping can occur, resulting in even greater cost (to someone) as well as more computer downtime.

Although repairs can be completed more quickly with on-call service, it is considerably more expensive, costing up to one and one-half percent per month of the total purchase price of the microcomputer system itself. McGrath (1982) recommends asking the dealer several basic questions about service prior to buying a microcomputer.

1. Is on-call service available? Some dealers provide such service only within a 30-mile radius of one of their stores.
2. Will all the components be covered by the same service agreement? Sometimes different service agreements (and repair personnel) are required for the terminal and, say, the disk drive or printer. Also, some dealers will service only their own brand-name products. If the terminal is purchased from one company and the printer from another, the buyer might have to make two separate service agreements.
3. What is the guaranteed response time? That is, when buyers inform the dealer they have a problem, do they wait an hour, a day, or forever for a call from the repair people? Guaranteed response time is only a guarantee concerning the time it takes to acknowledge the call, not a guarantee that the repair person will be in the office within a specified time.
4. Is the buyer entitled to a replacement system while the equipment is down? (One rarely is, but it never hurts to ask.)

Compatibility

As mentioned, a microcomputer system that readily accepts peripheral components from other manufacturers increases its owner's flexibility.

Another factor in this regard is the existence of other microcomputer systems in the workplace. There are obvious advantages in buying all microcomputers for a given setting from the same manufacturer, especially if identical models can be used (compatibility between the various models of a single manufacturer cannot be guaranteed). Uniformity allows software programs to be used on any available unit.

Hardware Considerations

Certain issues related to the microcomputer system components themselves bear comment because they frequently surface at some point in the selection process.

First, although the amount of memory a microcomputer possesses varies from unit to unit, an initial memory size common to many is 64 kilobytes, or 65,536 bytes. A byte is composed of 8 bits, a bit being the smallest piece of information used by a computer. Each byte represents either a number or a letter. The memory capacity of a microcomputer is determined on the basis of how many bytes of information it contains.

Most of the microcomputers on the market today have an 8-bit microprocessor that can handle 64 kilobytes of user-programmable memory. If more capacity and speed are needed, a 16-bit system becomes necessary. Programs written for a computer having a 16-bit processor can hold more information and run faster than a similar program written for a computer with an 8-bit microprocessor. Until more software becomes available for 16-bit computers, however, the 8-bit microprocessor will continue to dominate the market.

For most ordinary functions 64 kilobytes of memory will be adequate. If the system is to be used extensively for business purposes, however, more memory will be needed. Memory can be added either by purchasing a machine that already has a larger memory, or by increasing the capacity of a microcomputer having too little memory with an expansion card.

Insurance

Many public institutions such as colleges and public schools do not carry insurance on buildings and their contents because of the great expense involved. Therefore, when insurance is desired for a special item such as a microcomputer, it must be obtained separately. Other agencies and businesses should check their casualty and theft policies to determine whether their coverage extends to their microcomputer. If not, several insurance companies offer casualty and theft policies for microcomputers.

Also, it should be noted that the typical homeowner's insurance policy does not cover units used at home for business purposes. A separate insurance rider is necessary and is available at a modest cost from most insurance companies.

ERGONOMICS

Seemingly obvious, but all too frequently overlooked, are considerations of physical location and operator comfort. Ergonomics is the application of engineering data to problems between humans and machines.

Employees working with microcomputers in today's electronic office can develop an assortment of physical ailments, including eyestrain, headaches, stiff necks, and back pains. To reduce eyestrain resulting from prolonged microcomputer use, it is advisable that (1) the chair be positioned a comfortable distance from the viewing screen, (2) head movements be minimized by strategically locating reference materials nearby, (3) the viewing screen be shielded adequately from glare, and (4) brief rest periods be interspersed throughout long periods of use.

Neck and back strain can result from maintaining a static posture for hours at a time. When the video display and the keyboard are joined together in one unit, variation in body position is limited. A simple solution to this dilemma is to purchase a microcomputer system with a detachable keyboard. By separating the video display from the keyboard, one can position them independently. Locating the screen at eye level usually reduces neck and back strain to a minimum. Also, the ability to tilt and swivel the screen is a standard feature on some of the better-quality monitors.

Prior planning of suitable space eliminates a host of potential problems. For the sake of the operator and his or her neighbors, the microcomputer system should be situated in a relatively isolated space with good lighting and ventilation. Because the microcomputer console and printer can generate a considerable amount of noise (e.g., clicking keys and fan noise), physical separation is desirable so that persons in accompanying work spaces are not distracted.

Manufacturers are producing computer-oriented furniture in an impressive assortment of configurations. The customer has only to determine which arrangement will best accommodate his or her system.

The furniture should house the microcomputer system in an efficient and practical manner. A standard desk is not appropriate because it is too high (28 to 30 inches) to type on comfortably. Instead, a two-level desk that has a 27-inch-high surface for the keyboard and a regular 30-inch-high surface for other office functions is preferred. Also, a conventional desk top is not large enough to accommodate peripheral equipment—such as a monitor, printer, and several disk drives—that may be part of the system. Finally, adequate drawer and cubbyhole space is desirable for the storage of office supplies and other computer-related materials.

Because a microcomputer system routinely includes a number of different components, all of which run on electricity, the workplace must have an adequate number of outlets. When insufficient outlets are available, the existing space can be modified by the installation of a power outlet strip that houses multiple outlets along a single bar. Moreover, to protect the equipment from damage caused by spurious power surges, the multiple-outlet bar should contain a power-surge circuit breaker.

Even static electricity created by user contact with carpeting can generate a charge strong enough to alter information stored on a magnetic diskette or similar device. This problem can be easily prevented, however, by the purchase of a relatively inexpensive anti-static floor mat.

As shown in Figure 2-3, a comfortable chair that provides good back support is of paramount importance. If the system is to be used by several different operators, a swivel chair is recommended so that each person can adjust it to the proper height.

FUTURE DIRECTIONS

Constantly changing computer technology makes it difficult to plan a system with future developments in mind. In fact, it may be wiser to ignore the future and recognize that rapid change in this industry is inevitable and, to some extent, unpredictable.

The next generation of microcomputers probably will offer more memory, better graphics, and greater computing speed as standard features.

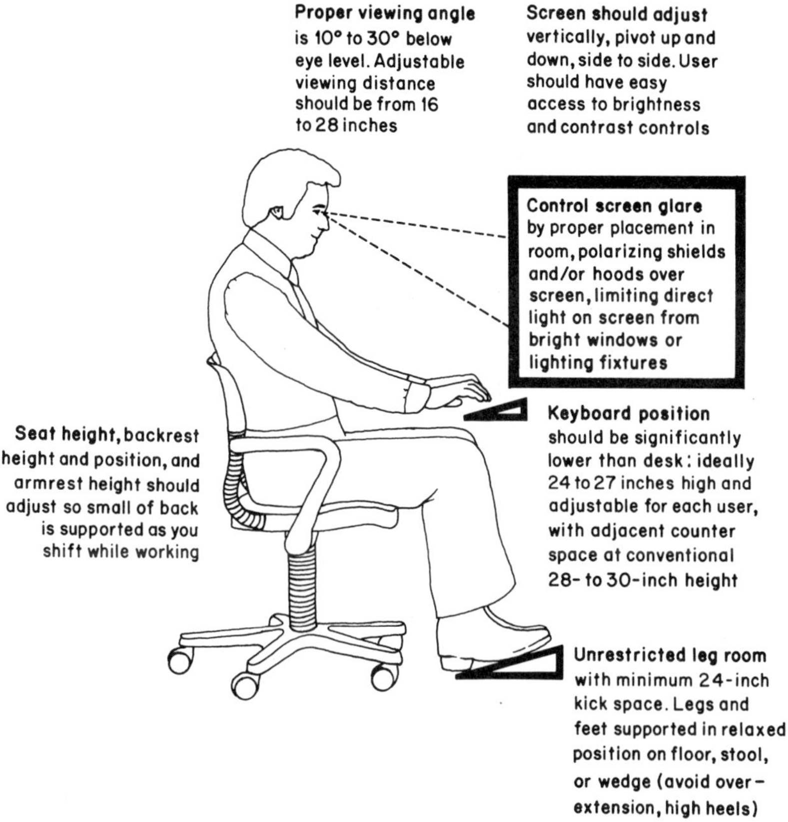

Fig. 2-3. Some basic relationships between microcomputer and operator that can minimize physiological stress associated with extended use. (Adapted from Sunset Magazine, *May 1984, p. 124.)*

The manipulation of information in the microcomputer will be accomplished routinely through some type of "mouse," touch-screen, or light-pen arrangement. Massive quantities of software will be available and will be usable on an increasing variety of different models and even brands of microcomputers. Low-cost printers will work more rapidly and produce higher-quality output. The end result of these developments will be increased computing power and versatility at an amazingly low price.

REFERENCES

Farmer, L. *Home Computers.* University of Tennessee Agricultural Extension Service publication No. 1080 (no date).

Goodman, D. *A Parent's Guide to Personal Computers and Software.* New York: Simon and Schuster, 1983.

McGrath, J. An introduction to computers. *Hear. Aid J.* 35:11–14, 1982.

McWilliams, P. A. *The Personal Computer Book.* Los Angeles: Prelude, 1982.

Rodwell, P. *The Personal Computer Handbook.* Woodbury, N.Y.: Barron's, 1983.

Staples, B. Which computer is for you? *Creative Computers Buying Guide,* Ahl Publishing Co., 1983, pp. 6–8.

3

Basic Operations of Microcomputers

William A. Yost

From our cars, to our offices, to our homes, and even to our places of recreation, the Computer Age has made an impact. The stampede of computers into every corner of our lives is primarily due to the introduction of the microcomputer. Like most technological breakthroughs, the conception of microcomputers was preceded by important technological discoveries: the invention of the transistor, and then the introduction of integrated circuits (IC) containing transistors and other electronic components. This miniaturization has reached a sophisticated stage, making massive electronic capability available at low cost, in small packages, and drawing little electric power.

The birth of microcomputing might be traced to 1946, when John Bardeen, Walter Brattain, and William Shockley invented the transistor. Following the diode and the transistor, the concept of the integrated circuit resulted in a quantum leap in the application of microelectronics to research and to practically all other aspects of society. The IC is a single sheet of semiconductor material that is functionally equivalent to a number of discrete electronic components (resistors, transistors, etc.) and their interconnections. Thus, the function of an amplifier, a flip-flop, or now the entire central processor of a computer can be performed by a single monolithic (system contained on one chip) IC.

The technology of the IC was enhanced even further by MOS (metal oxide semiconductor) technology. The MOS chip allowed for an increase of several orders of magnitude in the number of circuit elements that could be functionally contained on a small chip of metal oxide. This increase in circuit-element density was accompanied by a much lower need for power by the MOS chip than by the previous ICs.

The MOS chip is based on unipolar-field-effect transistor (FET) technology, whereas most ICs are based on bipolar junction-type transistor technology (hence ICs are sometimes labeled bipolar ICs). An MOS chip can contain 15,000 or more FETs, which require far less power than junction transistors.

With the use of film hybrid technology all the advantages of MOS and IC circuitry can be enclosed in a single, sealed unit. The thin- and thick-film types of hybrid microelectronic circuits are made by bonding conductors and resistors, many ICs, MOS subsystems, and discrete components to a system of metallic film. These parts are all assembled on an

This chapter was written with help from Pat Harder and research support from the National Science Foundation. The present chapter is an update and revision of a chapter I wrote in 1976–1977 for the book *Microcomputers in Sensory and Information-Processing Research*, edited by M. S. Mayzner and T. R. Dolan (Hillsdale, N.J.: Lawrence Erlbaum and Associates, 1978). The basic format as well as Figures 3-1 and 3-2 and part of Figure 3-3 are derived, with permission, from that earlier version.—W.A.Y.

Table 3-1. Hardware options for microcomputers

Microprocessing Unit
8, 12, 16, or 32 bits.

Memory
RAM, ROM, PROM, EPROM, bubble, semiconductor, core.

Input/Output Circuitry
PIA, DMA, multiplexed port, RS-232 port, digital port.

Peripherals
Inputs: keyboard, mouse, digitizing pad, touch screen, voice, analog-to-digital converter, digital input, image processing.
Outputs: CRT, television, printer, plotter, graphics terminal, terminal, digital-to-analog converter, digital output, voice, video.
Communications: modem, facsimile, network.
Mass Storage: memory, floppy disk (from 3¼ to 8 inches), cartridge disk, fixed disk, video disk, magnetic tape, cassette tape, cartridge.

Abbreviations: RAM, random-access memory; ROM, read-only memory; PROM, programmable read-only memory; EPROM, erasable programmable read-only memory; PIA, peripheral interface adapter; DMA, direct memory access; CRT, cathode-ray tube.

insulated substrate of metal oxide. At this stage an extremely reliable large scale integrated (LSI) circuit is achievable in an incredibly small package, saving space, power consumption, and, therefore, cost of the system.

The basic microcomputer has four parts: (1) the microprocessing unit (MPU), (2) memory, (3) input/output (I/O) circuits, and (4) peripherals. Quite often the MPU, the memory, and the I/O circuits make up the *microprocessor* part of the microcomputer. The addition of peripherals makes the microprocessor a usable computer. Table 3-1 provides a list of some common options that exist for these four parts of the microcomputer. These items describe the hardware. The other ingredient for a workable computer is the *software*, the programs that control what the computer does. There are two basic types of software for microcomputers, (1) operating systems and (2) programs. Table 3-2 lists many types of programs that can be used on a microcomputer. These hardware peripherals and software programs will be described later in this chapter.

The basic unit of a computer is the *bit*. A bit is either on or off, much like a switch. A bit has a value of one when it is on and zero when it is off. A *word* is a string of bits, that is, a string of ones and zeros. The pattern of the bits (0s and 1s) in the word determines the nature of the message the computer sends or receives. Thus, each instruction is a different string of zeros and ones, that is, a different word. These words are between 4 and 32 bits long in microcomputers. The information in a word is sent along I/O, data, or control lines, and it is stored in registers, buffers, or memories. While the information is stored in a register, other words of information can be combined with the already existing word. Control logic routes the words to the appropriate lines, registers, or memories. The computer operates according to the rules of Boolean logic (*and*, *or*, etc.). These logical operations are performed in the registers. Once the desired operation is completed, the result is stored in memory. The software program determines the sequence in which these logical operations are performed and

Table 3-2. Basic software for microcomputers

Operating Systems

Operating systems are specific for the type of microprocessor unit or for the particular microcomputer.

Programs

Assemblers, compliers, higher-order languages, word processing, text editing, data bases, spread sheets, integrated software, communications software, graphics, games, educational software, special-task software (financial, engineering, statistical, record keeping, calendar, etc.)

when and where to send or receive the appropriate word. This general mode of operation is common to all computers, not just microcomputers.

HARDWARE

Figure 3-1 is a general diagram of a microcomputer with the MPU, two types of memory (Read-Only Memory [ROM] and Random-Access Memory [RAM]), and I/O circuits and lines. The peripherals to the computer are controlled by the I/O lines. The *data lines* are I/O lines that move information among the parts of the computer, while the *control lines* provide the logical sequencing of this information according to the instructions received from the software. It is the very small size of the microprocessor that has brought about the microcomputer revolution. The MPU, memories, and I/O circuits can all be placed on a single board the size of a postcard. This package can contain as many as a million circuits. The technology is on the verge of placing over a billion circuits on one IC half the size of a postcard. Along with the reduction in size, there is a reduction in the power required to operate the microprocessor. Many microprocessors could run on a solar cell. It is the peripherals (monitors, disks, printers, keyboards) that take up the space, require the power, and usually keep the price of the microcomputer from being even lower than it is.

Microprocessing Unit

Basically, the MPU contains registers and controls logic to read and write to the memory according to a sequence of instructions stored in memory and timed by a clock. Figure 3-2 shows some of the major elements and organization of a basic MPU. In general, the instructions and data are controlled by the program counter (PC), which keeps track of which instruction was just performed and which instruction should be executed next. The PC receives and sends data and instructions from memory via the address and data registers. The instruction decoder (ID) then interprets the instruction. The arithmetical and logic operations to be performed on the data are carried out in the accumulator (ACC) or accumulators. The status registers (STATUS) help determine what is happening in the accumulator. The data register (DR) and the address register (AR) help route data and instructions between the MPU and the memory. The control unit coordinates the activity within the MPU. A clock pulse and its support logic time the sequence of instructions in the correct order and manner. Thus,

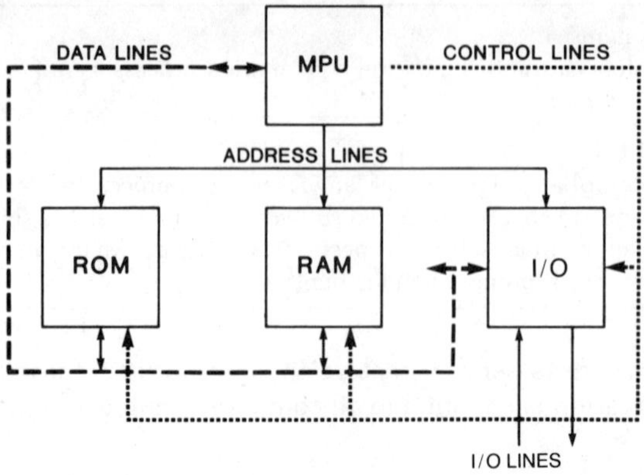

Fig. 3-1. The typical layout of a microprocessor. MPU, microprocessing unit; ROM, read-only memory; RAM, random-access memory; I/O, input and output devices.

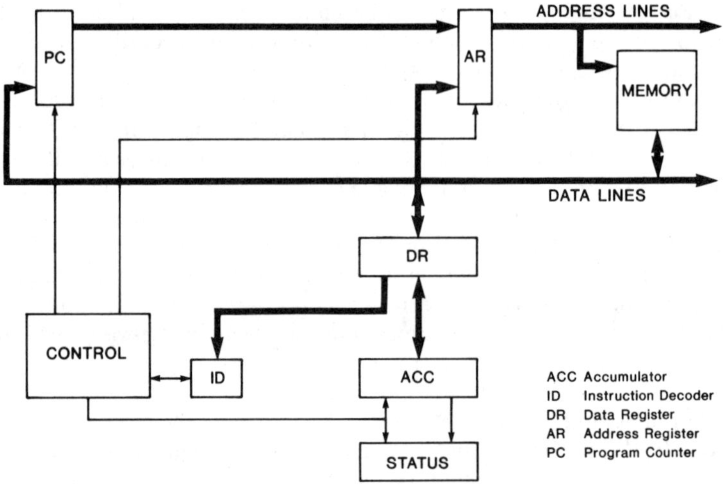

Fig. 3-2. The layout of a microprocessing unit (MPU). See detailed description in the text.

data are manipulated in the accumulator, and these manipulations are determined by the instructions in a memory and are deciphered by the instruction decoder. The PC, AR, DR, STATUS and CONTROLLER help in bookkeeping and in timing so that every operation is performed quickly, in the right order, and so that the user can interrogate the MPU to determine what is happening at any particular time. The time it takes to transfer data from register to register is often referred to as the *cycle time* of the MPU. The cycle time imposes a limit on the time required for one instruction to be executed and, thus, how fast the computer operates the software.

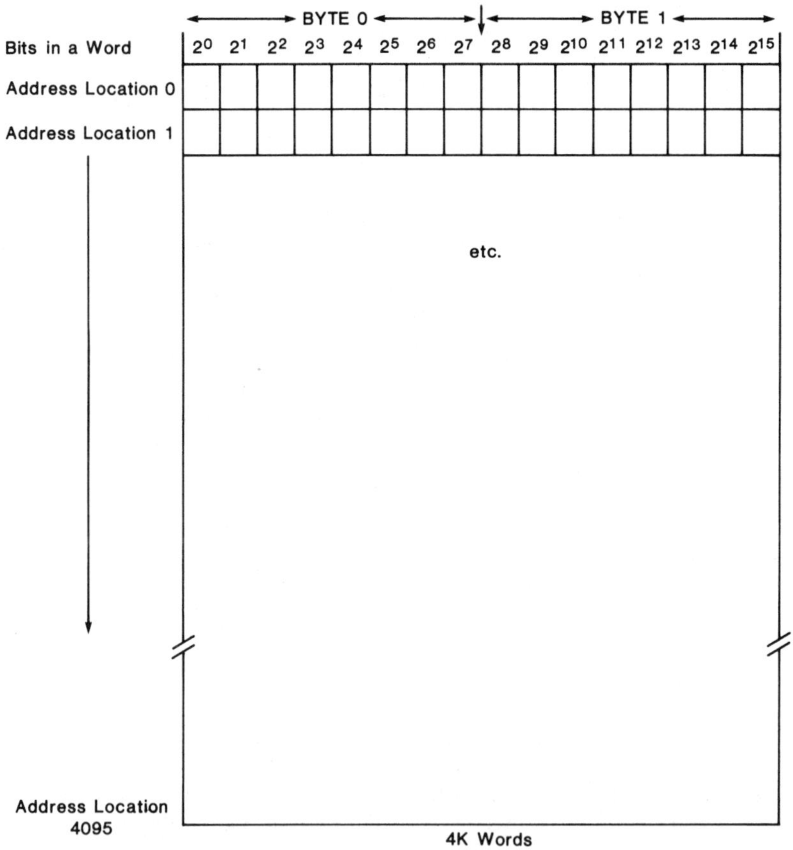

Fig. 3-3. The way in which memory is typically organized. This example is for an 8-bit word, 4K memory unit.

Memory

The device for storing information is the memory. Locations in memory are called addresses, and each address is N bits long (in microcomputers N is usually between 4 and 32 bits). Figure 3-3 shows how memory is typically organized. Each row in the memory represents one *word*, a word being 4 to 32 bits long depending on the "word size" of the microcomputer. The memory size is represented by the number of rows—that is, by the number of words. Microcomputers can have memories that contain thousands (256K = 256,000 words, for instance), or even a million (1 mega = 1,000,000 words) or more words. Sometimes a word is broken into *bytes*. (For example, a 16-bit word might be divided into two 8-bit bytes as shown in Fig. 3-3.) Thus, the number of bytes of memory will be larger than the number of words of memory. Dividing a word into bytes allows for devices (including two different microcomputers) with different word lengths to be interfaced with each other as long as the devices all use the same byte length (usually 8 bits). The addresses may be accessed randomly by the MPU, in which case the memory is called a random-access memory, or RAM. Other memories are fixed; that is, the code at each address within the memory cannot be changed. These are called read-only memories, or ROMs.

Most RAMs in microcomputers hold data on a "volatile" basis, which means that the stored information is lost when power is removed. RAMs can be dynamic or static. In dynamic RAMs, the information is stored at each address as an electrical charge on capacitors of MOS transistors. The charge will leak if it is not occasionally replenished, which can be accomplished by periodic memory-refresh pulses derived from the MPU clock. Static RAMs store the information permanently, so that special memory-refresh logic is not required. Static and dynamic RAMs differ in the amount of power and support circuitry required to operate them. Static RAMs use more power but have less control circuitry than dynamic RAMs.

ROMS are also usually semiconductor integrated circuits, in which the data are fixed and, therefore, not volatile. They are usually used for special purposes and within the MPU. ROMs are usually programmed at the time they are fabricated, and they cannot be changed. ROMs whose data can be altered—that is, whose memories can be programmed *once* by the user—are called programmable read-only memories (PROM). Once a PROM is programmed, however, its data are fixed. Some ROMS can have their memories altered more than once, but the process of rewriting the memory is slow and costly. Hence, these erasable programmable read-only memories (EPROMs) are typically used only for prototyping microcomputer systems.

RAMs and ROMs are often used together in microcomputers. For instance, a particular program may exist as a set of fixed instructions on a ROM. (Such programs stored permanently in ROM are sometimes referred to as *firmware*.) The data that will be analyzed by the program are stored on a RAM. The MPU reads the data from the RAM and the program instructions from the ROM and performs the arithmetical and logic operations necessary to provide the analysis.

Input/Output Circuitry

The I/O devices transfer data to and from the microprocessor and the various parts of the computer, including the peripherals, as well as sending or receiving control signals. The device to which or from which the data or signals are coming is usually called a peripheral. Typically, the microcomputer is designed to have special I/O interfaces to handle particular peripherals (e.g., a special connection or port for a keyboard through which programs or data can be entered, or a disk for storage of data).

In addition to these special-purpose I/O interfaces, a microcomputer might have general-purpose I/O lines that the user accesses through I/O ports or connections. These general-purpose lines, which can be connected to a variety of peripherals such as printers and modems, allow information to flow between the peripheral and the computer. A number of I/O ports can exist on a single computer, or special hardware (multiplexers) can be added to allow many peripherals to share a single I/O port. In most microcomputers, the exact operation of the port is specified by the software program, usually as part of the operating system.

The data can be transmitted along the I/O lines to a peripheral as bits of information. Although this type of *digital I/O* is used, it is a very inefficient way to transmit data because it takes one line for each bit of information to be sent or received. Thus, a variety of other forms of sending and receiving digital information have been developed. The RS-232 interface uses current to transmit the information. These transmission methods involve techniques for coding and decoding a message using a few transmission lines. Obviously, it is important that the microcomputer and the peripheral device agree on the type of I/O transmission interface each device uses.

Most computers treat many of the I/O interfaces as memory locations. This treatment enables the MPU to control directly the peripheral devices. Microcomputers also have a structure for communicating with I/O devices—that is, a structure for interrupting MPU activity to allow the MPU to communicate with an I/O device. Sometimes priority-interrupt options are available that enable the microprocessor user to determine which I/O device should be serviced first, second, third, etc.

General-purpose I/O devices, such as direct memory access (DMA) or peripheral interface adapters (PIA), are also used with some microcomputers. DMAs help speed the transfer of information between the various elements of the microcomputer. PIAs are usually general-purpose devices that lie between some peripheral device and the MPU. The PIA acts as a register, usually with some storage (memory) capacity. Thus, the PIA can route data to the MPU under MPU program control, storing some data if they are not needed at that particular time.

Often the computer sends information along the I/O lines faster than the peripheral device can use it. For instance, a printer cannot print information as fast as the computer can send it because the printer is a mechanical device and thus inherently slow. Under these conditions, either the computer can send its information at a very slow rate, or there can be a form of communication called *handshaking* between the computer and the peripheral that allows the information to be sent at a faster rate. The advantage of handshaking is that the computer is free to do other things as the peripheral device is accepting the data. The basic means of handshaking involves the peripheral device having a small amount of memory, usually called a *buffer*. The information is sent to the buffer at a fast rate and then is read from the buffer to the peripheral device at the slower rate required by the device. When the buffer is full, a signal is sent to the computer to stop sending data; when the buffer becomes empty (usually half empty), a signal is sent to the computer indicating that data can be sent again. The rate at which the data are sent is called the *baud* rate, and baud rates range from 150 to 9600. Many an owner of a new computer has been frustrated putting the computer system together because the handshaking and baud rates of all the devices have not been coordinated. This is especially true for systems consisting of parts from different manufacturers.

The I/O and the memory are considered in terms of the word length (number of bits in a word) of the computer. The major differences among microprocessors are word length, byte size, and how the data are sent along the I/O lines and circuits. If these three properties match, there is a good chance that the components will be compatible, although there might be considerable hardware and software effort required to make the complete system operational.

PERIPHERALS

Peripheral devices are apparatus that connect to the computer (via the I/O lines) to perform certain tasks. Perhaps the most often-used peripheral device is a keyboard to enter programs and data into the microprocessor. Many personal computers have the microprocessor and keyboard attached together. Other computers have a detached keyboard, and the microprocessor is with the monitor (another peripheral) or with the disk-drive unit (another peripheral). In all cases the input from the peripheral (e.g., the keyboard) to the microprocessor or from the microprocessor to the peripheral (e.g., the monitor) is controlled by the I/O lines and circuitry. Peripherals have been divided into four classes: (1) those that mainly provide input for the microprocessor, (2) those providing output, (3) those that aid in communication with other devices and computers, and (4) those for additional storage of information (in addition to the memory in the microprocessor).

Input Peripheral Devices

The most important input device is the keyboard. It provides the primary means of entering information into the microprocessor. Keyboards come with a variety of options. The basic keyboard has a typewriter layout of the alphabet and numbers. Many keyboards have a key pad (usually on the right side of the keyboard) through which numerical data can be entered efficiently. Some computers have special keys that perform explicit functions for the microcomputer—for example, a key for saving information on a disk and another key for printing the information seen on the monitor. In addition, a keyboard might also contain a series of programmable keys, the function of which can be determined by the user. For example, in word-processing software the user might program one of these keys to delete a line of text. Often the command to delete a line takes two or more keystrokes to execute. By programming the programmable keys, the user can save one or more keystrokes.

A variety of other input devices are available for microcomputers. A *digitizing pad* is a popular way to enter complex information such as a drawing. Anatomists and artists are making excellent use of these input devices. The digitizing pads consist of a surface and an electronic pen. The surface contains a matrix of sensors. As the pen is used to draw a picture on the surface, each cell in the matrix that the pen touches sends a message to the computer to store a bit in a map of the surface stored in the computer's memory (or on a disk). With a color monitor or printer, color can be specified either by using the keyboard or through some special function on the digitizing pad. These systems usually demand considerable memory and storage because the matrix must have a lot of cells to represent a picture faithfully.

The *mouse* is a shortcut to the digitizing pad. The mouse is a small wheel that is rolled across a surface. As it rolls, it moves a point, usually called the *cursor*, on the monitor screen in the direction the mouse is moved across the desk top. The mouse can be used to position the cursor at a particular location on the monitor screen or to draw a picture.

Sometimes a light pen used in conjunction with a specially developed monitor screen serves the same function as a digitizing pad. In this case, the light pen is moved across the monitor screen, and the special screen senses the location of the pen and translates its position to information usable by the software program. These devices are very useful for tasks demanding pictorial input.

Larger systems may use other forms of digitizing pictorial information, such as image processing technology in which the information captured by a television camera is converted to digital information and relayed to a computer. These systems usually demand more memory and faster computer speeds than those found in microprocessors.

Certain devices allow analog input to be converted to digital bits for computer use. These devices, called analog-to-digital converters (AD devices), are the basic hardware ingredient of the new voice-interactive devices. The speech input is divided into tiny temporal segments, and the voltage of each segment is converted to a number, which is read in sequence by the computer. Eventually, the AD converter and the software might enable the computer to recognize verbal commands. At the moment, most AD devices used in microcomputers sample sounds for computer analysis, such as a speech spectograph (see Chapter 12).

Output Peripheral Devices

The CRT (cathode-ray tube), or television monitor, is a major output device for the basic microcomputer. Most monitors use the same technology found in television. In the future some microcomputers will use liquid crystal display or plasma technology because of their low power consumption and high resolution. At present a television is often used as the computer's monitor. All that is required is the RF (radio frequency) connector that carries the correct signal to the television. The main options in monitors are color (black on white, white on black, green screens, complete color, etc.), refresh rate, and resolution. All CRTs work by sending a signal to a screen via a "gun" or "guns." As the gun moves across the screen, it leaves a mark. The rate at which the guns sweep across the screen determines the refresh rate, and the accuracy of the placement of the guns determines the resolution. The clarity of the characters and speed of the character change are determined by the refresh rate and the resolution. Thus, for word processing, a low-resolution screen might be adequate, whereas for detailed anatomical or graphic uses a screen with very high resolution might be needed. (Monitors rather than terminals are discussed in this chapter because terminals are usually connected to computer systems larger than the personal microcomputer.)

The printer is another important part of a useful microcomputer system. Most printers used with microcomputers fall into one of two broad categories: impact or dot-matrix printers. Impact printers are similar to typewriters and produce letter-quality print. They operate by having the symbol strike the paper through a ribbon. Dot-matrix printers use a matrix of pins (Fig. 3-4) that strike the paper through a ribbon. The combination of pins activated determines the symbol. The dot-matrix printer allows the use of an infinite number of symbols (only the number of pins in the matrix limits the possibilities). Different types of symbols are referred to as *fonts*. Because the printing head does not move, the dot-matrix printer can be very fast. Nevertheless, the dots used to construct the symbols can usually be seen, and thus the print quality is low, especially when the material is photoreproduced (as in photocopying or offset printing).

Although a dot-matrix printer can be used to plot figures and draw pictures, these printers are slow and difficult to use as plotters. Numerous

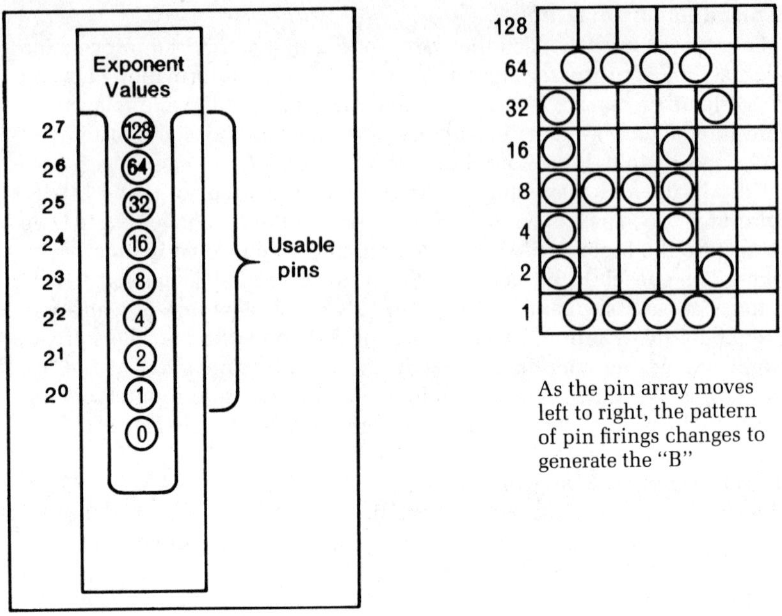

Each pin in the vertical array coded by a bit

As the pin array moves left to right, the pattern of pin firings changes to generate the "B"

Fig. 3-4. Example of the pin matrix for a dot-matrix printer. The combination of pins that fire determines the symbol, as shown at right.

plotters are available. Most are of one of three types: X-Y plotters, digital plotters, or video-copy plotters/printers. The X-Y plotter moves a pen (or pens) along either the horizontal or vertical axis. Diagonal lines are difficult to draw accurately, but X-Y plotters are simple devices and therefore inexpensive. The digital plotter can move the pen to any point on the paper (the resolution of the possible number of points is a distinguishing feature among plotters). The video-copy plotters/printers actually copy, via a photocopy or electrostatic technique, any image that is on the computer monitor. These plotters/printers often require special paper, ink, and toners for proper use and high-quality reproduction.

The speed at which a printer can print (as opposed to the baud rate) is measured in either characters per second (cps) or lines per second (lps). Printers have many options to increase their speed. Some print heads can print in both directions (bidirectional printing), thus saving the time of a return; blank spaces or lines can be efficiently passed over; special page formats can be programmed; etc. Thus, the actual speed at which characters can be printed is difficult to define exactly.

As was the case with input, analog output data can also be generated on a microcomputer. In this case a digital-to-analog converter (DA converter) takes a sequence of numbers and turns it into a sequence of voltages. With proper filtering a realistic analog signal can be generated. Hearing and speech scientists use DA conversion to generate simple and complex sounds, including speech, as described in Chapter 12.

Communication Peripheral Devices

The most often used communication device is the *modem*. The modem allows signals to be sent to and from two computers over the telephone lines. The rate of transmission is relatively slow (150, 300, or in some cases 1200 baud). A popular use of the modem is to allow a microcomputer access to a large data base stored on some other computer. The phone number of the data base is dialed (in some microcomputers, the computer might actually do the dialing) and the modem connected. With the proper instructions the data in the data base are available to the calling computer. For instance, many of the references in the National Library of Medicine are available on a data base called MEDLINE. Subscribers to MEDLINE can obtain information about certain references via the computer and the modem. The reference material can then be stored on the microcomputer so that the user can generate his or her own special reference library.

Mass Storage Peripheral Devices

The memory of the microprocessor usually is relatively small, and in most cases the contents of the memory are lost when power is turned off. Thus, if one needs to store large amounts of information for long periods of time, mass storage devices are required. The typical devices are cassettes, floppy disks, and fixed or hard disks. (In game-type computers both the program and some storage capability may reside on a plug-in module, but these are not often used in personal microcomputers.) In the near future bubble memory and products involving laser technology (as is used in video recorders) will be available for microcomputers.

The floppy and hard (fixed) disks are the most powerful mass storage devices for microcomputers. The amount of information that can be stored may be expressed in bits, bytes, or words. The disk is like a record, and the information is stored by magnetizing certain portions of the disk's surface. The *disk controller*, which resides in the microprocessor and communicates with the disk drive through I/O lines, aids the microprocessor in reading and writing information to and from the disk and memory. That is, the disk communicates directly with memory. The information is sorted on the disk by the use of timing tracks. These tracks help the microprocessor access the information quickly. The microprocessor interrogates a particular track for the directory of programs or files on the disk. The directory tells the disk controller which track to go to to find the information. Different computers sector their disks with different types of tracks. Thus, two computers are often unable to read each other's disks. When a disk is purchased it usually does not have any timing track. The tracks must be put on the disk by a program that *formats* the disk.

Floppy disks are portable and inexpensive but do not hold a tremendous amount of data (usually less than a megabyte). Hard disks can store large amounts of data, but they are fixed into the unit and cannot be moved. A common practice is to use a hard disk as the main mass storage device and a floppy disk drive as a backup device to obtain copies of programs or files. The floppies can also be carried from machine to machine.

Many microcomputers share the same hard disk in a *network*. Such networks require handshaking software and hardware so that more than one computer can access the same disk or program. With these shared systems, the more computers there are in the network, the longer it takes to execute a program, especially if all computers are using the same program or peripheral device.

SOFTWARE

The variety of hardware options described for microcomputers also applies to software. The basic program instructions for microcomputers are similar to those used by minicomputers, basically because the hardware architecture of microcomputers is modeled after that of minicomputers. As stated earlier, there are two basic types of software used by most microcomputer users: operating systems and programs. Nevertheless, all software eventually must communicate with the microprocessor in the language of the binary bit. This is the *machine language* of the computer that can often be programmed with the aid of a type of software referred to as the *assembler.* The assembler translates the software instructions directly into binary bits and allows variable names to be used rather than only bit codes. Many operating systems are written in some form of assembler language, and programs are written in all types of languages. Most non-assembler-language programs rely on a *compiler.* A compiler takes a program written in high-level English-like languages (e.g., BASIC, FORTRAN) and translates the instructions into binary bits, the language of the microprocessor.

Machine Language and the Assembler

The basic language of the computer is the setting of binary bits. Thus, programming begins with the manipulation of binary numbers. All programs and software must eventually be translated into binary bit code. This task is made easier by representing binary numbers as octal numbers (base 8) or sometimes as hexadecimal numbers (base 16). Certain combinations of bits are interpreted by the microcomputer software system. The instructions are symbolic or mnemonic codes. These instructions are translated into the machine language of binary bits by the assembler program. The number and type of instruction vary greatly from one microcomputer to another.

A string of binary numbers can be divided into groups of four bits for a hexadecimal number. Table 3-3 shows these types of conversions. Programming in octal or hexadecimal is easier than in binary, but still inefficient.

Operating Systems

When someone sits down at a computer, he or she wants to be able to enter, store, or print information. In general, the user wants to input information, have the computer perform some type of operation with it, and then provide an output. For instance, in word processing, the secretary wants to be able to type in a letter, make changes in it, print it, and save it on a disk for future reference. Somehow the computer must be able to perform all these tasks quickly and with a minimum of user intervention. In addition, the computer should be capable of performing identical tasks in the same way, independent of the particular program a user is executing. That is, storing data on a disk or printing on a printer should be per-

Table 3-3. Decimal, octal, binary, and hexadecimal conversions

Decimal	*Octal*	*Binary*	*Hexadecimal*
0	00	0000	0
1	01	00001	1
2	02	00010	2
3	03	00011	3
4	04	00100	4
5	05	00101	5
6	06	00110	6
7	07	00111	7
8	10	01000	8
9	11	01001	9
10	12	01010	A
11	13	01011	B
12	14	01100	C
13	15	01101	D
14	16	01110	E
15	17	01111	F
16	20	10,000	10

formed by the computer no matter what program is being used. The *operating system* is the software that arranges for these basic operations of the computer.

Some operating systems are unique to a particular computer, whereas others can be used on all computers that have the same basic microprocessor. Most operating systems assume that all the items to be used by the computer will be listed as files. Files can be programs, collections of data, letters, manuscripts, or an inventory. These files are stored on some type of mass storage device or media such as a disk. The operating system provides (1) a way to store these files on the disk and to keep track of where the various files reside, how much space is being used, and other "statistics" about the files and the computer; (2) a way to move the information in the files from the disk to the memory, the printer, another disk, or some other peripheral; (3) a way to change the information in a file or delete a file; and (4) usually an editor and an assembler. An editor is a program that allows the user to write a program. (Editors and word processing will be discussed later.) For instance, in some operating systems, the command DIR allows one to list all the files on a disk (i.e., to list the DIRectory of the disk); the command ERA allows one to ERAse a file from the disk, while SAVE saves a file, and TYPE types the contents of the file either on the monitor screen or on a printer (or some other peripheral), and REN allows one to REName a file. If each program or file is like a different instrument in an orchestra, then the operating system is like the conductor. It is the operating system's responsibility to make sure everything runs smoothly and in harmony.

Programs

Most microcomputer programs are used for computation, word processing (or text editing), data-base management, spread sheets, graphics, communications, additions to the operating system, and various combinations of these options.

Computation programs include BASIC, FORTRAN, PASCAL, etc. These programs were originally designed to aid in basic computations by computers. The ease of using the English-like language of BASIC has made it the main language for many computers. Some computers provide BASIC as part of the hardware in the microprocessor, whereas most programs must be read into the microprocessor from some mass storage device.

A wide variety of word-processing software is on the market. These products enable the user to type text and then to change the text material in very flexible ways. With the inclusion of programs that correct spelling and grammar and those that allow one text file to be combined with others, the microcomputer becomes a powerful office machine. Many word-processing programs also provide a wide variety of options concerning the format and form of the printed text. Some computers are designed only for word processing, and they should not be confused with word-processing software, which is one of many programs that might be used on a general-purpose microprocessor.

Text editing should not be confused with word processing. A text editor is a program that allows one to enter and change text material, but the commands that enter or change the text do not cause the material on the monitor to change. That is, in a word processor a command to move to the next word will cause the cursor to move to the next word. In text editing this same type of command does not move the cursor on the screen, but the software has moved to that location in memory. Thus, any additional material will be entered at that point even though the user will not immediately see the results on the screen. Editors are efficient programs that do not require much memory of the computer but a lot by the user.

Data-base management and spread sheets are two variations on a theme. The theme is the efficient processing of data or information files. Languages like BASIC allow data to be stored on files and for these files to be recalled at some later time. However, many commands in the program are required to accomplish this task, and files with similar information are difficult to access in an identical manner. Data-base management programs are very efficient for entering and retrieving large amounts of data. They are used for keeping inventories, doing accounting, keeping reference lists, storing tabulated data, etc. Many data-base management programs allow for sophisticated compilation of information in the data-base files. For instance, in a data base for references all the books with *hearing* in the title can be found in a matter of seconds or fractions of a second. If word lists are stored, the program might allow for all words with certain frequency of use or structure to be provided. A data-base program could be used to store information in a budget. However, if the budget is changed, the user does not immediately see the effect of the change on the entire budget. This immediate feedback is an advantage spread sheets offer over data bases. A spread sheet is a matrix of entries, such as a budget, with the various expenses listed by month. A change in one entry—for instance, the change in a secretary's salary—can be entered, and the effect of this change on the entire budget over the various dates involved can be quickly determined. Many scientists use spread sheets for performing simulations or modeling of complex systems.

The ability to draw graphs is often contained in a program such as BASIC, a spread sheet, or a data-base management system. However, special-purpose graphics-program packages are also available. The major requirement is that the monitor (and if hard copy is desired, a printer or plotter) be capable of drawing graphs. Many monitors do not have this capability because of the way in which the screen is refreshed or the way in which a character is placed on the CRT screen.

Software is available to aid in using the computer to communicate with other computers via a modem. These programs help establish the handshaking between the two computers; allow the transmitted data to be stored on the host computer's mass storage device, or printed, or sent to some other peripheral device; coordinate the retrieval of the communicated information with other software, such as word processing; and, if the hardware is available, may dial the number from a stored list of phone numbers or from a number entered at the keyboard.

A wide variety of other software is available to the microcomputer user, such as software that integrates many different programs. For instance, data from a data-base management file can be read into a spread sheet and then into a table in a word-processor file. Fancy calendars with memo and reminder options can be integrated with other programs. Graphics can be tied to the operation of a spread sheet or a data base. Special programs are available to recover files that were deleted by accident, to obtain detailed information about the status of the computer, and to identify where problems might be when things do not work. If you can think of some need for a program, someone has probably already developed it.

Programs are used in one of three general ways: a program is written, special instructions are used, or a menu supplies options. BASIC is an example of software that usually requires the user to write a program (a sequence of instructions) in order for the desired task to be performed. For some software (such as for the operating system described previously) the task can be performed by typing a single instruction. For instance, in a data-base management system the instruction *create* might begin a file for data, while *append* would allow one to enter data into the file. A popular means of executing a program is through a *menu* of options. A series of options appears on the screen; the user chooses one, and its function is performed. In word processing the menu might contain *D* for open a file, *X* for exit the program, *Y* for delete a file, *O* for copying a file from one disk to another, and *E* for renaming a file. The user types the letter of the option desired. Quite often additional menus appear until the task is accomplished. Computer manufacturers have been clever in designing menus and providing ways to make a choice. The menu options might be pictures (called pixels) rather than words (a picture of a file drawer instead of the word *file* or a trash can instead of *delete*). Keypads, special-function keys, a mouse, a touch screen, and soon voice may be used to choose the particular option. These gimmicks make the chore of going through the menu less tedious, they make learning the system fast and fun, and they reduce the amount of material to be learned. However, the experienced user may find these menu gimmicks cumbersome and slow.

4
Microcomputer-based Client-Record Management

Gary E. Rushakoff

In the clinical practices of speech, language, and hearing, it is customary to maintain information on each person for whom services are provided. This is done in order to document the services rendered to an individual and to provide information on that individual with which to make clinical decisions. This information is put on paper, stored in a manila folder, and placed in a file cabinet. This is an *archival* record-keeping system, a place where information is *kept*. Archival file systems are useful for storing information on many people but not for comparing and processing information *among* people or generating summary information about the types of services provided by a clinic.

It is often necessary to draw information from this archival storage system. When attempted manually, the task can be laborious, time-consuming, and occasionally impossible (Fig. 4-1). Once client records are stored on a microcomputer, however, clinicians have quick access to information that can be used for (1) administrative reports, (2) grants, and (3) budget justification for personnel, equipment, materials, and training (Rushakoff and Lombardino, 1984). With a computer-based client-record system, more specific information on clinic needs is available, and it is possible to plot changes in the distribution of clients being served. Computerized data allow clinics to plan and justify projected service needs.

Several studies have documented the development and benefits of record keeping in speech and hearing facilities using main-frame computers (Elliott, Vegely, and Falvey, 1971; Kamara and Kamara, 1976; Harden, Harden, and Norris, 1977; Peterson, 1977; Rushakoff et al., 1979), and microcomputer-based client-record systems (Jackson, 1983).

Computer-based records often help with daily clinical needs. As a personal example, another clinician and I were the only two clinicians working at one of the largest residential institutions for mentally retarded individuals on the East Coast. The file contained over 2000 records, even though there were only about 1400 residents at the facility. One day we were asked for a list of those residents between the ages of 3 and 18 years who had not had a speech-language evaluation within the past year. Since we were both new to the facility, we first had to spend many hours purging the file of inactive records. We then had to obtain a list from the administration of individuals between the ages of 3 and 18. It was then necessary to check each client record on the list for the date of his or her last evaluation. This process, which took several days, could have been accomplished in minutes with a computer-based system.

A more subtle example of the need for computerized records occurred at this same facility when a cottage aide called to say she had found a hearing aid in one of her resident's dresser drawers. She had not seen him

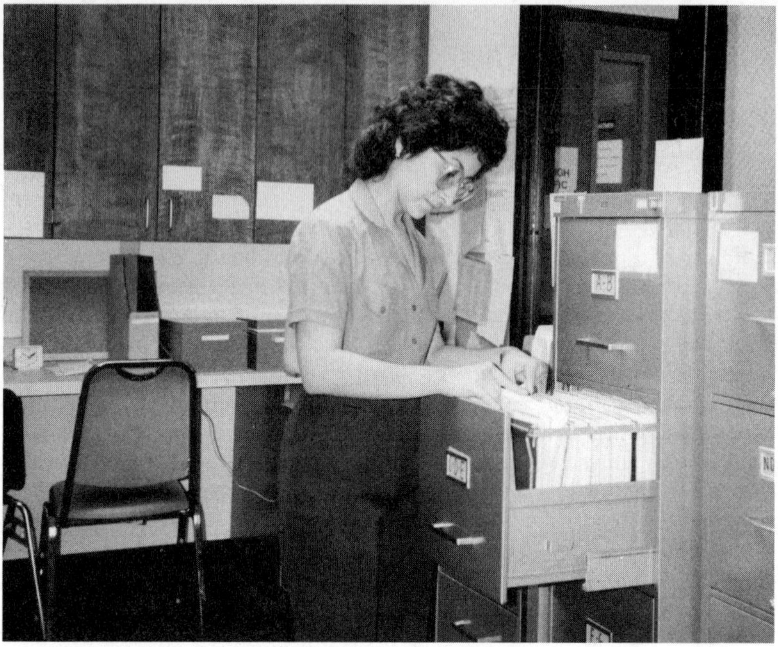

Fig. 4-1. Standard paper file systems are designed for storage and retrieval of information on individuals, but not for generating information about them collectively.

wear it for the year she had been there. Although the only problem in this case was the need for a new battery, it occurred to us that there might be many other residents who had hearing aids that might be sitting in dresser drawers with dead batteries. Calling the various cottages to ask who had a hearing aid would not identify those with long-unused aids. Once again it was necessary to search the file manually for those individuals with hearing aids, a process that would have taken the computer a few minutes.

Computer-generated client data can show trends in needs and services that are so subtle they are not noticed by the clinicians. For example, after computerizing 50 pieces of speech, language, and hearing information on 1200 individuals at a residential facility for mentally retarded individuals (Rushakoff et al., 1979), it was found that 67% of the residents did not or could not communicate through speech. This figure provided a strong budget and grant justification for more communication devices, materials on Blissymbols and sign language, and in-service training funds, and also identified specific skills needed in new speech and hearing personnel.

EQUIPMENT REQUIREMENTS

Most of the more widely used microcomputer systems allow client-record keeping through *data-base software*. In order to maintain the largest amount of information in the computer file system and to have it operate at the fastest rate, it is advisable to get the maximum random access memory (RAM) available. Since loading information from a disk is a time-consuming operation, some programs allow the use of a *RAM disk* (disk emulator), which is a firmware card filled with RAM chips. Depending on the size of the RAM disk, the entire contents of a floppy disk may be loaded into this card. This allows immediate access to information that often takes quite a while to load from the disk drive. Since RAM disks can be used only for disks that are not copy protected, they are usually used for the data disk but not for the data-base program disk. A printer is necessary to provide a hard copy of the information generated. Also, some data-base software either requires or works faster using two disk drives.

For clinics that wish to maintain voluminous records on large numbers of people, it may be advantageous to use a *hard-disk drive*. Even though large data files can be placed on several floppy disks, the task of sorting is often unwieldy and frustratingly time consuming. A hard-disk drive can solve this problem, but it is expensive, costing at least $700. As it can be devastating to lose information from a hard disk, the majority of hard-disk owners still use 20 to 40 floppy disks as a backup system.

If a clinic has a hard-disk drive and several microcomputers, it is possible to hook all the systems to the hard-disk drive. This is known as a *local-area network* (LAN). It means that the computerized client records can be accessed by any microcomputer system in the building. The expense involves wiring all the microcomputers to the hard-disk drive and purchasing a controlling device for the LAN that allows only one microcomputer to access the hard disk at any one moment.

A *modem* allows the transfer of client data from one microcomputer to another over the telephone. This device can be used to transfer information regarding clients to funding and referral agencies. A modem can also be of value to clinicians who work in several locations, such as a school system or multiple private offices. A microcomputer with the data-base program and client-record disk can be located at one facility. The clinicians can operate that microcomputer and the data-base program using the microcomputer at other facilities via a modem. The clinician can call the secretary and ask to have the telephone hooked to the microcomputer. If the school system can afford to have an extra telephone line, the main system can be kept online, in order to bypass the secretary. The clinician need only have the computer dial the telephone number of the main microcomputer system. To ensure confidentiality, this type of setup requires a data-base program that allows the use of a password.

UNDERSTANDING DATA-BASE PROGRAMS

In order to decide which software to purchase and how to set up and use a client-records data base, it is necessary to understand some common terminology.

A *data base* is a collection of information (data) that may or may not be related. The most familiar data base is the library, which has information on thousands of topics available in books, newspapers, periodicals, records, films, and so forth. The encyclopedia is also a data base, that is, a collection of information.

A *file* is a collection of information that *is* related. The telephone book is a collection of information on almost everyone who owns a telephone

Table 4-1. Examples of data-base file structures

File: Client records
Record: Person
Fields:
1) Name
2) Address
3) Telephone number
4) Date of evaluation

File: Standardized assessments in clinic
Record: Test
Fields:
1) Name of test
2) Age range
3) How long to administer
4) Author
5) Year of publication
6) Publisher

File: Clinic inventory
Record: Item
Fields:
1) Item
2) Location
3) Condition of item
4) Tag number
5) Cost of item

in a community. A data base is made up of many files. For example, the telephone book (file) can usually be found at the library (data base). For clinical record keeping, the file may consist of all clients who have had, or are currently receiving, clinical services.

A *record* is a specific collection of information stored in a file. In a clinical record-keeping system each record would be of a different person. If a clinic is providing services to 80 people, there would be 80 records in the file. This terminology is different from terms usually used in the clinic. We often say, "Pull David's file from the file cabinet." If we were using a computer-based system, we would say, "Pull David's record from the file."

Each record is made up of specific pieces of information. Each piece of information is called a *field*. In a client record-keeping system the name, address, telephone number, date of birth, and so on are each known as a field.

To summarize, a file is made up of a number of records, and records are made up of a number of fields (Table 4-1). Virtually all data-base software is designed around these three building blocks, and understanding them helps one to understand the differences in the capabilities of various programs.

SETTING UP A DATA BASE

It is difficult to decide what information to collect on each client. Unlike the paper-record system, which allows the collection of any information the clinician would like to include, the computerized record system must be specific (see Table 4-2 and also Elliott, Vegely, and Falvey, 1971; Kamara and Kamara, 1976; Rushakoff et al., 1979). Some types of information lend themselves well to computer files, and others do not. For example, while it may be easy to indicate whether a client has a semantic language problem (1 = yes, 2 = no), it is not easy to computerize a lengthy description of that problem.

Clinicians should determine their current information needs before setting up a data base. For example, many clinics need to produce data regarding the number of clients evaluated or the number of clients in various age groups or communication-disorder categories. However, even though clinicians might not find a current need for knowing the hearing level of each ear of each client, this information might prove useful later. Information regarding the specific needs of a clinic may provide focus and justification for equipment, personnel, materials, and so forth. Many data-base programs allow the user to change the structure of the file at any time to reflect changes in data collection needs.

Choosing Data-base Software

It is almost never necessary for a clinic to write, or contract to have written, its own client record-keeping microcomputer software. I know of at least two clinics where sizable amounts of money and time were spent for programmers to write a record-keeping microcomputer program. Unfortunately, both clinics ultimately purchased data-base programs at their local computer store for $300–$500.

The data-base program should match the skill level of the user. In general, the easier a program is to learn and operate, the less flexible it turns out to be in performing complex data-base functions. The novice-oriented data-base program may be limited and include a number of compromises in order to keep the process simple. In most data-base systems, the user interacts with the program via a series of menus. While a menu-driven program is easier to learn and use than a command-driven program, it may take more time to operate, as each menu must be loaded from the disk each time a different function is selected.

One should give serious thought to data-base software that is totally *memory resident*. The term memory resident means that all the modules in the program are loaded into random-access memory (RAM). Programs that are not memory resident must go to the disk to load each module selected. Memory-resident software is appealing because the user can go from one application (e.g., data entry) to another instantly. The disadvantage of memory-resident programs is that they take up memory space that could be used to increase the file capacity of the program.

It might be difficult for the novice microcomputer user to select a data-base program. Often it is not until a program is used for a period of time that one realizes that critical features are missing. Also, computer store vendors may not be the best source of information. Dozens of data-base programs are available, and unless the clinician happens to be interested in the programs with which the computer store personnel are familiar, he or she is not likely to get clear answers to important questions. However, reliable vendors should be willing to let the clinician look at software documentation, where the answers to some questions can (sometimes) be

Table 4-2. Sample file structure of a client record-keeping system

SPEECH AND HEARING CLINIC

Filled out by: ______________________ Date filled out: __________

Name (Last name, first name) ______________________
Date of birth (e.g., 07/04/77) ______________________
Street address ______________________
City/State ______________________
Zip code ______________________
Home phone ______________________
Parent's name ______________________
File no. ______________________
School ______________________
Referred by (e.g., Smith, J., friend) ______________________
Sex (male/female) ______________________
Date of evaluation (or 1st Rx session) ______________________
Evaluation supervisor ______________________
What foreign language ______________________
Recommend for further therapy? (Y/N) ______________________

Primary complaint _____
Secondary complaint _____

Primary diagnosis _____
Secondary diagnosis _____
Tertiary diagnosis _____
Hearing screening (P/F) _____

Recommended for therapy? (Y/N) _____

Test 1: _____
Score: _____

Test 2: _____
Score: _____

Articulation _____	1 = problem
Language _____	2 = normal
Voice _____	3 = no information
Fluency _____	
Hearing _____	
Oral mechanism _____	

Hearing

Type of loss RE: _____	1 = normal
Type of loss LE: _____	2 = conductive
	3 = sensorineural
	4 = mixed
	5 = questionable
	6 = unknown type
	7 = insufficient data due to behavioral constraints
Degree of loss RE: _____	1 = normal
Degree of loss LE: _____	2 = mild
	3 = moderate
	4 = moderately severe
	5 = severe
	6 = profound
Discrimination RE: _____	1 = excellent
Discrimination LE: _____	2 = fair

Table 4-2. (continued)

	3 = poor 4 = questionable 5 = insufficient data
Impedance pattern RE: _____ Impedance pattern LE: _____	1 = normal 2 = middle ear 3 = cochlear site 4 = 8th nerve pattern
Tympanogram RE: _____ Tympanogram LE: _____	1 = A 2 = A shallow 3 = A deep 4 = B 5 = C 6 = could not test

found. Data-base programs must be easy to use. Most people do not want to know *how* a specific program works; they just want to be able to put in data and get processed information out in clear formats.

File Managers

File managers are the computerized version of the metal file cabinet. In general, most file managers are easier to use than the more powerful relational data-base program. All file managers allow the user to set up a client file, enter information, and, to some degree, sort and search these records and print them.

There is a special type of file manager, the *dedicated* file manager, that is already set up. In other words, the program designer has already decided which pieces of speech, language, and hearing information will be collected. In a communication-disorders context these types of dedicated file managers may have a generic name like, "A Computer Program for Record Keeping in a Speech and Hearing Clinic." A problem arises if the clinician wants to collect a piece of information the author did not allow space for, such as social security number, test score, referral source, and tympanogram result. Also, dedicated file managers do not have as powerful data-processing functions as do general file managers.

Relational Data Bases

Relational data-base programs have the same features as file managers but often provide a greater ability to manipulate the data. However, the major feature of relational software is its ability to compare, manipulate, and merge data from separate files. For example, the speech pathologist may have one file of students receiving speech services. The occupational therapist may have a separate file, and the physical therapist a third file. With a relational data-base program the clinicians would be able to ask questions such as, "Which students between the ages of 6 and 18 are receiving speech therapy, occupational therapy, *and* physical therapy?" A relational data base could process that information by looking through all three files in one operation. A file manager does not have this capability.

Relational data-base software can also be used to simplify a clinic's client-records system. For example, many clinics have one small index-card file with the client's name, address, and a number that matches the number of their record in the large file cabinet (Mueller and Peters, 1976). This card system is a small file that allows access to the main file. This strategy can also be used in a computerized version that keeps *two* files for client records.

In general, relational data-base programs are considered more difficult to learn and use than file managers. Some relational data-base programs are not menu-driven and require the user to create a program in order to set up a file. dBASE II is one of the most widely used relational data-base programs for microcomputers; however, for all its power, some users find it expensive and difficult to use.

Integrated Software

It is often necessary or advantageous to include information drawn from a client-records data base in an administrative report, grant request, or research paper. In 1982 and 1983, several programs were designed so that data from a specific data-base program could be transferred easily to a file in a word-processing program. By 1984, integrated software had been developed, which enabled two or more "applications" to operate within the same program. Usually this means that one software package can contain a data-base program, a word processor, and a spread sheet. The information from the spread sheet or data base can be transferred easily to a word-processing file. This flexibility can be useful when the information generated from the data-base module needs to be inserted in the middle of an administrative report or grant. The other advantage to integrated packages is that they have a similar command structure, so one set of commands operates all modules. Although consumers may spend less money buying all three applications in one package (e.g., word processing, data base, spread sheet), there are those who believe that integrated software programs may be less powerful than individual programs.

CAPABILITY OF DATA-BASE SOFTWARE

Dozens of data-base programs are available for the more widely used microcomputer systems, and more are being introduced every year. They can vary in cost from $20 to $700. In general, the differences among these programs can be described in terms of (1) capacity, (2) data entry, (3) data retrieval, and (4) report generation.

Capacity

Only a limited number of words can be typed on a piece of paper, a finite number of pages can be placed in a manila record folder, and only a limited number of folders can fit in a single metal file cabinet. These limits also hold true for computer record-keeping software. In order to determine what capacity is needed, the clinic should first set up the client record file on paper (see Table 4-2).

1. *Number of characters per field:* Many programs limit the length of any particular field. For example, a program that limited the field length to 12 characters would not hold most people's names. Neither would it hold most city and state information. Although it is true that one can

Table 4-3. Data-base software decision-making form

Features	*File Handler*	*Relational Data Base*
Characters per field	_____	_____
Characters per record	_____	_____
Fields per record	_____	_____
Records per file	_____	_____
No. of fields sorted (no. of keys)	_____	_____
No. of fields in multilevel sort	_____	_____
No. of fields searched	_____	_____
Memory requirements	_____	_____
Custom report generator (Y/N)	_____	_____
Restructure file (Y/N)	_____	_____
Password security (Y/N)	_____	_____
Menu-driven (Y/N)	_____	_____
Hard-disk capability (Y/N)	_____	_____
Custom data entry screen (Y/N)	_____	_____
No. of open files	_____	_____

set up one field for the last name and a second field for the first name, this strategy may be more work than it is worth. Other strategies for reducing the number of characters needed is to use a code system so that instead of requiring a long field for "name of test," the clinician can just enter a two-digit code.

2. *Number of characters per record:* By definition, the record is all the information on a particular individual. Most programs limit the total number of characters that can be used in each record. For example, some programs limit record length to 1000 characters or less. Programs that allow for a very limited number of characters per record can present problems. A program may indicate that a record can have up to 70 fields, *but* only 280 characters per record. That means the average length of each field is only 4 characters!
3. *Number of fields per record:* The number of fields per record defines the total number of specific pieces of information (fields) each individual can have. A program with a limit of ten fields per record would barely get past the name, address, telephone number, and date of birth. The paper version of the file will indicate how many fields are required. With relational data-base software, a dual-file strategy can be used to increase the total number of fields for an individual.
4. *Number of records per file:* Just as a limited number of manila records can be placed in a metal file cabinet, the number of records is also limited in a computer file. Since it may be of value to keep both active and inactive records in the computer file, a clinic should estimate the number of people they will provide services for during the next 5 years. Although some software may indicate that it can hold 65,000 records per file, this number may not be reached because of the limits of the computer memory or the storage limits of the disk.

Data Entry

Data entry refers to the ease of (1) setting up a file, (2) changing a file, (3) entering data into a record, and (4) changing information in a record.

1. *Setting up a file:* Once the file structure has been developed on paper, it can be entered into the data-base program. Most programs do this interactively by asking the user to type in the name of field #1, which could be "Name." It may then ask how long this field should be. Most individuals' last and first names require 20–30 characters. When all the fields are entered, the file is set, and data can be entered.
2. *Changing a file:* It is possible that when files are initially set up, information is not included that one wishes to add later. Some programs do not allow the user to change or add new fields after the file has been entered; other programs allow the user to change, delete, and add new fields at any time.
3. *Entering data:* Most programs allow easy entry of record data. Some programs enable the data entry screen to be customized, which can be especially useful when there are many clinicians entering data. For example, without this feature a program in the data entry mode might just say, "Name ________________." A program that allows the user to design the data-entry screen could say,

> Type in the name: Last name, first name
> (for example: Smith, David) ________________

This feature can also be useful when codes are used to enter information, for example,

> Speech Intelligibility Level (enter the number) ________________
> 1—normal
> 2—mild
> 3—moderate
> 4—severe

Most programs have two methods of correcting an error in data entry. If the user has just entered a mistake, a "backup" can be initiated to that field in order to enter the correct information. When all the data for a record have been entered, the program often displays the information, with the instruction to press the return key if the information is correct, or to enter the number of the field that has a mistake. Some programs protect against errors in data entry. For example, in the illustration above on intelligibility, the program would allow the user to enter only 1, 2, 3, or 4 and would not accept any other number. Programs should also allow the user to change data easily at a later time. The clinician should not have to reenter the entire record but be able to change only the data in specific fields.

DATA RETRIEVAL

The ability to reorganize and process information is the heart of data-base programs. This ability is the key that separates it from archival paper-record-keeping systems. There are three main processing functions of data-base software: (1) sorting, (2) searching, and (3) frequency of occurrence.

Table 4-4. Example of a multilevel sort first by disorder, then by last name

Disorder	Name	Date of Birth	File No.
Aphasia			
	Carr, Dennis *	09/12/39	5.0295
	Duffey, Mary	02/04/27	5.0167
	Gordon, David	11/22/32	5.0746
	Jenkins, Stuart	09/03/23	5.0285
Articulation			
	Barry, Richard	03/12/63	6.1823
	Martin, Jack	11/02/57	6.2295
	Pierce, Robert	03/09/80	6.1090
	Sullivan, Walter	12/24/81	6.2551
	Thompson, Shelly	09/22/82	6.8461
Cleft palate			
	Cooper, Julian	02/22/79	1.0827
	Denney, Charles	04/08/80	1.0602
	Harden, Linda	11/14/74	1.8482
Developmental language			
	Allen, Michael	06/14/81	3.0112
	Cannon, Jill	11/03/82	3.0330
	Ferguson, Kent	03/09/79	3.0202
	Stone, Raymond	10/30/81	3.0939

* All names used in these examples are fictitious.

Sorting

Sorting organizes *all* of the records in a file either alphabetically or numerically. While the most common way to keep records organized is alphabetically by last name, it might prove useful at times to have the file ordered by date of evaluation, date of birth, primary disorder, and so forth. A *single-level sort* organizes all the records based on the information in one field. It is also possible for programs to accomplish a *multilevel sort*. For example, we could use an alphabetized list of all clients in each disorder category (see Table 4-4). The program would first sort all the records by disorder and then, within each disorder category, sort the names alphabetically. Some programs allow multilevel sorts using several fields at once. It is important to realize that not all programs allow the user to sort or search any field. For example, a program may allow 50 fields per record, but when the file is first established, only 5 fields can be chosen to sort or search. Those fields that are chosen by the user to be sorted or searched are called *keys*.

Searching

Unlike sorting, which affects all the records in a file, searching finds only those records that meet one or more conditions. Single searches are used to find records based on information in one field. For example, the program could be told to find the record of *Smith, David*, and that this information will be located in the *name* field. If it is not possible to determine the first name, most programs will allow a partial search of a field; for example, find everyone whose last name is "Smith." There are many applications for the search capability other than just finding an individual's record. It is

Table 4-5. Multilevel search information requested: Males between the ages of 6 and 21 years with an articulation deficit who have normal hearing in both ears and were evaluated within the past 3 years.

Date of Birth	*Name*
03/12/65	Barry, Richard
09/03/65	Glover, Jerry
12/02/65	Diamond, Arthur
06/10/68	Sayre, Chris
01/22/69	Brown, David
11/19/72	Wright, William
06/30/74	Meyer, John
06/02/76	Simpson, Harlan

possible to find all the records of people who were given a particular language test, or to find all those with a voice disorder, or all 4-year-olds. One of the more exciting capabilities of data-base software is the *multilevel search*. This capability allows the retrieval of records of individuals who meet a series of criteria (see Table 4-5). For example, the program could find individuals who are "male, between the ages of 6 and 18, dysfluent, have normal hearing, and live within city limits."

Another capability of the search procedure is to create a separate file for records found in the search. The search procedure could identify individuals who meet specific requirements and then store their records on another disk, creating a new file.

Frequency of Occurrence

The frequency of occurrence function answers questions related to "how many." For example, it could print a list of all the primary disorders in the computer file of clients and indicate how many people have each disorder. This capability allows clinics to produce percentages of clients in each disorder category. It can also determine the number of clients in each age assessment category.

Report Generation

While processing data is the heart of data-base software, the manner in which the data are printed is also important. Inexpensive programs often do not allow any customized output, but instead just print the data in one long column. Flexibility in formatting the printout varies greatly and is a very important consideration. Printing flexibility should allow the user to (1) define left, right, top, and bottom margins, (2) print headers and footers (i.e., titles, footnotes, etc., on the top and bottom of the form), (3) put the date on the page, and (4) number the pages. It also should allow the user to save the format so a new one does not have to be created each time a report is needed.

CONFIDENTIALITY AND SECURITY OF RECORDS

Communication-disorders clinicians need to be concerned about the loss of client records and confidentiality of recorded information. Although it does not happen often, it is possible to lose client-record information stored on disks. Archival paper records are indeed more resistant to loss. There are several reasons why it is not recommended that microcomputer-based client-record systems replace standard paper records. While it is possible to include summaries of various aspects of a case on a computer-based system, it is usually not possible to include the breadth of information or the other documents often found in patient records traditionally stored in a paper-record system. There are two ways to protect against loss of microcomputer disk records: (1) making a duplicate or backup disk of the data, and (2) keeping printouts of the disk records.

Clinicians must also be concerned about confidentiality of client records. An easy way to ensure confidentiality is to restrict physical access to the disks by locking them up. If the disks must be left out and accessible during the day, many data-base programs allow the precaution of requiring a password to access the data on the disk. When necessary, the password can be changed. The password feature should not give clinicians a false sense of security, however. Many inexpensive programs are available that will scan any disk and show the user all the information on it, including the password!

Microcomputer-based client-record keeping systems allow clinicians to collect and display data, to provide information needed by others, and to provide information for decision making considerations. The computer file system can provide information and population characteristics which can be used to improve quality and quantity of clinical services. The major limitation of microcomputer-based files is the file and record capacity limits imposed by the floppy disk. New data-base software is being developed that is more powerful and easier to use. As clinics around the country begin to maintain client information on the microcomputer, a large data base will be formed of individuals with communication disorders. This data base will open new avenues of research.

REFERENCES

Elliott, L., Vegely, A., and Falvey, N. Description of a computer-oriented record-keeping system. *ASHA* 13:435–443, 1971.

Harden, R. J., Harden, R. W., and Norris, M. Computer program for the analysis of clinical enrollment. *ASHA* 19:472–474, 1977.

Jackson, C. O. Use of microcomputers for school hearing screening and evaluation records. Presented to the American Speech-Language-Hearing Association Annual Convention, Cincinnati, 1983.

Kamara, C., and Kamara, A. Computer billing, service analysis, and financial reporting in a hearing and speech agency. *ASHA* 18:229–231, 1976.

Mueller, P., and Peters, T. A clinical record-keeping system. *ASHA* 18:352–353, 1976.

Peterson, H. A. More about computer assisted clinical record keeping. *ASHA* 19:617–618, 1977.

Rushakoff, G. E., Vinson, B. P., Penner, K. A., and Messal, S. A. Clinical decision making through electronic information processing. Presented to the American Speech-Language-Hearing Association Annual Convention, Atlanta, 1979.

Rushakoff, G. E., and Lombardino, L. J. Microcomputer applications. *ASHA* 26:27–31, 1984.

5

Microcomputer Applications in the University Setting

Jackson Roush and Yoshiyuki Horii

The recent application of computer technology to the field of communication disorders is already having a substantial impact. Some speech pathology and audiology training programs have acquired their own minicomputers, although cost is still a prohibitive factor for many. Fortunately, advancing microprocessor technology is quickly diminishing the differences between mini- and microcomputers. As this trend continues, affordable computer technology is becoming increasingly available to university training programs. A recent survey of microcomputer use in the academic setting revealed that nearly half the speech and hearing departments or clinics responding to the survey had at least one microcomputer (Rushakoff and Lombardino, 1984). Most respondents listed word processing and maintenance of client records as their highest priorities for microcomputer utilization. We predict that in the coming years, the number of university programs utilizing microprocessor technology will increase dramatically and those already equipped with microcomputers will apply them with greater diversity and creativity.

MICROCOMPUTER TEACHING APPLICATIONS

Computer-Assisted Self-Instruction

Now in its second decade of development, computer-assisted instruction (CAI) has evolved from early systems requiring special languages and expensive computer hardware to highly flexible and affordable microcomputer systems. Most currently available instructional software or "courseware" is no longer coded in a special CAI language but rather in the popular interactive computing and display language known as BASIC. Huntington (1980) discusses several advantages and disadvantages of BASIC in developing CAI systems for microcomputers: (1) There is a low initial investment in programming. (2) Instructors can easily learn the language. (3) Instructors can revise their own courseware. (4) Courseware development time lag is relatively short. (5) Programming flexibility is high. (6) Support for BASIC is widespread, permitting maximum sharing. Among the limitations of using BASIC in this context are (1) all scoring must be programmed, (2) answer analyses must be programmed uniquely, (3) storing of numerous responses necessitates the creation of separate files, (4) pathing analyses require the use of counters, (5) logical section steps (present query/analyze response) must be repeated continuously, (6) cumulative record-keeping is difficult, and (7) input/output capabilities are currently limited to video or printed display, and a keyset. Despite these limitations, most users appreciate the extensive flexibility and control afforded by programming in BASIC.

Computer-assisted instruction software can also be programmed for microcomputers using an "authoring system." Instead of requiring that each line be programmed separately, authoring systems provide a series of questions permitting the instructor simply to type in the desired sequence of interactions. Recently, the creation of special authoring languages such as Super PILOT have provided substantial assistance to CAI developers. Rushakoff (1984) notes that Super PILOT is relatively easy to learn, less time-consuming than BASIC, and more amenable to combining color graphics and text than is BASIC. He also notes, however, that courseware developed using Super PILOT results in a slower response time for each frame and significantly less disk-storage capability. Given the growing availability of relatively low-cost, high-volume disk-storage systems, the latter problem is likely to be ameliorated in the future.

Regardless of the computer language employed, creators of CAI software must decide among a variety of options for the design and formatting of their instructional materials. Will the program employ graphics or will it be limited to printed text? If graphics are to be used, will they appear in color or monochrome? Each of these features may enhance or detract from the effectiveness of a program depending upon the specific courseware objectives. Another important consideration is feedback to the student. Feedback modes include audible beeps indicating a correct or incorrect response, specific scores indicating ongoing or final performance, and detailed explanations as to why a response was incorrect. An option known as *branching* allows the student to access additional information in a problem area. Instructors electing to create their own CAI programs, as well as those electing to purchase commercially available materials, need to consider each of these features as they relate to specific instructional objectives.

Existing CAI Software

For nearly 20 years CAI has been used extensively in a variety of contexts ranging from elementary school applications to advanced medical training. The field of communication disorders has only recently begun to employ the microcomputer for instructional purposes. At the time of this writing, most CAI materials are designed for instructional applications in audiology, although materials for teaching anatomy and physiology as well as language analysis have also emerged. Figure 5-1 is from a series of CAI materials developed by Rushakoff et al. (1984) for teaching anatomy and physiology of the speech and hearing mechanism. Described as a microcomputer-assisted "study partner," the programs are designed to serve as a self-instructional supplement to traditional classroom and laboratory presentation. Figure 5-1A is a schematic diagram of the vocal mechanism accompanied by a multiple-choice question. Figures 5-1B and 5-1C, respectively, show response frames for an incorrect and correct response to the question presented in Figure 5-1A. Along with the instructional unit on phonation, from which Figure 5-1 is taken, CAI programs covering the speech mechanism, respiration, neurology, embryology, and the hearing mechanism are also included. These programs provide useful examples of how interactive CAI materials can be applied to the field of communication disorders. If color monitors are available, the value of using color when combining text with graphics is also apparent. Although the programs can be used with a monochrome monitor, the overall

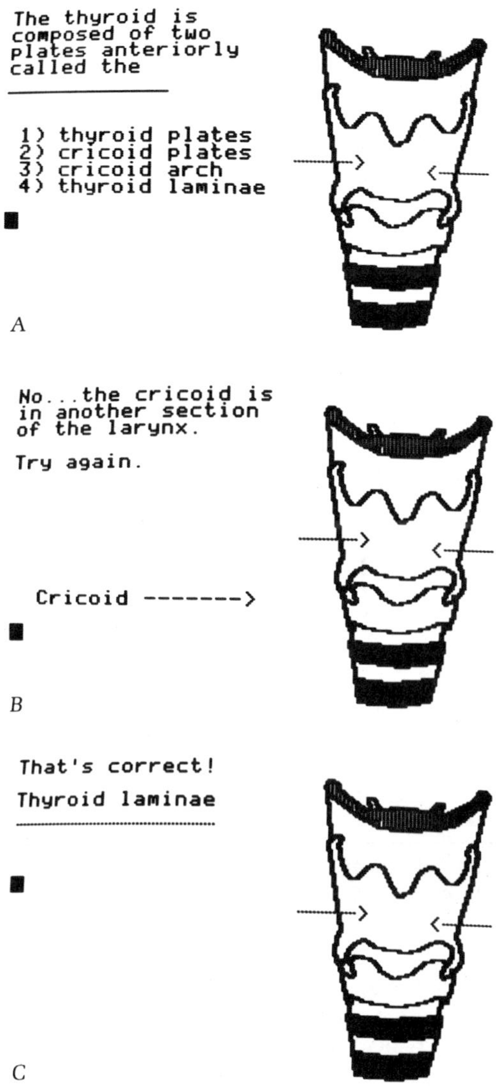

Fig. 5-1. Video terminal displays showing question and response frames from computer-assisted instruction unit on anatomy of speech mechanism. (From Rushakoff et al., 1984, with permission.)

presentation is greatly enhanced by using color to highlight the anatomical descriptors and their corresponding subdivisions. It is also interesting that the authors of this CAI package elected not to include "scoring" for student feedback, noting that many students find it beneficial to occasionally select a "wrong" answer to determine why it was incorrect. Again, we see that courseware design is determined by the specific instructional objectives of each application.

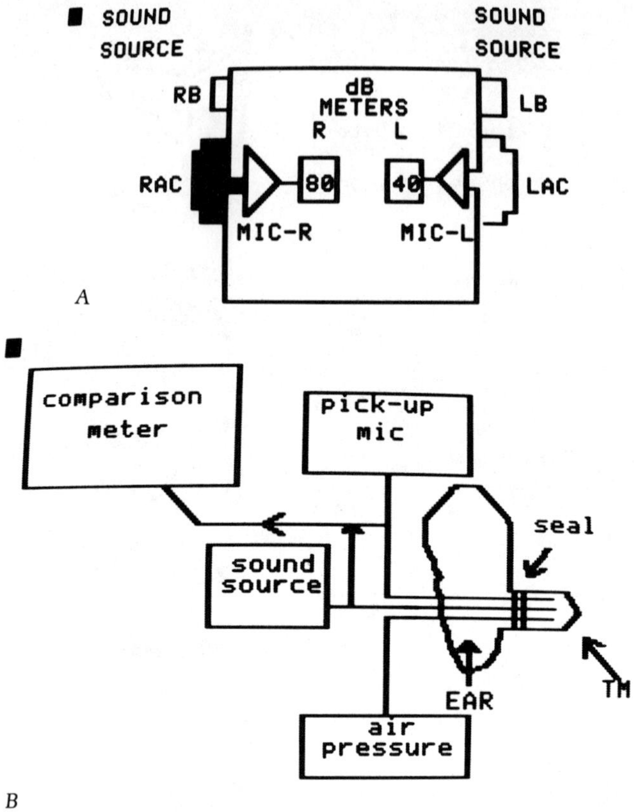

Fig. 5-2. Video terminal displays from a computer-assisted instruction program on basic audiologic concepts. (From Rose, 1984, with permission.)

In another example of CAI courseware, Figure 5-2 is from a set of materials recently developed by Rose (1984) for teaching basic audiologic concepts and test procedures. The schematic in Figure 5-2A depicts interaural attenuation as related to masking for pure-tone audiometry; Figure 5-2B is a sample display from the unit on acoustic immittance. Following an orientation to the graphic displays and a brief tutorial on each of the topic areas, a series of question/response interactions is initiated. The program indicates the accuracy of a response through explanatory text. Also included are programs for instructional assistance in electronystagmography, hearing aids, decibel notation, and test battery interpretation.

Another CAI package, designed to provide practice in the administration of pure-tone audiometry and masking, is the Computerized Audiometric Programmable Simulator (CAPS) developed by Zimmerman (1983). A sample display from the program is shown in Figure 5-3. In this example, a bone conducted signal is presented to the right mastoid while an earphone delivers masking to the left ear. As shown, the client responds by raising a finger on the right or left hand. The frequency and intensity of stimulus and masking, displayed at the upper right, are controlled from the computer keyboard. Thresholds generated by the student are displayed in the lower left quadrant, and immediate feedback as to the accuracy of a masked threshold is provided in the evaluation matrix shown at the lower right. The CAPS simulator, written in BASIC, is supplied with a file containing nine audiograms. Additional audiometric configurations can be programmed by the instructor or purchased separately. The simulator also allows for recording of student responses for later evaluation by the instructor.

Several other microcomputer-assisted instructional packages are currently under development. A new series by Lotterman (1984) will include tutorials and clinical simulations related to basic audiologic principles and test interpretation. Johnston (1984) has developed a series of programs designed to provide instructional assistance in the area of language analysis. CAI materials for editing of children's language transcripts, recognition of inflectional morphemes, and calculation of mean morphemes per utterance have been completed and development of additional units on other aspects of language-sample analysis is currently underway. Based on several semesters of experience with graduate and undergraduate students, the authors report that results are encouraging, both in terms of student acceptance and performance (Johnston and Backler, 1984).

The overall effectiveness of computer-assisted instruction in the training of speech pathologists and audiologists has not yet been systematically investigated. Nevertheless, based on its success in other fields and favorable preliminary reports from practitioners in the field of speech and hearing, computer-based instructional techniques are likely to play an expanding role in future years. Levitt et al. (1978) note that university training programs have traditionally found themselves in a professional dilemma because of the need to provide high-quality training experiences while maintaining equally high standards for clinical service. Computer-assisted instruction offers a variety of options for facilitating the transition from classroom teaching to clinical practice. However, despite this

Fig. 5-3. Video terminal displays from a computerized audiometric simulator. (From H. Zimmerman, CAPS: Computerized Audiometric Programmable Simulator. *Las Cruces, N.M.: Audiosoft, 1983. With permission.)*

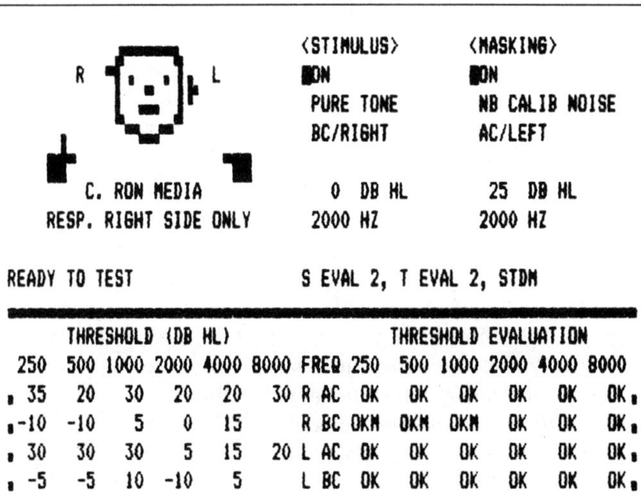

enormous potential, discretion must be exercised in the design and implementation of computer-based instructional materials. Arons (1984), in an insightful review of computer-based instruction, notes that many CAI programs are merely "page turners" for material better suited to text presentation. He suggests instead creative use of the "Socratic dialogue," a series of questions carefully chosen to lead the student into self-discovery through logic and reasoning. Viewed accordingly, the challenge in developing useful instructional materials lies more in the design of effectual dialogues than in their programming and technological preparation. Arons also cautions against overuse of CAI materials, noting that even the most impressive computer-assisted training materials will never supplant the essential classroom dynamics of discussion, argument, and verbal interaction.

USE OF MICROCOMPUTERS IN CLASSROOM TEACHING AND DEMONSTRATION

In addition to providing self-instructional applications, the computer-assisted programs described previously can also be used to enhance conventional didactic presentations or laboratory demonstrations. For example, programs permitting the display of a complete audiologic battery allow the instructor to present a profile of test results, illustrating the effects of various auditory pathologies. A variety of clinical cases can be conveniently displayed for presentation and discussion. Universities able to afford the new large-screen video terminal displays can provide viewing by an entire class at once. Microcomputer instructional assistance can also be applied to the presentation of course content that traditionally has been difficult to carry out in a classroom because of constraints on time, instrumentation, or student background. The microcomputer's flexibility and high-speed processing capability permit convenient implementation of many laboratory demonstrations that were inconceivable a few years ago.

Acoustic Theory and Electrical Analog

The acoustic or source-filter theory of speech production and the electrical analog simulating these theories have been systematized by Dunn (1950), Chiba and Kajiyama (1944), Stevens, Fant, and Kasowski (1953), and others. Typically, students in master's-level speech pathology and audiology training programs lack the mathematical and engineering background needed to readily understand these theories. With the aid of a microcomputer, however, it is quite easy to replicate Dunn's two-, four-, or eight-section vocal tract model, Stevens's and others' 35-section model, or even the three-parameter descriptions of Stevens and House (1955). The microcomputer procedures required to accomplish these replications involve calculation of response characteristics of a transmission line having impedances appropriately chosen to simulate the human vocal tract. Once iterative routines are established to calculate the response magnitude for pulse inputs, extension to 10, 20, or 35-section models is quite simple. Many fundamental concepts can be effectively illustrated in this manner. For example, students can be shown what happens when vocal tract constriction is moved from back to front, or the result of gradually enlarging the pharyngeal cavity while holding all other variables constant. In the past, these basic principles could not be effectively demonstrated in the classroom. With the microcomputer, however, illustrative examples can be provided easily and efficiently. As a result, students more readily acquire the concepts needed to understand these important fundamentals. Furthermore, results presented in the literature can be verified and elaborated upon.

Aerodynamic Analysis

Airflow and pressure studies provide further examples of topics involving constraints on instrumentation and measurement procedures that have made it difficult to provide effective classroom demonstration and laboratory exercises. Traditionally, a face mask with a pneumotachograph and associated pressure transducers and bridge amplifier have been required to measure airflow signals, while a catheter and pressure transducer have been used to obtain pressure (oral and nasal) measurements. The signals are then displayed on a printer or optical device such as a visicorder or oscilloscope. In order to calculate volume of air inhaled from the flow signal, it has been necessary to first demarcate the inhalatory segment and then integrate the flow signal to obtain a volume measure. To obtain average volume-velocity, it has been necessary to divide the measured volume by the time interval of the segment. These procedures, in addition to being time-consuming, require frequent calibration for accurate recording. The procedural complexities have been known to inhibit semester-long projects, let alone single laboratory demonstrations. With a microcomputer, the laborious and time-consuming aspects of converting traces to volume, velocity, or flow can be accomplished immediately. For example, RESPAN (Horii and Cooke, 1975) is a program for respirometric analysis that operates on airflow function during speech obtained through a pneumotachograph pressure transducer system (Hardy, 1965; Isshiki and Ringel, 1964). The program accomplishes derivation of all data conventionally obtained by visual inspection and hand measurement of oscillographic records. Statistical data (histograms and the mean and standard deviation of instantaneous volume-velocity) are also printed out. With the availability of online analysis and immediate results of comprehensive aerodynamic measures during connected speech, illustrative data can be easily provided for instructional purposes. Examples of actual use of this program may be seen in Horii and Cooke (1978) and Itoh, Horii, Daniloff, and Binnie (1982).

Another example from the aerodynamics of speech production can be drawn from Warren's calculation of the velopharyngeal orifice area using oral and nasal pressure and nasal airflow measurements (Warren and DuBois, 1968; Lubker, 1969). The physical relationship of these variables to the velopharyngeal orifice size is given as:

$$\text{Orifice area} = \frac{\text{Rate of airflow through orifice}}{2\sqrt{\left(\dfrac{\text{Orifice differential pressure}}{\text{Density of air}}\right)}}$$

Thus, one can theoretically obtain the size of the velopharyngeal orifice by obtaining the values of these three variables. Before applying it to human subjects, Warren and DuBois (1968) tested the formula using an analog vocal tract with an adjustable velopharyngeal opening. Replication of these studies provides an excellent opportunity for students to learn how theoretical models and empirical findings can disagree and how limitations of theoretical models and assumptions can affect interpretation of the measurements derived.

In order to provide such a laboratory experience, a demonstration program was written to calculate velopharyngeal orifice size from measured airflow and pressure within the nasal cavity. With this program, both airflow and pressure are sampled and quantized using a 12-bit analog-to-digital converter, and then translated into appropriate physical units. The estimated velopharyngeal opening is then calculated using the formula given previously. In one laboratory session, both the Warren and DuBois (1968) and Lubker (1969) studies can be successfully replicated by students. Use of the microcomputer in this manner not only facilitates replication of airflow-pressure studies reported in the literature, but also allows one lecture and demonstration to accentuate several important concepts related to normal and pathologic speech production. In addition to these specific examples, it should be noted that statistical analyses which once required that data cards be punched and submitted to university computing centers for analysis can be carried out easily and quickly by microcomputer. It has been our experience that the immediate availability of statistical results in the classroom or laboratory increases student interest in research projects and research methods courses (see Chap. 14).

REPLACEMENT OF TRADITIONAL INSTRUMENTATION BY MICROCOMPUTERS

In recent years microcomputers have begun to replace traditional analog devices for teaching, research, and clinical application in the university setting. Before discussing the use of microcomputers in this context, we must first examine the nature of analog and digital devices and how they relate to microcomputer applications.

Analog-to-Digital and Digital-to-Analog Conversion

Analog devices generally deal with continuous electrical or mechanical signals. Voltmeters, audiometers, oscilloscopes, tape recorders, sound spectrographs, and delayed-auditory-feedback devices are some examples of analog devices commonly found in the speech and hearing clinic or laboratory. Digital devices convert continuous signals to a numerical representation, which is then used for storage, display, and analysis. In the speech and hearing laboratory, analog-to-digital (AD) and digital-to-analog (DA) converters form an essential link between the microcomputer and analog instruments. Use of these converters distinguishes microcomputer applications in the laboratory setting from those typical of home or business applications. In essence, the AD converter changes electrical signals to a series of fixed numbers at a fixed rate. In contrast, the DA converter changes a series of numbers to corresponding voltages.

It is important to note two basic features of AD and DA converters. One feature is conversion rate. Conversion from AD or DA takes place at a fixed rate (e.g., 1 time per second, 10 times per second, or 1000 times per second). The other feature, quantization level, refers to the amplitude resolution of the converter. The amplitude resolution is determined by the maximal input range and the maximal number of different amplitudes the

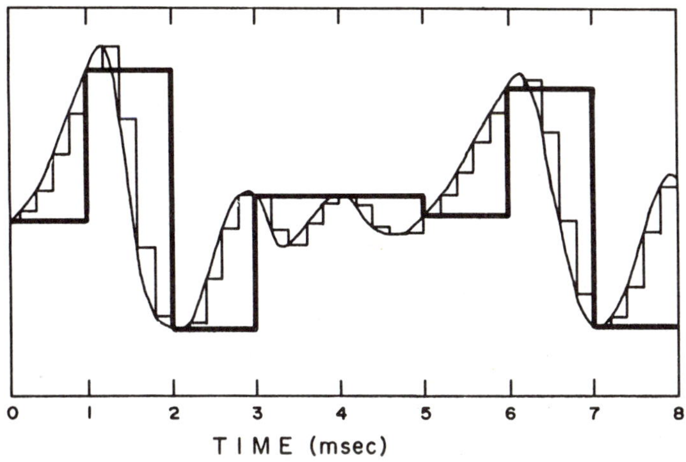

Fig. 5-4. The effects of conversion rate on the accuracy of digitally represented signals. The bold line depicts the waveform sampled at 1000 conversions per second; the thin line is the waveform obtained at 5000 conversions per second.

converter can represent accurately. The maximum number of levels the converter can represent is 2 to the power of the bit length (e.g., 2**2=4 for a 2-bit converter; 2**12=4096 for a 12-bit converter, and 2**14=16,384 for a 14-bit converter).

The effects of conversion rate and converter bit length on the accuracy of digitally represented signals are illustrated in Figure 5-4. In this illustration, approximately one glottal cycle of the phoneme /a/ is shown as produced by a normal adult female. The bolder line depicts the waveform sampled at a rate of 1000 conversions per second; the thinner line is the sampled waveform obtained at 5000 conversions per second. It can be seen that the latter representation is a "stair-step" function with considerably better approximation to the original resulting from the faster sampling rate.

Obviously, it is desirable to sample the signal at the fastest rate possible; however, if the converted numbers are to be stored in computer memory or other mass storage device, rapid conversion rates will quickly deplete the available memory. Applications requiring fast conversion rates, therefore, need careful consideration of memory limitations. In general, the conversion rate should be at least twice as fast as the highest-frequency component in the signal. For example, if the highest-frequency component in a given sound is known to be 2000 Hz, then the sampling rate should be at least 4000 times per second. This rate, referred to as the Nyquist rate, is particularly important when conducting spectral analyses. If the highest frequency in the signal is not known, low-pass filtering can be used to provide a cutoff frequency well below half the sampling rate.

Effects of limited amplitude quantization levels are illustrated in Figure 5-5. In this example, the phoneme /a/ is shown using two different converters: a 2-bit converter having four quantization levels, and a 4-bit converter having sixteen quantization levels; a sampling rate of 1000 times per second was used for both. As seen in Figure 5-5 the numerical repre-

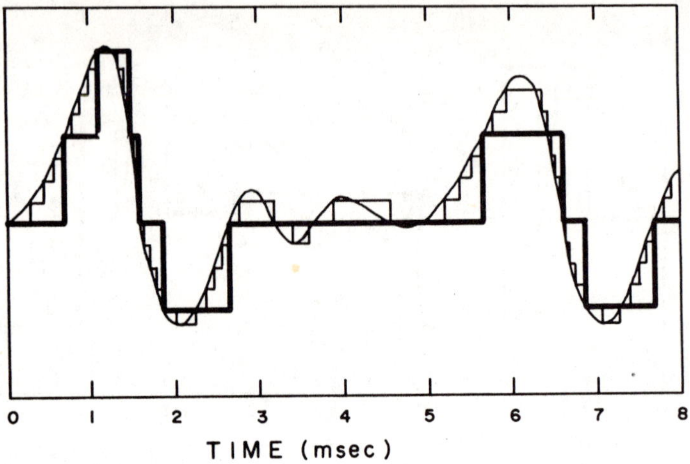

Fig. 5-5. Effects of limited converter-bit length on amplitude quantization levels of the sampled waveform. The bold line depicts the waveform sampled with a 2-bit converter, and the thin line shows results with a 4-bit converter.

sentation is closer to the original signal with a 4-bit converter than with a 2-bit converter. It should be noted, however, that in this example the signal amplitude covers the full range of the converter. If the signal were very low in amplitude, such that it covered only four different amplitude levels near zero, the resulting numerical representation would have been very poor, even if a high conversion rate were used. The choice of sampling rate, filtering, and conversion resolution depend on how the data are to be used. Sampled data may be used for digital recording of speech intended for reconversion to sound; for such purposes relatively high sampling rates are required, and the AD and DA converters should have at least 12-bit resolution. Furthermore, high-quality anti-aliasing filters are required, and pre-emphasis/de-emphasis filtering should be employed.

Other important uses of sampled data include measurement functions, such as using the microcomputer as a digital meter or for measuring utterance and pause durations. In such applications much lower sampling rates can be used, and some forms of distortion (such as aliasing, which would be very unpleasant if played out as reproduced sound) are not problematic as long as the sampled data are used only for analysis. If expense of perceptual hardware and storage is no object, a high-resolution digital recording system can be used for most applications. However, since data sampled at 10 kHz will fill a 10-megabyte hard disk with less than 10 minutes of speech, a laboratory interested in analyzing pause and utterance durations for hour-long periods would be well advised to consider a lower sampling rate.

Voltmeters

The use of a microcomputer to replace a conventional voltmeter illustrates one of the more straightforward applications of the AD converter. For example, suppose that 0, 10, and −10 volts correspond to numerical values of 0, 2046, and −2046, respectively. The measured voltage is simply converted to its numerical equivalent and divided by 204.6 to determine its corresponding voltage. The result can then be printed out. The microcomputer can perform this conversion at the user's command, or it can be programmed to do so at fixed intervals.

Additional applications of the digital voltmeter include absolute average and root mean square (RMS) voltage measurements. Absolute average voltage measures are frequently made for AC electrical signals. In this case, fullwave rectification is first needed in order to change all negative values to positive values; an average is then computed. If the square root of the squared and averaged values is then calculated, the result is the RMS voltage. The averaging interval can be made short to simulate a fast-responding voltmeter or long to simulate a slower response.

DC Power Supplies and Function Generators

A power supply (voltage source) can also be replaced with a microcomputer equipped with a DA converter. When the number corresponding to a given output level is known, the desired voltage can be calculated. Modifications to such a program allow the computer also to serve as a waveform generator. The typical analog waveform generator allows the user to set amplitude, frequency, and waveshape. Such a device can be simulated completely within the limitations of temporal and amplitude resolution and the inevitable harmonic distortion produced by a stair-step approximation.

Oscilloscopes

The oscilloscope is one of the most important instruments in the speech and hearing science laboratory. Most oscilloscopes are capable of accepting either AC or DC electrical signals as inputs, which are then displayed on a phosphor screen. The sweep speed and the vertical scale can be adjusted independently. Often, two separate inputs can be accepted, one for vertical and the other for horizontal inputs; many oscilloscopes also have the storage capacity to allow a fixed display. This capability is especially valuable, if not essential, for signals that are not continuous and repetitive, such as words or syllables. The functions of the oscilloscope can be easily simulated on a microcomputer equipped with either a digital interface or an AD converter. If the converter has at least two channels, two different signals can be sampled and their digital values transferred to the computer's graphic memory locations. Depending on the particular microcomputer employed, determination of these locations may involve some rather tedious programming. Once programmed, however, the only difference between the traditional oscilloscope and its digital counterpart is the "discreteness" of the waveform produced. In addition, the memory size allocated for the horizontal locations of high-resolution graphics limits the visual resolution of the waveform on a video screen. Of course, the standard video monitor can be replaced with a higher-resolution graphics terminal.

Delayed-Auditory-Feedback Devices

Adjustment of the distance between the record and playback heads of a tape recorder can produce delayed auditory feedback (DAF) between the input and output of an auditory signal. DAF units are currently used for stuttering therapy and occasionally for audiologic evaluation of pseudo-

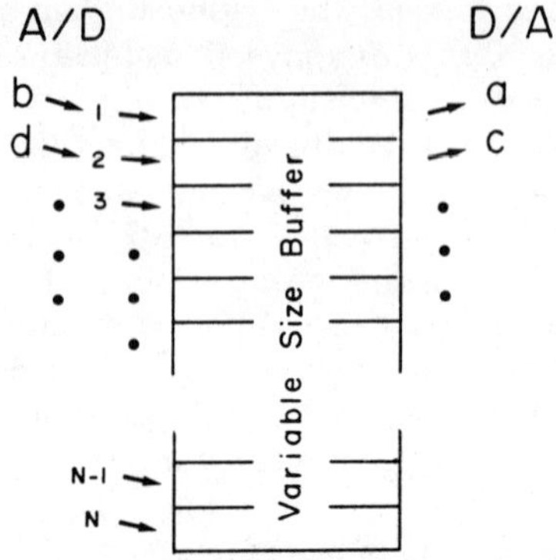

Fig. 5-6. Illustration of the basic concept of a delayed-auditory-feedback device simulated by microcomputer.

hypoacusis. The most important feature of a DAF unit is its ability to store auditory signals for a desired time interval. A microcomputer equipped with AD and DA converters is capable of providing such memory and delay (Horii, 1974b).

Figure 5-6 illustrates the basic concept of DAF simulated by microcomputer. In essence, the original signal is sampled and stored in memory until the allotted memory is consumed. The memory allocated is determined by the desired time delay and sampling rate. As soon as the memory reaches capacity (the bottom of the buffer in Fig. 5-6), the computer begins to output the sampled value from the top through the DA converter (*a* in Fig. 5-6). From then on, for each output a new input is sampled (*b* in Fig. 5-6) and stored in the memory location just vacated by the DA converter. When the bottom of the buffer is reached, the process repeats itself from the top. As an example, consider a sampling rate of 10,000 conversions per second with a memory buffer of 20,000 words; if the entire buffer were used, the delay produced would be 2 seconds. To obtain a 0.2-second delay, the size of the buffer would be changed to 2000 words, and so on. Since the maximal delay at a given sampling rate and memory size is limited, the sampling rate would need to be reduced if longer delays were needed.

Filters

Another commonly used analog device is the filter. In the speech and hearing laboratory, filters are typically used to condition signals and to modify their spectral characteristics. With a microcomputer, these functions can be carried out with digital filtering techniques. One of the simplest digital filters is the *running-average* filter. Figures 5-7A and 5-7B illustrate how a source signal consisting of high-frequency components riding on a low-frequency component can be low-passed with a running-average digital filter. As seen in Figure 5-7, the high-frequency components, evidenced by the peaks and valleys, are smoothed in the output. Another example is the high-pass filter. Figure 5-7C shows the results obtained when a running difference is taken from sampled values. In comparison to the original signal (Fig. 5-7A), the output of the difference

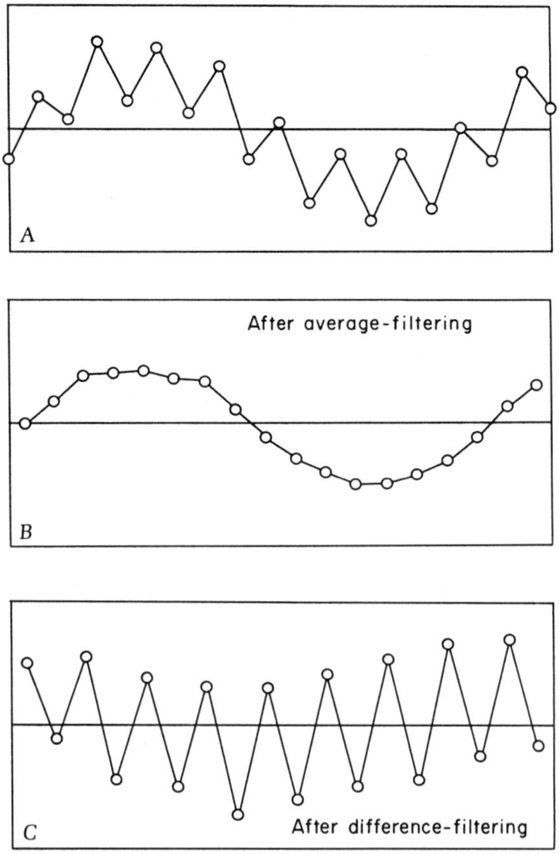

Fig. 5-7. Illustration of how a source signal consisting of high-frequency components riding on a low-frequency component (A) can be low-passed with a running-average digital filter (B) or high-pass filtered with a running-difference digital filter (C).

filter shows exaggerated high-frequency components and reduced low-frequency components. Finally, Figure 5-8 presents a mathematical flow chart of a bandpass filter with a 6 dB per octave rolloff, with center frequency and bandwidth specified numerically. Bandpass filtering involves sampling and delaying of signals by up to two sampling intervals. More than one digital filter can be easily implemented for such applications as vowel synthesis. For example, cascading three digital bandpass filters will result in three-resonance vowels. A more detailed discussion of digitally produced synthetic speech is presented in Chapter 12.

Sound Spectrographs

Many phonetic studies of normal and pathologic speech have been conducted using a sound spectrograph. Sound spectrography can also be achieved with a microcomputer. The most essential function of digital sound spectrography is the Fourier analysis of a sampled waveform. Discrete Fourier transforms applied to digitized speech produce spectral

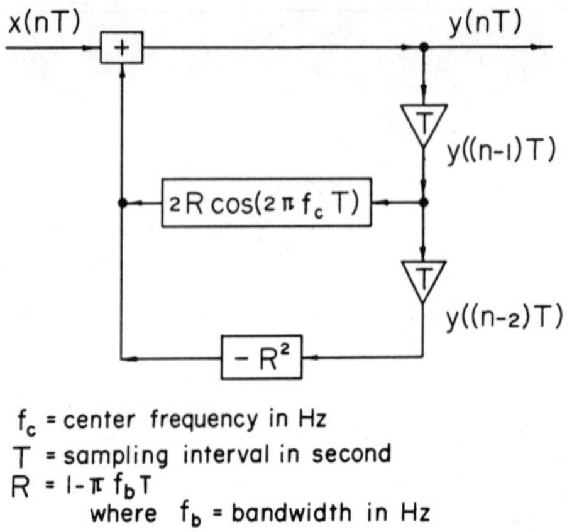

Fig. 5-8. A diagram illustrating a mathematical flow chart of a bandpass filter with a 6 dB per octave rolloff, with center frequency and bandwidth specified numerically.

density functions of the signal over a frequency region from zero to one half the sampling rate. The computer program SSPEC. (Horii, 1974a) employs the fast Fourier analysis technique described by Cooley and Tukey (1965) and the CEPSTRUM techniques described by Noll (1964) and Schroeder (1968) to generate digital sound spectrograms with simultaneous plottings of intensity level. If voicing is present, a fundamental frequency for connected discourse is also generated. To use that particular program, the user initially specifies three threshold values—a threshold for silence, a threshold for possible voicing, and a threshold for definite voicing. The other input to the program consists of speech waveform data sampled and digitized at 10,000 samples per second. A set of 512 data points (which correspond to 51.2 msec with the 10-kHz sampling rate) constitutes a *time segment* and is first analyzed for intensity. If the segment has intensity above the given threshold for silence, the 512 values are weighted and are submitted to fast Fourier analysis. From the sine-cosine magnitudes returned by the fast Fourier analysis, amplitude levels of the spectral components are calculated, and special printing characters are selected according to the energy levels present in the frequency region of the time segment. If the spectral ratio is greater than the given threshold for definite voicing, the fast Fourier analysis is again applied to the logarithmically converted amplitude values (now reduced to 216 points), and a peak-picking technique on the resulting outputs determines the fundamental frequency for the segment. If the spectral ratio is between the threshold of possible voicing and definite voicing, the program provides a calculated fundamental frequency in hertz. If the overall intensity level of the time segment is below the user-given threshold of possible voicing, however, the second Fourier analysis is bypassed. In any case, the program provides the results of spectral, intensity, and fundamental frequency analysis for this time segment in a printout similar to standard sound spectrograms but with simultaneous plottings of intensity and, if the segment is voiced, fundamental frequency. In the final sequence, the

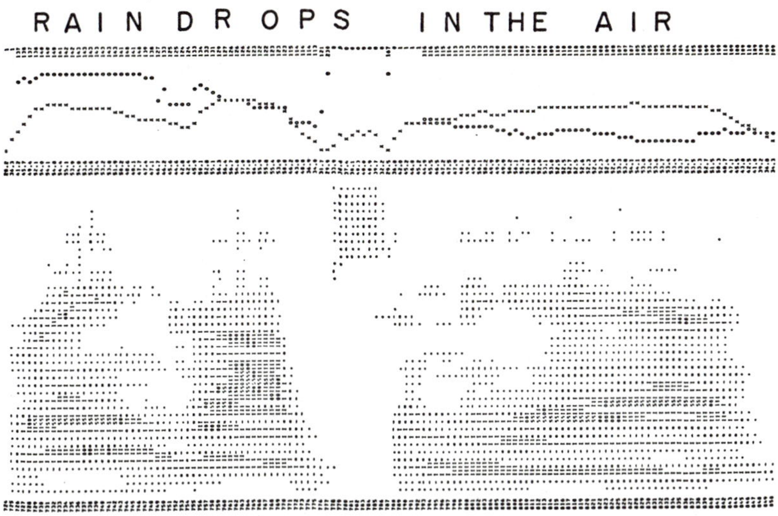

Fig. 5-9. Sample output from a digital spectrogram. Upper segment of the display shows intensity and fundamental frequency; the lower segment shows spectral characteristics.

program uses the last 412 data points in the previous time segment plus the following 100 data points as a new time segment; that is, the time window of 51.2 msec is moved by 10 msec to obtain the new time segment. An example of the output is shown in Figure 5-9.

ENHANCEMENT OF LABORATORY MEASURES WITH MICROCOMPUTERS

In addition to replacing traditional instrumentation in the speech and hearing science laboratory, microcomputers can be used to enhance or simplify conventional instrumental measures. Several examples of such applications are presented in this section.

Evoked-Potential Applications

In recent years, there has been growing interest in studying the brain's electrical activity in response to auditory or visual stimulation. Most evoked-potential analyses involve synchronized recording of electrical events obtained from surface electrodes placed on the scalp. Many signal-averaging systems are now equipped with a digital interface that allows microcomputer control and storage of waveform data and patient information as well as convenient labeling of waveform peaks and stimulus parameters. In addition, evoked-potential waveforms transferred to the microcomputer can be added, subtracted, smoothed, and inverted, and unique programs can be written to access a variety of patient data or to generate complete clinical reports. Figure 5-10 illustrates a summary report obtained from a microcomputer used in conjunction with a clinical signal averager. Use of the microcomputer in this manner allows not only greater clinical convenience and flexibility, but also a variety of teach-

NICOLET EVOKED POTENTIAL LABORATORY

PATIENT NAME: Tom Williams
PATIENT NUMBER: 341-4462-903
TEST: ABR
TEST DATE: 9/17/83

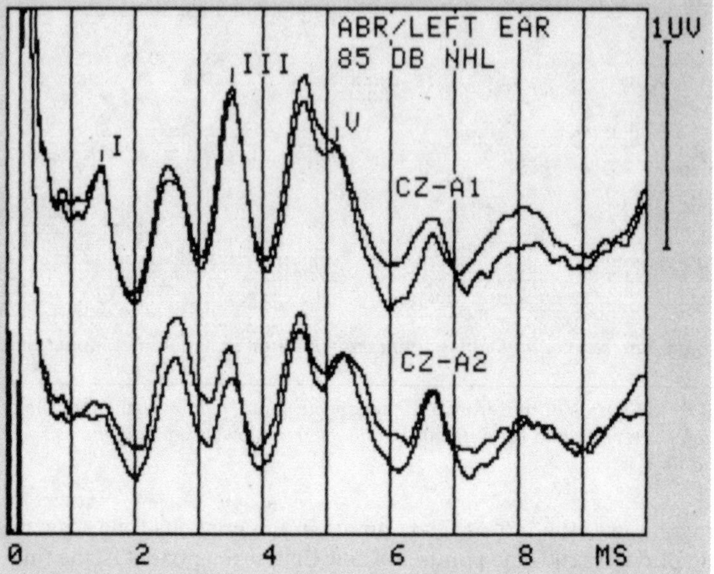

REMARKS:
A two channel ABR was recorded to left ear stimulation. The stimulus intensity was 85 db nHL. The subject was cooperative. All responses replicated well.

WAVEFORM LATENCIES

I	(1.9)	1.48
III	(4)	3.52
V	(6)	5.16
I-III	(2.4)	2.04
III-V	(2.2)	1.64
I-V	(4.4)	3.68

NICOLET EVOKED POTENTIAL LABORATORY

PATIENT NAME: Tom Williams
PATIENT NUMBER: 341-4462-903
SEX: Male
BIRTHDATE: 4/21/44
TEST: ABR
TESTED BY: Terry Williams
TEST DATE: 9/17/83
REFERRED BY: Robert Kelly, M.D.
REMARKS:

CLINICAL IMPRESSION:

The inter-wave and absolute latencies of the ABR waveforms recorded all fell within normal limits. This is suggestive of normal peripheral and central auditory function. Should the patient continue to have complaints, he should be retested in six months.

Fig. 5-10. ABR waveforms and summary report generated by the Apple IIe computer used in conjunction with the Nicolet CA 1000 clinical averager. (From Nicolet Biomedical Division, with permission.)

ing applications for university training programs equipped with microcomputers but not with signal-averaging systems.

In a recent experiment, we used a clinical signal averager in a tachistoscopic test of cerebral dominance comparing cortical responses obtained from the left and right sides of the brain. This study required the random presentation of single words to either the left or right visual field. Since the signal averager was not able to accommodate the presentation of words as stimuli, we used a microcomputer to generate the visual stimulus and to produce a trigger pulse at the instant of each visual stimulation. The order of visual-field presentation (left or right) was randomized in advance and programmed into both the signal averager and the microcomputer. As a result, the averager knew when to sample brain activity and where to store it for later analysis. In this example, we see how two microprocessors can be used in synchrony to accomplish a specific task.

Prosodic Analysis of Connected Speech

Intonation and intensity analyses are often desired for comparative study of normal and pathologic speech. The Visi-Pitch, manufactured by Kay Elemetrics Corporation, for example, can be interfaced with a microcomputer to accomplish fundamental frequency and intensity measures more efficiently and conveniently than is possible through conventional use of the instrument. The Visi-Pitch appears to be gaining in popularity as a teaching device and clinical tool for analyses of voice, intonation, accent, and emotion. It is a portable device providing extraction and display of fundamental frequency (Fo) in real time, from either a live voice or a tape recording. Four different filters are available for analysis, depending on the frequency range of the subject's voice. The extracted Fo contour is displayed on a storage oscilloscope, and a continually variable electronic cursor allows the selection of any point along the contour. A digital readout of Fo values is provided in Hertz.

For many clinical and research applications, the manual recording of the digital readout is overly tedious and time-consuming. By interfacing the Visi-Pitch with a microcomputer, it is possible to transfer period and frequency information for computer analysis. Once coupled to the computer, period data are generated after each period, and frequency data are generated every 0.5 seconds. Clearly, the rate of frequency data generation is too slow for most applications, whereas the use of period information in real time requires considerable programming effort. Fortunately, continuous analog output (DC signal proportional to Fo) is also available from the Visi-Pitch and is readily amenable to displaying an intensity trace either separately or simultaneously with Fo.

Fingertapping as a Test of Cerebral Dominance

Hemispheric specialization for language processing has been investigated using a variety of behavioral tests including dichotic listening and dichotic and time-sharing tapping-talking tests. In general, these tests have indicated that the left cerebral hemisphere is dominant for language processing in most right-handed individuals. Fewer than one half of left handers show left hemispheric dominance. Abnormal hemispheric dominance for language processing has been hypothesized as a cause of language-learning disabilities, stuttering, and other communicative disorders.

Klingman and Sussman (1983) state that the time-sharing tapping-talking tasks originally developed by Kinsbourne and Cook (1971) are easy to administer and high in validity and repeatability. The subject is instructed to fingertap a switch as rapidly as possible while talking and again without talking. The task is repeated for the right and left hands. Disrupting effects of talking on fingertapping are then compared for the right and left hands. The cerebral hemisphere contralateral to the hand showing the greater disrupting effect is considered the dominant one for language processing. This procedure may prove useful for clinical and research purposes, but only if it can be conveniently administered and interpreted. In an effort to develop a practical means of collecting fingertapping data, two simple programs were written for our microcomputer (Horii, 1983c). The first program is a timer-counter, and the second is a hemispheric-dominance index calculator. The timer-counter program starts a 15-second timer as soon as the keyboard space bar is pressed. The computer then monitors the number of times the space bar is pressed during the 15-second interval. When executed, the timer-counter program prints out the number of taps occurring in a sampling interval and awaits the next trial. The index calculator program waits for the user's keyboard inputs indicating the number of taps made by the right and left hands while the subject is talking and during silence. The program then calculates the index of disruption and prints out the inferred dominant cerebral hemisphere. Application of the microcomputer in this manner allows fingertapping data to be collected and analyzed almost instantaneously.

Pause-Utterance Length and Frequency Analysis

Analysis of duration and frequency of occurrence of pauses and utterances is often desirable in the study of pathologic speech. Such measures are also of interest in the analysis of communicative interactions between mother and child, clinician and client, and teacher and student. Initially, automatic analysis of utterance and pause may appear quite simple. *Pause* has been defined as any segment of the smoothed speech signal having an amplitude of x mvolts or less and a minimum duration of y msec; *utterance* was then defined as all nonpause segments (Rochester, 1976).

Application of these definitions, however, immediately reveals that pauses are often segmented into smaller units because of brief ambient or instrumental noise bursts. Raising the amplitude threshold in an attempt to avoid the noise bursts results in systematically underestimating utterance durations while overestimating pause durations. Thus, it is critical to adopt a strategy that allows rejection of transient noises during otherwise unitary pauses without raising the amplitude threshold. A programmed microcomputer permits convenient implementation of such a strategy. Assuming that noise transients during pauses are, in fact, brief in comparison to real utterances, the basic definitions can be modified to include a noise-rejection criterion that allows utterance segments of less than a given duration to be reclassified as pause segments.

Figure 5-11 shows the instrumental setup used in our laboratory for calculation of pause and utterance length and frequency-of-occurrence analysis (Horii, 1983b). The initial stage involves signal conditioning with a rectifier-smoother. The rectifier-smoother extracts amplitude envelopes of the speech signal by full-wave rectification and low-pass filtering. The extracted envelope signal is then AD converted at a sampling rate of 1000 Hz. A program written for our microcomputer keeps track of occur-

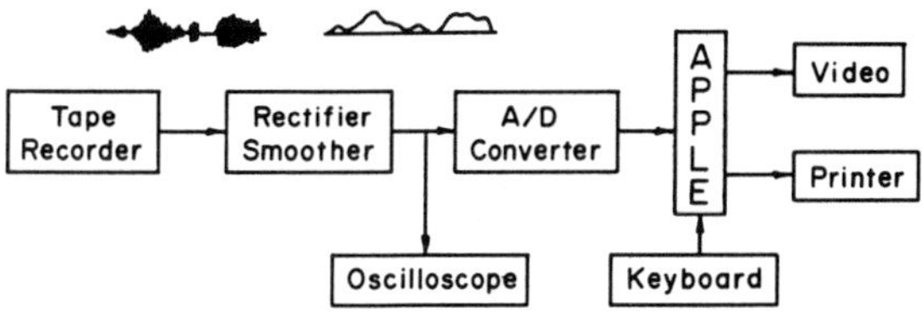

Fig. 5-11. Instrumental setup used for calculation of pause and utterance length and frequency-of-occurrence analysis. The amplitude envelopes of a speech signal are extracted by full-wave rectification and low-pass filtering and digitized via an AD converter at a sampling rate of 1000 kHz.

rences and durations of the segments above and below the amplitude threshold specified. A sampling interval is terminated by pressing the keyboard space bar. The program then scans and, if necessary, collapses the segmented data using the durational criteria specified initially. The printout shows the utterances and pauses (in milliseconds) in order of occurrence, along with the means and standard deviations of their durations.

MICROCOMPUTERS IN THE UNIVERSITY SPEECH AND HEARING CLINIC

Among the first computer applications to interest speech pathologists and audiologists were those of clinical management and record keeping. These applications have been of particular interest to those in university and audiology training programs because of the extensive management and record-keeping tasks unique to this setting. These tasks include organization and administration of student practicum requirements and record-keeping activities required for various clinical and educational certification standards. The American Speech-Language-Hearing Association (ASHA) requires graduate students in speech pathology and audiology to engage in clinical activities involving both evaluation and intervention with clients having a variety of communication disorders. A minimal number of clock hours is designated for each activity and disability area. Whereas scheduling of academic requirements is easily synchronized, students typically vary in their clinical practicum status. Consequently, the task of organizing and assigning clinical placements is a tedious one needing revision each semester.

In recent years, several authors have reported ways of computerizing student practicum records. Most of the management techniques reported to date have not been designed for microcomputers but for large time-share systems (Mahaffey, 1973; Harden, Harden, and Norris, 1977; Peterson, 1977). For example, Harlen and Hasegawa (1976) describe a program written in FORTRAN IV for use with a minicomputer. Each semester, a student's clock-hour status is entered on punch cards. The computer assigns clinical experiences to appropriate categories, updates the file, and provides printouts for the clinical director, the faculty supervisor, and the student. Such a system has obvious advantages in maintaining the organization, records, and prioritization of clinical placement.

Another record-keeping activity unique to the university clinic is that of evaluating and recording student practicum performance. Oratio (1979) describes a FORTRAN program developed for analysis of client-clinician interactive behaviors during therapy. From numerically coded input, the frequency and percentage of interactive behaviors is determined from a range of fifty interaction categories. The system can be used effectively as an observational tool with students enrolled in prepracticum coursework or as a means of objective behavioral analysis for the clinician and supervisor.

As noted at the beginning of this chapter, recent technological advances have resulted in rapid expansion of microcomputer capability. In fact, most of the computer-based management tasks described can now be handled conveniently and cost-effectively with a microcomputer. At the University of Colorado we have used APPLEWORKS to create a variety of programs for clinical report writing and record keeping. The spread-sheet and data-base management components are used to create files containing each student's practicum and clock-hour record. Also included are students' academic records and class schedules, allowing clinical assignments to be made on the basis of priority and compatibility with client schedules. Files are updated each semester and printouts are provided to students and relevant department members. Externship placement sites are also fully catalogued, and information needed by the clinical director, such as off-campus supervisors' ASHA certification numbers, is readily available. Information of interest to students, such as general descriptions of the practicum sites, is also provided. A feature permitting the merger of mailing lists simplifies the distribution of written materials required for each off-campus placement. Finally, the APPLEWORKS word-processing package enables students to prepare their own clinical reports using diskette storage. The student and supervisor then meet to examine each report, and revisions are incorporated as needed. Students inexperienced at writing reports can refer to a file containing a variety of sample reports. Following review by the student and supervisor, a letter-quality printer generates the finished product along with an appropriate cover letter. We find this system greatly enhances student feedback while substantially reducing secretarial demands.

Advances in computer technology will profoundly influence future academic practices. From instructional applications to research, computers will enable students and professors alike to achieve far greater productivity and efficiency. Although there will be concern on the part of some who feel that expanded computer application threatens the interpersonal qualities of our profession, it is our belief that advances in computer technology will permit greater freedom to explore professional creativity and innovation. Of course, there is always the danger that some students will become overly enamored with the methodology, losing sight of their original interests in clinical service or research; computers seem to be especially potent seducers in that respect! For those able to maintain an appropriate balance, however, we can expect a burgeoning of new microcomputer applications.

Computer technology will continue to expand dramatically. The most successful practitioners will be those able to adapt the computer to their own individual needs. Only by providing students with the training needed to enable competent computer application and innovation, while at the same time preserving their clinical interest and creativity, will we ensure that this new technology is used to its fullest advantage in the field of communication disorders.

REFERENCES

Arons, A. Computer-based instructional dialogues in science courses. *Science* 224:1051–1056, 1984.

Chiba, T., and Kajiyama, M. *The Vowel, Its Nature and Structure*. Tokyo: Tokyo-Kaiseikan, 1941.

Cooley, J. W., and Tukey, J. W. An algorithm for the machine calculation of complex Fourier series. *Mathematics of Computation* 19:297–301, 1965.

Dunn, H. K. The calculation of vowel resonances, and an electrical vocal tract. *J. Acoust. Soc. Am.* 22:740–753, 1950.

Harden, R. J., Harden, R. W., and Norris, M. Computer program for the analysis of clinical enrollment. *ASHA* 19:472–474, 1977.

Hardy, J. C. Air flow and air pressure studies. *ASHA Reports* 1:141–152, 1965.

Harlen, N., and Hasegawa, A. Computer processing of graduate student clinical clock hours as needed for ASHA certification. *ASHA* 18:295–298, 1976.

Horii, Y. Digital sound spectrograms with simultaneous plotting of intensity and fundamental frequency (abstract). *Behav. Res. Methods Instr.* 6:55, 1974a.

Horii, Y. Variable delayed auditory feedback (abstract). *Behav. Res. Methods Instr.* 6:55, 1974b.

Horii, Y. Some voice fundamental frequency characteristics of oral reading and spontaneous speech by hard-of-hearing young women. *J. Speech Hear. Res.* 25:608–610, 1982.

Horii, Y. Automatic analysis of voice fundamental frequency and intensity using a Visi-Pitch. *J. Speech Hear. Res.* 26:467–471, 1983a.

Horii, Y. An automatic analysis method of utterance and pause lengths and frequencies. *Behav. Res. Methods Instr.* 15:449–452, 1983b.

Horii, Y. A forum on computer applications in speech physiology: Interactive versus automatic voice fundamental frequency analysis. *ASHA* 25:97, 1983c.

Horii, Y. Repeatability of the maximum fingertapping rate as hemispheric lateralization index (abstract). *ASHA* 25:138, 1983d.

Horii, Y., and Cooke, P. Analysis of airflow and air volume during connected speech. *Behav. Res. Methods Instr.* 7:477, 1975.

Horii, Y., and Cooke, P. A. Some airflow, volume and duration characteristics of oral reading. *J. Speech Hear. Res.* 21:470–481, 1978.

Horii, Y., and Hughes, G. W. Speech analysis by computer. In *Proceedings of the 28th Annual National Electronics Conference*, Chicago, Ill., 1972. Pp. 74–149.

Horii, Y., and Ramig, P. R. Stutterers' hemispheric dominance: Fingertapping rate during speech and silence. *ASHA* 25:133, 1983.

Huntington, J. F. Microcomputers and university teaching. *Improving College and University Teaching* 28:75–77, 1980.

Isshiki, N., and Ringel, R. L. Airflow during the production of selected consonants. *J. Speech Hear. Res.* 7:233–242, 1964.

Itoh & Horii (in press).

Itoh, M., Horii, Y., Daniloff, R. G., and Binnie, C. A. Selected aerodynamic characteristics of deaf individuals during various speech and nonspeech tasks. *Folia Phoniatr.* 34:191–209, 1982.

Johnston, J. *Calculatory MLU.* Bloomington: Indiana University, 1984.

Johnston, J., and Backler, M. Language sample analysis: computer assisted instruction. Presented at a conference of the American Speech-Language-Hearing Foundation: The Personal Computer as a Professional Tool, Las Vegas, Nev., Feb. 1984.

Kinsbourne, M., and Cook, J. Generalized and lateralized effect of concurrent verbalization on a uniform skill. *Q. J. Exp. Psychol.* 23:341–345, 1971.

Klingman, K., and Sussman, H. Hemisphericity in aphasic language recovery. *J. Speech Hear. Res.* 26:249–256, 1983.

Levitt, H., Slosberg, R., Hawie, D., Mazor, R., and Rosenstein, M. Computer-based techniques for enhancement of clinical techniques. *ASHA* 20: 398–402, 1978.

Lotterman, S. *Introduction to Audiology.* San Diego: College Hill, 1984.

Lubker, J. F. Velopharyngeal orifice area: A replication of analog experimentation. *J. Speech Hear. Res.* 12:218–222, 1969.

Mahaffey, R. B. A computerized procedure of keeping student records for ASHA-CCC requirements. *ASHA* 15:590, 1973.

Noll, M. A. Short-time spectrum and 'cepstrum' techniques for vocal-pitch detection. *J. Acoust. Soc. Am.* 36:296–302, 1964.

Oratio, A. Computer assisted interaction analysis in speech-language pathology and audiology. *ASHA* 21:179–184, 1979.

Peterson, H. More about computer assisted clinical record-keeping. *ASHA* 19:617–618, 1977.

Rochester, S. R. Defining the silent pause in speech. *J. Ont. Speech Hear. Assoc.* 8:1–4, 1976.

Rose, D. *Computer Assisted Instructional Program for Audiology.* San Diego: College Hill, 1984.

Rushakoff, G. E. Microcomputer assisted instruction in communication disorders. *J. Childhood Commun. Disorders* 8:1, 1984.

Rushakoff, G. E., and Lombardino, L. J. Microcomputer applications for speech-language pathologists and audiologists: An introductory course of instruction. *ASHA* 26:27–31, 1984.

Rushakoff, G. E., Jackson, C., Farmer, S., and Farmer, J. *Microcomputer Assisted Study-Partner in Anatomy and Physiology of the Speech and Hearing Mechanism.* San Diego: College Hill, 1984.

Schroeder, M. R. Period histogram and product spectrum: New methods for fundamental frequency measurement. *J. Acoust. Soc. Am.* 43:829–834, 1968.

Stevens, K., and House, A. S. Development of a quantitative description of vowel articulation. *J. Acoust. Soc. Am.* 27:484–493, 1955.

Stevens, K. N., Kasowski, S., and Fant, C. G. M. An electrical analog of the vocal tract. *J. Acoust. Soc. Am.* 25:740–753, 1953.

Warren, D. W., and DuBois, A. B. A pressure-flow technique for measuring velopharyngeal orifice area during continuous speech. *Cleft Palate J.* 52–71, 1968.

Zimmerman, H. *CAPS: Computerized Audiometric Programmable Simulator.* Las Cruces, N.M.: Audiosoft, 1983.

6

Microcomputer Applications in Speech Pathology

R. Ann Howard

Speech-language pathologists across the country are responding to the use of the computer as a clinical tool in rapidly increasing numbers. Many hope this new high-tech appliance will perform the miracles of increasing the number of clients that can be seen in a given amount of time, releasing the clinician from routine tasks and thus providing more time for creativity, shortening preparation time, and ensuring the preservation of effective techniques through storage capabilities. The computer is sometimes heralded as a distraction, a "new toy," and an injection of adventure for both the clinician and, one hopes, the client. On the other hand, there is the hope that computer use will aid in standardizing clinical procedures and at the same time allow for better individualization of patient treatment.

For some speech-language pathologists the computer is able to fulfill many of these roles, while for many others, use of the computer is fraught with setbacks and pitfalls. Clinicians are dismayed to discover that programming all those creative ideas is difficult and extremely time-consuming. Even with high-level languages (BASIC, PASCAL, FORTH, etc.) and authoring programs such as Super PILOT at one pole and HARTLEY'S CREATE and SHELL GAMES at the other, programming takes study, skill, determination, and time. And then, the resulting program is only as good as the programmer. Also, due to the specificity of speech problems and the individual differences of the clients, many programs, whether purchased or self-produced, are only applicable to a small number of clients—sometimes as few as one. Herein lies the possible pitfall of "busy work." Each clinician must realize that computer use can actually decrease the spontaneity and intuitive direction of treatment. As for the hope that a computer will provide more free time, most programs now available for speech pathology practice still require the physical presence of the clinician.

THE COMPUTER AS AN EDUCATOR

Often the clinician must instruct or explain a concept that has been verbally presented many times before. Using the computer to present this type of material may be a real advantage, especially in light of the fact that most of what we learn is reinforced through the modality of sight. Presentations defining vocal abuse, effective voice usage, important facts about dysfluency, and the characteristics of normal and deviant swallowing all lend themselves to computer presentation.

Considerable counseling time is necessarily spent with the families of clients. Computerized presentation of pertinent material not only could save the clinician time, but also could give the families a better understanding of the problems and a guide for realistic expectations. For many families, a computerized introduction to speech pathology—including a job description, educational background, areas of expertise, specific office procedures, fees, billing procedures, services offered, and frequently asked questions and answers—would be extremely useful. In one computerized presentation, many concerns could be dealt with in an organized way so that no facts would be inadvertently omitted.

Computer presentation, besides being novel, has numerous advantages. It cannot be easily discarded or lost as is the case with written materials, although the client can refuse to absorb the information. Computerized material can be presented at a speed appropriate for each client. It can be immediately reverbalized by the client for clarification or emphasis. The program could be designed to require interaction and allow the client to indicate which areas he or she does not understand. The clinician could then provide an explanation or clarification. Another advantage of a computerized program is the ease with which information can be added, deleted, or revised without incurring additional printing costs.

The computer provides a realistic way to give families information on such areas as the developmental sequence of speech and language acquisition, the differences between delayed and disordered language, the commonly recognized elements of dysfluent speech and their ramifications in communicative behavior, and types of abuse to the vocal mechanism. The family that has some understanding of the development and ramifications of speech disorders seems, on the whole, less confused and guilt-ridden and more able to participate effectively in the therapeutic process.

Clinicians, too, could benefit from computerized instruction. Because of job changes or new clients, many clinicians experience loss of skill in treating disorders not dealt with on an ongoing basis. The clinician in this situation may feel inept, disorganized, and insecure. Learning new approaches and reviewing old therapies may be of value. Computerized educational material can be used effectively to reinforce feelings of competency and skills important to all clinicians. In the best of situations, we would all like to believe that we treat only those clients with whom we feel competent and confident. In reality, client choice is usually not an option, and support and reinforcement of our knowledge is imperative. An existing software program, *Competency Training Systems* (Filter) allows the clinician to rate severity, breathiness, and tension present in a series of speech samples. The clinician's rating is then compared with an expert's rating. A similar software program is offered for practice in rating levels of hypernasality.

The well-seasoned as well as the less experienced clinician is constantly searching for skill augmentation, new ideas, and new techniques to increase competency and to forestall boredom. The profession of speech-language pathology is relatively new, and totally new concepts are continually being developed. Clinicians must be aware of current developments and formulate a routine plan for incorporating new bodies of knowledge into their personal repertoire. A speech-language pathologist who completed academic preparation in 1966, for example, typically has no formal training in such areas as pragmatics unless he or she consciously incorporated means for professional growth through the years.

Terminology changes rapidly so that a relatively isolated clinician may no longer recognize current writings about familiar areas. Of course, the degree of knowledge lag has immense variation, and various clinicians experience it in different ways. Isolated practicing clinicians know that this is a real problem and generally welcome any means of raising their awareness and competency levels.

For the student of speech pathology, computerized learning provides many of the same advantages it holds for the certified clinician: a concise, well-organized review of salient points and a clear presentation of new ideas. Because computer programming of material demands well-organized, logical presentation, data can be presented concisely so that less time and effort are required to glean the critical information. For example, using a computer, a person could conceivably review an enhanced outline of this chapter and quickly get as much information as would be gleaned from reading the complete text. Other critical factors include the opportunity for the presentation of repetitive material and the interactive function of the computer, which has the advantage of compelling attention through asking for student responses. The interactive computer function serves the important role, often missing in education, of making one aware of what he or she does and does not know. The *Microcomputer Assisted Study Partner in Anatomy and Physiology of the Speech and Hearing Mechanism* (Rushakoff et al., 1984) provides a model for computer-assisted learning.

THE COMPUTER AS A SOURCEBOOK

For the efficient clinician, the use of a sourcebook is a necessity. Although usually held in reserve, the sourcebook proves its value on those days of blank mind, low energy, confusion, or boredom. Which sourcebook to use becomes automatic knowledge in the mind of the experienced clinician. The microcomputer provides the possibility for each clinician, with a minimal expenditure of energy, to compile his or her own personal sourcebook. How many times does a clinician search back through treatment records to glean some technique or series of presentations that seem to be called for by the client at hand? So many good and effective ideas are intuitively developed out of desperation and then soon forgotten. How often does a clinician find himself or herself developing material previously developed but no longer accessible? Using the personal computer, a clinician's material can be saved, categorized, and cross-referenced for easy accessibility. Lists of words with specific sounds, difficult-to-pronounce words, and sentences of varying length and complexity can all be stored on disks. Of course, with the use of a computer, such lists can be easily deleted, enhanced, or revised. Practice materials making reference to the Beatles or the Monkees can be updated to refer to Michael Jackson. Moreover, once instituted, this personal sourcebook allows time for the development of additional material as backup for the same level of presentation. Fewer clinicians need hear from their clients, ". . . but I did these sentences last time."

Computerized treatment and management outlines and flow charts provide logical order to material presentation as well as notes regarding treatment that can be stored. In short, the computer as a personal reminder system can help the professional provide a better-organized, more inclusive treatment program.

The sourcebook need not remain exclusively personal. At any stage of development there is the possibility of sharing developed materials with fellow clinicians. The organization of clinical users' groups is exciting, challenging, and stimulating.

Forever, clinicians have tried to share ideas, but with questionable success. Now, by sharing a software disk of material or providing a printout of pertinent portions of a file, materials can be shared efficiently, completely, and accurately, thereby avoiding much duplication of effort and adding greatly to treatment repertoires.

THE COMPUTER AS A CLINICIAN

Client knowledge that the speech-language pathologist utilizes a computer in treatment is often a great motivator. Although many clients, especially children, have some access to computers at school, the time they have with the computer tends to be limited. The prospect of using a computer without prior scheduling and waiting one's turn is a great motivator to attend therapy sessions.

Many of the tasks assigned to clients are predictable and repetitive. We have all prepared the same lesson plan in a variety of modes to compel attention and sustain interest. The computer allows another mode, which can be rejuvenating not only to the client but also to the clinician. Just as clients tire of responding in the same modes repeatedly, clinicians, too, profit from presentation of material in a new manner.

One highly motivating activity is to allow a client to prepare material (games, tasks, or tests) for another client. Willingness and enthusiasm flourish as the client draws on what he or she has learned and becomes the "fantasy therapist." Some of the simple authoring programs designed for the computer allow a client to design tasks for others with minimal difficulty.

Interest and attentiveness seem to increase in proportion to a client's active participation. The chance to chart one's own response and see it immediately displayed on the monitor is especially reinforcing. A wide variety of written statements, bells and other noises, flashes of color, and imaginative graphics can be utilized to indicate success or failure. Cues, clues, and encouragement to try again or to move ahead can be graphically presented. Rates of success can be counted and displayed numerically or by line or bar graphs. Individual records for single or cumulative performances can be structured and stored for future access. Records of one client can also be easily compared with those of others.

Microcomputers provide an invaluable asset to the speech-language clinic or private practice. They can be easily justified as a treatment tool, especially when their role in office management and family education is also considered. Nevertheless, these clinical settings—where time is money and cost effectiveness is imperative—continue to encounter hindrances to implementing computer usage. The first of these, obviously, is the budgeting of funds to purchase the basic computer system. Second, and more critical, is the fact that, at present, the majority of speech-language clinicians simply do not have computer skills. Perhaps the single most serious difficulty is that of software review and development. Time required for software review is extensive and costly. Computer software selection is much more time-consuming than leafing through a catalogue or packet of materials to determine their usefulness. With written materials, an experienced reviewer can usually tell from a cursory inspection whether the material is relevant for his or her treatment population. In the event that a purchase of written material subsequently yields only a limited amount of usefulness, the expense involved is usually manageable. To review computer software through purchase may be a costly mistake.

The clinician must consider the basic usefulness of the program. Does it purport to deal with an item necessarily dealt with in treatment, or is it only a novel idea, a diversion? Does the program require client response? Is the response mode workable for the client? How much response time is allowed, and can it be varied? Is the program clear and developed in depth? Is it developmentally programmed? Does the rate of presentation fit the client? Does the level of presentation meet the client's needs and abilities? Does it include reinforcement factors? In what ways are responses charted? Will the program be useful with more than one client?

In addition, the same cautions apply to the selection of computer software as to the selection of any treatment material. Clients' needs require individualization. Therefore, the clinician must be able to alter the software to meet specific needs and be willing to use it only when and where it will effect the desired changes in client behavior. One potential pitfall of computerized programs, once selected or developed, is that, because of their ease of use, they can become a substitute for clinician interaction and thereby become a poor solution to those tough Monday mornings and Friday afternoons.

In the current highly competitive software market it is frequently difficult for clinicians to secure computer software for complete review. Manufacturers of clinical software are aware of the possibility that unauthorized copies will be made during the "evaluation and review" process. Reviewing software in users' groups, software already purchased by other clinics, or attending computer meetings and workshops are partial solutions to the problem of keeping up with the latest offerings.

School systems are usually out in front with innovative instructional devices, and this is certainly true with computers. It is often possible for the speech-language pathologist to utilize the hardware and software already available in the schools. As with any technique or teaching material, care must be taken to use the computer wisely. In areas where the computer is not a viable approach to a problem, it should not be utilized. While microcomputers are becoming extremely useful to clinicians, they should not be treated as a cure-all. Computers are not clinicians. At this time they are very limited in their ability to make clinical judgments or to tailor their presentation for different individuals. They cannot provide emotional support to a client or understand the scope of a comprehensive treatment program.

All clinicians keep records of some sort. Most clinicians wish they had more extensive records. The capability of the computer for keeping clinical records is nearly limitless. Currently available are software programs with specific functions such as recording case histories of the child with speech-language disorders (Harlan) or client identification information plus summary results of testing (Harlan). Some available software file systems include client data, test results, treatment notes, goals achieved, and clinician comments (Schuldt). Some software programs are even more treatment oriented, allowing for filing of home assignments, vocabulary word lists, parts-of-speech word lists, or language and sentence pattern word lists (Schuldt).

Speech-language pathologists are often arbitrarily divided into two types: persons who are primarily interested in research, and persons who are clinicians and thus considered to be unprepared for, or disinterested in, doing clinical research. The "clinical" group seems to believe that they operate from an intuitive base and that detailed record keeping would interfere with their therapeutic style. The computer can do much to aid the clinical group in collecting and supplying information to the "research" group. Because treatment-oriented software can be programmed to count responses and modes of response, the clinician can acquire a large data base without undue expenditure of time and energy. Perhaps those more fitted for research will be able to design programs to allow the clinician to acquire meaningful data.

One solution to the problem of a staff without a computer expert is to encourage one or more staff members who are personally interested in computers and willing to devote some of their own time to them to supply the computer groundwork. Their research and enthusiasm can then be shared with their colleagues. An advantage of a setting with multiple staff members is that the chore of software review and development can be shared among several persons.

APPLICATIONS FOR SPECIFIC TREATMENT AREAS

At present, utilization of the microcomputer as a clinical tool for speech disorders is rather limited. A review of currently available software in the areas of articulation, fluency, and voice nets very few functional programs. The majority of available software deals with articulation disorders.

Articulation Disorders

Programs available for the evaluation of articulatory abilities rely on the speech-language clinician for accurate perception, transcription, and computer input. The majority of the programs display the target stimulus, such as a single word, phrase, or sentence. The clinician then reads this stimulus to the client and records the client's response. Programs such as *Lingquest 2* allow the clinician to select stimulus material including spontaneous speech samples. A number of these programs (Blache, 1982; Fitch, 1982; Harlan, C., 1982a; Parrot Software, Telage, 1980) evaluate articulation from the distinctive-feature viewpoint. Results of other assessment programs are reported as structural statistics and percentage of correctly produced sounds (Shriberg, 1984) or as level of phonemic development and level of severity (Blache, 1984). Harlan's program ranks errors in order of severity and arranges them in suggested treatment sequence. A second program by Schuldt not only assists in determining a specific articulation diagnosis, but also provides information about causes, associated conditions, treatment recommendations, and a bibliography relating to the selected disorder.

When the assessment of production is completed, and diagnostic results are printed out, some programs suggest treatment procedures. Haynes authored a software program designed to assist the clinician with paperwork. The clinician selects problem areas for each client, and the computer suggests a goal and 20 objectives for each problem sound. Appropriate word lists are offered by the PEPPER program from College Hill Press (Shriberg, 1984). Blache has authored a program that includes a tutorial introducing his diagnostic approach and that designs an individualized minimal word-pair treatment program for each subject analyzed. A program offered by Parrot Software helps determine goals for the client and then sets up an interactive game the client can play with letters and pictures on the screen. On a more limited basis, a program by McDermott (1982) stores a subject's phonemic repertoire, arranges it into one- or two-syllable words, and prints out lists of words by phoneme and indicates the position of the phoneme in the words. A similar generation of word lists containing consonants or vowels in the initial, medial, or final position has been authored by Schuldt.

Treatment programs for articulation disorders have been designed in varying modes. A program designed to be used by trained aides as well as clinicians presents stimulus items, provides reinforcement based on the clinician's judgment of accuracy, and advises the clinician when to adjust levels of difficulty (Fitch, 1982). An adventure-type game featuring speech-sound "monsters" in underground caverns provides motivation and practice for primary students (Blache). A type of program requiring less clinician participation is *The /S/ Meter* developed by Rushakoff, which provides visual feedback to clients attempting to maintain correct pronunciation of the /s/ phoneme.

Dysarthria

Computerized diagnostic applications for dysarthria are also available. One analyzes results of the *Frenchay Dysarthria Assessment* (Enderly and Roworth, 1984); the second analyzes 50 words and 20 sentences and quantifies single-word and sentence intelligibility and speaking rates (Yorkston, Beukelman, and Traynor).

Voice Disorders

Treatment of voice disorders has been approached in two distinct manners. The *Vocal Abuse Reduction Program* (Johnson and Child, 1984), a program for treating voice disorders arising from abuse or misuse, concentrates on clinician training as well as information assessment and intervention. The *Visible Speech Aid* system provides graphic displays of amplitude, pitch contours, and syllabic rhythms. These are traced on the monitor screen in response to signals picked up through the microphone. A client is able to compare his or her effort with a target pattern and receives instant visual feedback. A game encouraging practice in pitch control and sustained phonation is also contained in the program.

Microcomputer applications for the handling of dysfluency are not readily available. Although it is a fairly safe supposition that individuals have begun using the computer in some manner relative to dysfluency, as yet no programs are on record. Some attempts have been made to take subjective material and add objectivity to it in order to make it more scientific and less magic. Metz, Samar, and Sacco (1983) used the computer to quantify various speech parameters and how they were affected by treatment.

Augmentative Communication Systems

Augmentative communication systems supplement the insufficient speech of nonoral individuals. As computer technology increases, so does the availability and specificity of augmentative devices. In only a few years, technology has progressed from lap boards displaying pictures representing basic human needs to portable, computerized, communication systems featuring synthesized voices and computer printouts. Many of these can be adapted for use by severely motor-handicapped individuals.

Basically nonportable devices for clinical or home use have been developed by Rushakoff et al. and the Schneier Communication Unit. *Talk II* and *Quick Talk* couple an Apple II Plus microcomputer and disk drive with an Echo II speech synthesizer. The unit can be modified to accommodate the physically handicapped person, who can then generate his own personal dictionary of utterances.

All Talk, *Form-A-Phrase*, and *Vocaid*, all products of Adaptive Communication Systems, provide voiced communication in various portable forms. Also portable, but lacking voice, is the *Memowriter* by Sharp Electronics. This device prints up to a six-line message and stores commonly used words and phrases in each of the keys for easy one-key recall.

More sophisticated and expensive are devices such as *The Vois* from Phonic Ear. *The Vois* is operated from specially designed keyboards capable of producing a wide variety of single-word and connected utterances. *The Vois* is quite portable, as is the *Speech Pac/Epson* Notebook Computer, which combines the Epson HX-20 portable computer with a speech synthesizer and software program. It provides a printout as well as speech, and allows access to all standard Epson computer functions as well as serving as a communicator.

CONCLUSION

Recent advertising from Children's Television Workshop described the evolution of the computer from a "big, dumb adding machine" to what it is today. It stated that computers today ". . . can think, imagine, and, some say, feel and worry." What clinician would not be pleased to be described in such terms? The only essential factor missing from such a description is that of expertise. When more clinicians become "computer-friendly" and share their expertise with the machine, the two will find an efficient, compatible partnership that will increase over-all clinical effectiveness in terms of both treatment and time utilization.

REFERENCES

Blache, S. E. *Error Analysis Program* (2nd ed.), CUSH Software Registry, Nov. 1981.

Blache, S. E. *Comprehensive Phonemic Inventory for School-Aged Children*. San Diego: College Hill, 1984.

Enderby, P. M., and Rowarth, M. *Frenchay Dysarthria Assessment Computer Differential Analysis*. San Diego: College Hill, 1984.

Filter, M. *Competency Training Systems*. Harrisonburg, Va.

Fitch, J. L. *Communication Skill Builders*. CUSH Software Registry, 1984.

Harlan, C. L., Jr. *Computer-Assisted Distinctive Feature Analysis* (2nd ed.). CUSH Software Registry, Nov. 1982.

Harlan, C. L., Jr. *Computer-Assisted Articulation Error Analysis* (2nd ed.). CUSH Software Registry, Nov. 1982.

Harlan, D. *Speech-Language Diagnostic Test Summary (SUMS)* (3rd ed.). CUSH Software Registry, Nov. 1983.

Harlan, D. *Child Speech-Language Case History (KIDS)*. Apropos Systems, 227 Otis, Colorado Springs, Col. 80916.

Haynes, S. *The Articulator*. ATP Software, 20 Commercial Blvd., Novato, Ca. 94947-6191.

Johnson, T., and Child, D. *VARP: Vocal Abuse Reduction Program*. San Diego: College Hill, 1984.

Lingquest 2. Lingquest Software, Inc., Charles E. Merrill Test Division, Columbus, Oh.

McDermott, L. D. *Computer Aided Intelligibility* (2nd ed.). CUSH Software Registry, Nov. 1982.

Metz, D., Samar, V., and Sacco, P. Acoustic analysis of stutterer's fluent speech before and after therapy. *J. Speech Hear. Res.* 26:531–536, 1983.

Rushakoff, G., and Edwards, W. The /s/ Meter: A beginning for microcomputer assisted speech therapy. Paper presented at the American Speech-Language-Hearing Association Annual Convention, Toronto, 1982.

Rushakoff, G. *Microcomputer Assisted Study Partner in Anatomy and Physiology of the Speech and Hearing Mechanism*. San Diego: College Hill, 1984.

Shriberg, L. PEPPER: Programs to Examine Phonetic and Phonological Evaluation Records. San Diego: College Hill, 1984.

Schuldt, M. *CDTS Articulation Diagnosis and Treatment*. Harding and Harris Behavioral Research, Inc., Box 1599, Orem, Utah 84057.

Schuldt, M. *CDTS Client File*. Harding and Harris Behavioral Research, Inc., Box 1599, Orem, Utah 84057.

Schuldt, M. *CDTS Mini Client File*. Harding and Harris Behavioral Research, Inc., Box 1599, Orem, Utah 84057.

Schuldt, M. *CDTS Sound Search*. Harding and Harris Behavioral Research, Inc., Box 1599, Orem, Utah 84057.

Telage, K. A computerized place-manner distinctive feature program for articulation analysis. *J. Speech Hear. Disord.* 45:481–493, 1980.

Visible Speech Aid. Software Research Corp., 3939 Quandra, Victoria, B.C., Canada V8X 1J5.

Weiner, F. F. *Process Analysis Version 2.0*. State College, Pa.: Parrot Software, 1985.

Yorkston, K., Beukelman, D., and Traynor, C. *Computerized Assessment of Intelligibility of Dysarthric Speech*. C.C. Publications.

7

Microcomputer Applications in Aphasia and Head Trauma

Russell H. Mills

Speech pathologists and neuropsychologists are cognizant of the complex nature of the language and cognitive systems in both normal and disordered states. A direct consequence of this complexity is that most of the intervention applied has been provided in person by the clinician. Until recently only the most basic tasks of clinical evaluation and treatment have been instrumented. Still, in many clinics increases in case load have outpaced increases in staffing and have caused clinicians to seek ways of increasing both the quantity and quality of the services they provide to their patients. One approach to achieving these goals is through more extensive use of automated therapy.

The belief that aspects of language therapy for the aphasic patient can be automated is not new. In 1967 a device was conceived by Keith and Darley (1967) that could automate limited therapeutic tasks. Figure 7-1 shows the home-built device, called the *Electric Board*, which was battery-powered and capable of presenting a variety of matching tasks to the aphasic patient. An example was the matching of pictures and their associated printed names. When the patient placed a stylus in each of the proper stimulus and response holes, an electrical connection was completed between the stimulus word and its pictorial referent. A battery caused a bulb to illuminate, indicating a correct response. By changing the stimulus and response overlay sheets, the task could be changed. By manually changing the interconnections of the wires on the back of the device, the order of the correct responses could be changed. The device was an important development because it demonstrated that automation in therapy for aphasia could be advanced beyond that provided by audio recording and playback devices such as the *Language Master* (Bell and Howell Corp.). Still, the Electric Board was limited in utility because it (1) could not present spoken stimuli and reinforcement, (2) was hard-wired and not easily changed for alternative tasks, and (3) did not record the patient's performance for later inspection by the clinician.

During the 1960s and 1970s a relatively sophisticated electronic system called *logic circuitry* was employed in the study of speech and language pathology. This system was composed of a variety of discrete electronic modules interconnected by plug-in wires to perform a desired task (Fig. 7-2). Today logic circuitry continues in use, both independently and in conjunction with computers, but primarily for research purposes. Its use in day-to-day clinical tasks has been limited by its high cost and the difficulty encountered in rapidly reconfiguring it for the performance of alternative clinical tasks.

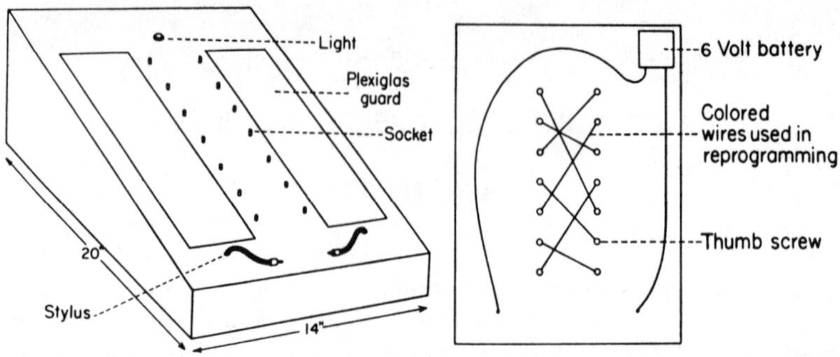

Fig. 7-1. Materials and procedures in the "Electric Board" of Keith and Darley (1976) designed to automate limited therapeutic tasks.

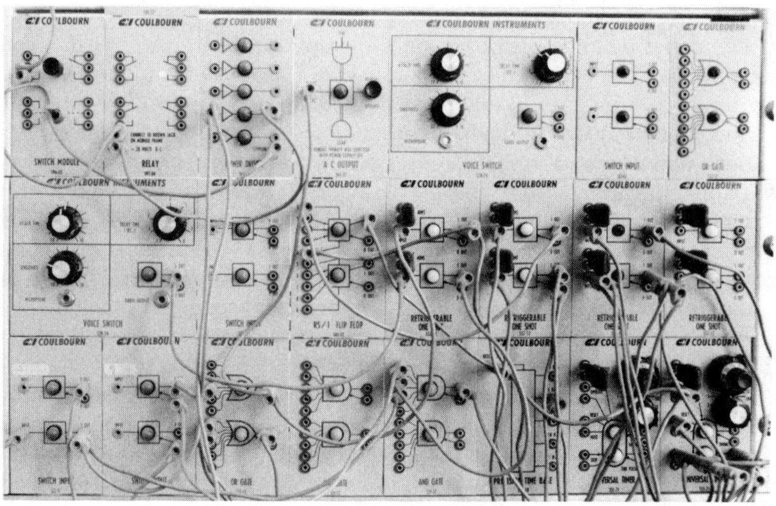

Fig. 7-2. Logic circuitry used in the 1960s and 1970s to study speech and language pathology.

BENEFITS OF MICROCOMPUTER THERAPY

The preceding overview of two early systems suggests that there are reasons for their failure to achieve widespread clinical use. If these limitations can be eliminated in future designs, then therapeutic automata may prove to be strong allies in the diagnosis and treatment of patients who exhibit aphasia and cognitive dysfunction. New systems must (1) be clinically flexible to allow the presentation of a wide variety of tasks; (2) be accessible to a wide variety of patients; (3) collect, analyze, store, and print response data; (4) produce highly intelligible speech; and (5) be cost effective. At present it appears that the microcomputer offers the best hope of achieving these goals of automated therapy. If microcomputers can automate selected portions of our clinical activities, three major benefits will ensue: increased stimulus control, increased precision of measurement, and increased clinical efficiency.

1. *Increased Stimulus Control.* Microcomputer technology provides the clinician with the opportunity to control a variety of stimulus parameters in the treatment room. The intensity and rate of auditory stimuli, and the size, location, color, and duration of text and graphics can be precisely controlled across repeated trials of a task. Beyond this, the computer can be called on to modify these parameters from within a treatment program. Finally, as software becomes more sophisticated, we will see more "intelligent" programs that learn from the pattern of a patient's performance (Rahimi, 1980). When programs become able to make complex clinical decisions at the prior direction of the clinician, they will be truly powerful allies.
2. *Increased Precision of Measurement.* When conducting live therapy clinicians frequently rate responses by the use of "plus-minus" scoring. This system was selected because it is workable; nevertheless, it is apparent that critical information may be lost. Microcomputers offer the opportunity not only to measure single parameters more precisely, but also to measure multiple parameters in a functionally simultaneous manner. Thus, in addition to determining that a response is incorrect, it is possible to collect data describing response latency, number of stimulus presentations required to produce the response, semantic relatedness to the target, and overall patterns of error.
3. *Increased Clinical Efficiency.* Many clinicians are experiencing a rapid growth in the demands for their professional services. Many also believe that the patients under their care could benefit from additional therapies. However, in many institutions an increase in the demand for services is not always followed by an increase in staff. Given the chronic shortage of clinicians in some institutions, the microcomputer can be seen as a means of delivering more clinic- and home-based therapy to a greater number of patients. The preceding statement is not an advocation of the position that the microcomputer can or should replace the clinician. Rather, today's computers are capable of presenting a variety of practice and drill tasks that do not require "real-time" problem solving and parameter adjustment by the clinician. The systems can also be assigned complex tasks, such as data collection and analysis, that would take excessive amounts of time if done manually. Such nonclinical applications, which are discussed elsewhere in the text, can have a dramatic impact on our clinical efficiency. That is, though some clinical tasks currently cannot be automated, the completion of nonclinical duties by the computer can free additional time for direct patient contact.

MICROCOMPUTER DEVELOPMENT

In 1971 the Intel Corporation released its first microprocessor (Willis and Miller, 1984). However, it was not until the third generation of microcomputers (e.g., the Apple, TRS-80, Ohio Scientific) had been on the market for several years that limited clinical applications began to appear (Gianutsos and Klitzner, 1981; Mills and Thomas, 1981). Over the past few years hardware and software technologies have advanced to the level where microcomputerized therapy is a very promising, albeit not satisfactorily proved, approach. Nevertheless, clinical applications exist for this technology that appear to be both useful and cost effective.

HARDWARE CONSIDERATIONS

Chapters 2 and 3 of this book cover the issue of hardware selection. Nevertheless, several considerations are of special importance when selecting a hardware system for use with aphasic or head-injured populations.

Availability of Software

The software to be used must be appropriate for the hardware system selected and for the patients who will use it. It is of little help to acquire a particular computer if software does not exist to perform the operations you wish. Consequently, in order to select a useful hardware system, it becomes necessary to evaluate the range of software that can be used for the evaluation and treatment of language and cognitive disorders. Although some programs have been developed from within the fields of speech pathology and cognitive psychology, much of what is available has been borrowed from the fields of education and special education. Therefore, a hardware system compatible with the general education software now being offered will also prove useful in therapy-related applications. This "software-first" approach to hardware selection is especially valid in a field where few clinicians will actually be involved in the production of the software they use.

Availability of Peripheral Devices

Many of the commercially available educational programs can be executed on an unadorned microcomputer consisting of a central processing unit, a data-storage device such as a disk drive, and a monochrome monitor. Many educational programs present information to the student as text or graphics, and the student responds through the keyboard. These methods of stimulus output and response input can be quite limiting when the same hardware system is used in language and cognitive rehabilitation. It is imperative that the system selected interface with a variety of peripheral devices. The most clinically useful are speech synthesizers, speech digitizers, hardware clocks, printers, joysticks, single switches, and graphics pads. The degree of expandability varies from one system to the next and is very important to the successful clinical use of the microcomputer.

Speech-Production Methods

Language therapy depends heavily on the spoken utterance. When computerized training in auditory comprehension is desired, production of computerized speech is, of course, mandatory. In other tasks spoken reinforcers and cues may be desirable. Clinicians interested in programs that talk will find a variety of technologies to choose from. These include cassette-tape interfaces, speech synthesizers, linear predictive coding, and speech digitization. These systems all have their own strengths and weaknesses (Mills, 1982). The two most critical factors in selecting a speech-production system are the quality of speech and the availability of software. The prospective purchaser should listen to the speech produced by the various systems under consideration before making a selection. When the speech will be used for the purposes of stimulus presentation, the critical factor is whether a patient with a neurologic deficit will be able to understand the mechanized speech produced. Live speech represents a relatively undistorted signal, the comprehension of which is often impaired in the aphasic. Therefore, for purposes of auditory comprehension training it would seem appropriate to select a system that produces speech of very high quality. However, when the speech-production system will be used as an augmentative communication device, the primary receiver is likely to be one who is neurologically normal. Thus, a speech-production system that produces speech of lesser quality may be adequate. Once a system of acceptable quality has been located, it is then necessary to determine what software is available to support the types of tasks the clinician wishes to present.

Response-Input Alternatives

Whereas the neurologically normal computer user can input information through the keyboard, alternative forms of response are often desirable for the neurologically impaired. A variety of forms are available, but the price tags vary greatly. Light pens, joysticks, single switches, and graphics pads are all available at reasonable prices. Touch-sensitive screens, while more desirable, tend to be too expensive for many clinic budgets. Due to technologic advances, however, the cost of touch-sensitive screens may come within the reach of clinic budgets in the near future.

Programs designed to train visual perception and fine motor control are frequently employed with head-injured patients. The usual means of response input for these programs is a joystick, which is actually more appropriate as an input mechanism than the keyboard. Joystick responding is more concrete and more like responses to a similar task in live therapy. Joysticks also have the advantage of being connected to the computer by a cord. The cord can allow a wheelchair-bound patient to sit at a distance from the computer, with the joystick affixed to a lapboard, and still be able to execute the computer program.

Alternative response input by aphasic patients requires one additional consideration. Patients of the Broca's type, who frequently exhibit a right hemiparesis, often cannot use a traditional joystick. The most popular design of joysticks places the fire button at the base of the stick, making its use a two-handed operation. It is desirable to acquire a joystick that has the fire button on the top of the stick so it can be used even by the hemiparetic patient.

PATIENT SELECTION CRITERIA

The selection of an appropriate hardware system will not ensure that all patients will be able to take advantage of microcomputerized therapy. As will become evident in the discussion of software, not all therapeutic tasks are equally possible with the microcomputer. Although the microcomputer easily processes typed input, it is very limited in its ability to process human speech. Therefore, at present, reading and spelling dysfunctions are more readily treated than dysarthria and dyspraxia. The specific deficits exhibited by a patient will, in part, dictate whether that patient is appropriate for computer-based therapy.

Visual and Auditory Processing Abilities

An important factor in patient selection is the ability of the patient to process visual information. Because aphasia most frequently results from strokes, which are most commonly experienced after the fifth decade of life, visual acuity problems may be present in this population. In addition, the neurologically impaired of any age may exhibit convergence and tracking problems that may confound microcomputer use. Thus, in both populations it is important to know the status of visual acuity, tracking, and visual perceptual abilities. Auditory abilities are less critical, but important. Although the information presented in many programs is issued in the visual modality, reinforcers are often presented in the form of computer-generated tones. While it is necessary that the patient be able to detect these reinforcers, many are dually encoded as on-screen text and graphic feedback. Auditory processing abilities are also important during computer-familiarization training, during which the clinician often provides verbal cuing as to the patient's interaction with the computer.

Memory Functions

A patient's recent memory processes are an important factor in determining whether he or she can learn to use the computer. Although performing computer-based tasks can be extremely valuable in rehabilitation, interaction with computers often requires more abstract skills than tasks presented in a "live" mode. For example, pointing to a picture that has been named by the clinician is a concrete task. Pressing a key on the keyboard to match a picture on the monitor screen to a printed or spoken word is more abstract. Some patients with memory impairments seem to have the most difficulty remembering unnatural extensions of the task, such as pressing the return key after making a response selection. The inability to remember all the elements of computer operation required for a program will limit the degree of independent use a patient can achieve.

Response-Input Capability

Many programs are designed to accept response information only through the keyboard. The vast majority of aphasic patients are, in fact, able to utilize keyboard response entry. On occasion it has been necessary to make modifications to accommodate selected patients. When a patient has difficulty locating the proper keys, the keys can be coded with colored stickers. If the problem continues, then a *keyboard mask* can be constructed. The mask is constructed of posterboard and is cut to expose only those keys required for the execution of a specific program. As was discussed in the section on hardware, many systems will accommodate alternative response modes, such as joysticks, touch screens, or single switches. However, the software must be compatible with the alternative-input device selected for use.

Patient Attitudes

A difficult consideration to quantify is the patient's attitude toward the technology. It is likely that the range of attitudes toward the use of microcomputer technology found in a population of speech-language pathologists and neuropsychologists is, along one dimension, similar to that expected in a population of brain-damaged clients. That is, in both groups we might find responses ranging all along an acceptance-rejection continuum. At one extreme are those clinicians and patients who are decidedly opposed to the use of the computer. At the other extreme are those who have embraced the technology, sometimes to an unrealistic degree. In the middle range lie the majority, who have some positive expectations coupled with some reservations about what microcomputers can accomplish. Experience indicates that the brain-damaged population is skewed in the positive direction. Very few patients have rejected treatment by use of the microcomputer. Most are very excited about the prospect. In some cases they have had expectations that are unrealistically high—a reaction for which the clinician must be prepared. The majority fall in the central group. However, the quality of early experiences with computerized treatment can move a patient to either extreme.

Patient-Software Match

In determining candidacy for computerized therapy, the "patient-software match" is a critical factor in determining successful use of the system. Clinicians responsible for the selection of the hardware and software systems are frequently most concerned with the selection of the "right" microcomputer and peripheral hardware. Software acquisition often takes a back seat. A sure way to convince a patient that the microcomputer is not appropriate for her or him is to have an inadequate software library that forces the patient to use inappropriate software. This type of misapplication of technology can move a patient from the positive end of the continuum to the negative end very quickly.

The patient-software match must be based on the results of the patient's speech, language, and cognitive evaluation and must consider the elements in patient selection listed previously. When these factors are considered in light of a clinic's existing hardware, software library, and staff expertise, it can be determined whether this new technology has anything substantial to offer a given patient.

SOFTWARE

Acquiring software that is appropriate to the needs of a given patient population, meets the clinician's treatment expectations, is compatible with a particular hardware system, and is within the clinic's budget is a complex task. Multiple factors have been identified that should be considered in selecting software for use with patients who exhibit cognitive dysfunction and aphasia (Wilson, 1983).

Control of Parameters

Programs useful for a large number of patients allow control of parameters such as grade level of stimuli, rate of speech, base-line test versus treatment mode, selection of cues, and trials allowed before the correct response is given. Control of these parameters may not be of critical importance with a neurologically normal population. However, when used with those who have experienced brain damage, a minor alteration in the operation of the program can determine success or failure, learning or frustration.

Alternative Response Input

Programs that limit patient responses to the keyboard may preclude their use by certain of the patients in these populations. Where possible, programs for these populations should allow joystick, graphics pad, and single-switch input. For patients with severe motoric involvement, computer utilization may be precluded without the option of single-switch input. It is not sufficient that the microcomputer be equipped with these input devices. It is also necessary that the software in question be prepared to accept the input.

Base-line Test Mode and Treatment Mode

Determination of the effects of treatment depends on accurate base-line, probe, and post-treatment evaluations. Without the ability to collect these data in the absence of cues, it is difficult to determine the effect of any given program on the patient's language or cognitive abilities. Therefore, a program that provides a menu-selectable base-line mode would be highly desirable.

Stimulus File Entry

When only the programmer's stimuli can be used, it is not possible to individualize the task for a given patient. The inability to do so may prove critical with certain programs. For example, for a given patient it may be important to focus spelling drills on family names, or vocabulary exercises on employment-related words. However, in other programs (e.g., a video game provided to a head-injured patient for the improvement of motor control and visual perception) this may not be a critical limitation.

Data Collection, Storage, Analysis, and Reporting

Currently, few programs fully tap the potential of the computer for data collection and analysis. Many "game" programs collect little data, fail to store it, and refuse to print it. Thus, it is necessary for the clinician or patient to read the data from the cathode-ray tube (CRT) and record it by hand. A surprising number of educational programs in use collect and report only marginally useful response data. Even programs marketed by clinicians often fail to measure powerful variables, such as response time, or to analyze response data for patterns of error. These failures to report adequate data do little to help achieve the goal of improved clinical efficiency. The clinician who bases clinical decisions on the collection of extensive patient response data will be disappointed by many of the current software programs.

Error Trapping

Most programs operate flawlessly when the user performs as the program expects. However, when a patient inputs an unexpected response some programs may "hang" or "crash." That is, if a program expects a single-digit input, it may stop executing if a letter or the space bar is pressed. Such inappropriate responses are fairly common in the brain-damaged population, especially during early microcomputer training. Thus, when previewing a program it is necessary for the clinician to input unexpected responses. If the program fails, then it will not be appropriate for independent patient use. It may also prove to be frustrating for the patient, even when monitored by the clinician.

SOFTWARE REVIEW

During the past 2 years a large number of software packages have become available. Some have been borrowed from the special education and general education markets. Others have been produced by speech pathologists and cognitive psychologists specifically for use with special populations. In this chapter it is not possible to review all the current offerings, but only to review a representative sampling of the programs available.

Software for the Evaluation of Aphasia

At present there are two ways in which the microcomputer can assist in the evaluation of aphasia. The first is in *direct evaluation* of patient responses, and the second is in *patient data analysis* applications.

DIRECT EVALUATION

It is well established that the disorder of aphasia crosses modalities (Darley, 1977). Thus, it follows that the evaluation protocols in use will sample behaviors from a wide variety of tasks in the several modalities (Kertesz, 1979). From the discussion of various hardware components elsewhere in this text, it becomes apparent that certain modalities are more easily tested than others. For example, the evaluation of reading comprehension requires no sophisticated peripheral component, merely an unadorned microcomputer and appropriate software. The evaluation of auditory comprehension, on the other hand, requires the use of a speech-generation system that produces speech of acceptable quality. The evaluation of writing is limited to the evaluation of typed responses owing to the computer's difficulty in evaluating the extremely complex graphic patterns present in handwriting samples. Finally, the evaluation of spoken utterances produced by the aphasic patient (i.e., speech recognition) is at the far edge of current technology and not yet ready for widespread clinical use.

Given that testing in each of the modalities is not equally possible with our current hardware limitations, it comes as no surprise that no microcomputerized "aphasia evaluation" exists. The bulk of the direct evaluation usage of the microcomputer with this population is made by the pre- and post-testing of treatment software. The use of single-subject designs is appropriate with the presentation of traditional evaluative measures to assess the generalized effects of treatment.

PATIENT DATA ANALYSIS

When the microcomputer is used for patient data analysis, it is for the purpose of analyzing responses that have been collected previously by the clinician. Two language-sample analysis programs are *Lingquest-1: Lan-*

guage *Sample Analysis* by Lingquest Software, Inc., and *Systematic Analysis of Language Transcriptions* (SALT) by Miller and Chapman (1982).

Lingquest-1 analyzes a transcribed sample of 50 to 100 utterances that are input through the keyboard by the clinician. The program reports opportunities for occurrence, instances of correct usage, percentage of correct usages for a variety of grammatical forms, phrase structures, sentence structures, and verb tenses. It also reports type-token ratio and mean length of utterance.

SALT also requires keyboard entry of a speech sample and provides similar, though not identical, data to the clinician. In addition, *SALT* contains a search routine that can retrieve discourse elements or whole utterances based on clinician-specified parameters. This search routine allows the retrieval of specific linguistic elements that might be required in the formulation of a language diagnosis or treatment plan.

At present the microcomputer does not analyze speech-sample data accurately. Nevertheless, Kearns (1980) has shown that there may be value in speech-sample analysis in the evaluation and treatment of apraxia of speech. There are currently several programs that will provide an analysis when phonologic information is typed into the computer. Telage (1980) described a program that evaluated input from *A Deep Test of Articulation* (McDonald, 1964). Also, *Lingquest-2: Phonological Analysis* is a program that evaluates the results of an articulation test or a free-speech sample. The program then calculates and reports consonant and vowel usage and patterns of omission and substitution, and performs a phonologic process analysis. The results of either program may be valuable in the evaluation and planning of treatment for patients exhibiting phonologic dysfunction.

Although no microcomputerized battery of tests for aphasia exists, one program is available that assists the clinician in the calculation of test data. A major contribution to the field of aphasiology was the development of the *Porch Index of Communicative Abilities* (PICA) (Porch, 1967). The powerful multidimensional scoring system employed has a negative feature, however. The calculation of test data is a time-consuming task. Recently, Porch and Katz developed a program called *PICAPAD* that employs the computer to compile the PICA data. When the clinician inputs the raw scores the program calculates subtest means, percentile scores, high-low gap values, high overall average prediction (HOAP) slopes, and other descriptive scores.

Software for Treatment of Spelling Deficits

The treatment of spelling disorders is a natural for the computer. It usually requires that stimuli be presented in text form on the CRT and that responses be input through the keyboard. Such a program requires no sophisticated hardware and straightforward programming skills. In fact, the development of a spelling program was the subject of an early report (Seron et al., 1980). This task utilized a minicomputer to present a spelling task to five subjects. During the task the clinician and patient were seated at the computer terminal. The clinician dictated the word to be spelled, and the patient typed it on the keyboard. To guard against the patient learning incorrect response patterns, the computer displayed only those letters that were correctly typed. The authors reported that all five subjects who received computerized spelling practice made substantial gains. However, the gains were only partially maintained at 6 weeks post-treatment.

The Seron et al. (1980) study was important because it demonstrated that the computer could have a positive effect in language rehabilitation. Nevertheless, their program had a major limitation. The fact that the clinician was required to dictate the words negated any opportunity for individual practice or increased clinical efficiency. One might question whether the task could have been equally effective as a paper and pencil exercise. Recognizing this limitation, the authors modified the program to make use of pictures instead of clinician dictation to present the words (Katz, 1984).

Because spelling is a skill frequently addressed in general education, there are many programs from which to choose. Some programs such as *Spelling Bee*, by Edu-Ware, present stimuli as high-resolution pictures. *Compu-Spell*, also by Edu-Ware, uses an incomplete-sentence format. The *Create It–Spell It* program by Hartley Courseware takes a different approach. It uses a cassette control device to present the words via cassette tape. In all these programs, responses are input through the keyboard. Additional programs, such as those produced by the Minnesota Educational Computing Consortium (MECC), provide spelling drills in formats such as crossword puzzles, word searches, hangman, and anagrams. Because the approach of a program may be appropriate for one patient but not for another, many clinics have several spelling programs on hand.

Software for Treatment of Reading-Comprehension Deficits

Like spelling, reading-comprehension training is a natural for the microcomputer. There are a large number of programs available in the general education market that address this area. However, because many were developed for the neurologically normal elementary student, they often have features that make them inappropriate for the adult aphasic patient. For example, a program may present material at an appropriate reading level but use juvenile subject matter. Pacing of the programs has also been found to be too rapid, and often critical parameters are not under clinician control. Because of these limitations, it is encouraging to find that sets of reading-comprehension programs are being marketed by clinicians, who may have a better notion of the requirements of the aphasic population.

Using programs they developed, Katz and Nagy (1982) evaluated the effects of microcomputerized reading-comprehension treatment with seven chronic aphasic subjects. Their programs consisted of test and treatment elements. The treatment elements included identification of the functions of objects, question words, grammatical structures, and the comprehension of short paragraphs. The five subjects who completed the study showed only small gains in reading comprehension. The methods used in the study were not dramatically different from those used in live therapy. Therefore, the results may only confirm the resistance to change frequently encountered in the chronically brain damaged.

Katz followed the development of these public-domain programs with an offering of three reading-comprehension programs through Sunset Software. The programs are titled *Understanding Questions*, *Understand-*

ing Sentences, and *Understanding Stories*. The programs offer some of the features clinicians look for, including menu selection, immediate versus delayed presentation of test questions, data collection, data analysis, CRT display of response-data graphics, and across-session data analysis. A nine-diskette series, *Computerized Reading for Aphasics*, is produced specifically for the aphasic population by SLP Software. These programs provide drill and practice in the comprehension of synonyms, antonyms, questions, modifiers, definitions, and so forth. The SLP programs offer random stimulus presentation and response alternatives, base-line mode, response-time measurement, and the ability to enter the clinician's own stimulus files.

A series of programs from Media Materials, Inc., allows treatment of higher-level reading deficits. Their programs *Keys to Sequence* and *Building Inference Skills* require the reader to detect detail, draw conclusions, make inferences, etc. Media Materials has also released programs based on specific functional skills, such as banking and auto repair. The reading-comprehension programs discussed in this section are all available for the Apple microcomputer.

Software for Improving Semantics and Syntactics of Language

Some text-based programs have improved reading comprehension as their goal. The programs in this section require reading, but attempt to train specific linguistic processes. A series of these programs is marketed by Hartley Courseware, Inc. The names of the programs reflect the area of language addressed by each. Hartley produces programs such as *Verbs; Pronouns; Who, What, When, Where, Why;* and others. The typical Hartley package provides 15 to 20 separate programs on each disk. For example, in the case of *Verbs* the clinician has multiple programs at different levels of difficulty to teach different aspects of verb comprehension and use. This feature is very useful, as it allows the clinician to select those programs that will best ensure mastery of the concept. File-building routines are also provided.

Software for Treatment of Auditory-Comprehension Deficits

Auditory-comprehension training with the microcomputer requires a method that produces high-quality speech. Mills (1982) reported the results of the use of digitized speech with a chronically aphasic male in a single-subject design. The results indicated that the subject improved his performance on the computer program, Token Test measures, and PICA auditory-comprehension subtest scores after treatment. The digitized speech production method is now in use by Brain-Link Software, which produces three software packages designed for use in auditory-comprehension training of aphasic patients. The three packages are *Word Recognition, Function Recognition*, and *Preposition Recognition* and are used to train clients to comprehend sequences of one to three spoken nouns, verbs, and prepositions. All programs provide extensive control of treatment parameters, data collection (including response times in milliseconds), data analysis, and hard-copy output.

The technology of mechanized speech continues to advance. Recently, a method of speech production called *linear predictive coding* (LPC) has become commercially available. This technique allows speech of better quality than synthesized speech and requires less of the computer's RAM than digitized speech. One LPC system is used in the *Ufonic Speech System* produced by Borg-Warner Corporation.

Software in the Treatment of Cognitive Dysfunction

In addressing the subject of treatment of those with cognitive dysfunction, Bracy (1983), stated that, ". . . we must enhance the processes of monitoring sensory input, selectively attending, maintaining attention for extended periods, discriminating stimulus attributes, initiating responses, inhibiting responses/making differential responses, generalizing stimulus properties and generalizing responses." Although the computer cannot replace the critical human intervention provided by the clinician, it can provide extensive practice and drill to address many of the deficits cited previously. Finally, the microcomputer offers the possibility of home-based treatment and thus increases the amount of intervention available to head-injured patients.

The computer software required to address these areas is wide-ranging. Lynch (1983) stated that commercial game programs such as *Pong*, *Super Breakout*, and *Caverns of Mars* are appropriate for the training of attention, concentration, memory, reaction time, visual tracking, and eye-hand coordination. Most of the popular game programs are available for use with inexpensive computers.

In addition to using game programs, neuropsychologists have begun to produce software for the treatment of the head-injured population. Bracy produced an extensive array of programs reflecting his orientation to the treatment of head-injured patients. These programs, available through Psychological Software Services, come in collections representing selected areas, such as *Foundations Skills*, *Visuospatial Skills*, *Conceptual Skills*, *Memory Skills*, *Auditory Skills*, and *Problem Solving*. A variety of individual programs are also available. Because one of Bracy's goals is to allow home-based treatment, the programs were prepared to operate on inexpensive computers.

Over a period of years, Ben-Yishay (1982) developed a wide-ranging noncomputerized approach to the treatment of cognitive deficits secondary to head injury. Activities for the improvement of attention, learning, and integration have now been provided in a computer format, *Orientation Remedial Module*.

Harley Courseware has released a package titled *Cognitive Rehabilitation*. It is a four-diskette series that addresses categorization, sequencing, association, and memory. An additional *Authoring Program* allows the clinician to create his or her own treatment programs. The programs provide random or sequenced stimulus presentation, "hint" frames preceding responses, and "explanation" frames following incorrect responses. Response data are collected and stored.

One final application to the problems of the head injured reflects an entirely different use of the microcomputer. The concept of microcomputer "orthosis" is being applied to the management of the memory problems of the cognitively impaired (Kirsch and Levine, 1984). A unique feature of this application is the use of the microcomputer as an assistive, rather than an instructional, device. The objective of orthosis is to place the microcomputer in the patient's home where it continually executes a background program. Contained within the background program are critical events that must be remembered and performed at specific times throughout the day (e.g., the patient's medication schedule). Simultaneously, the computer may also execute a foreground program that prompts the patient's memory in the performance of some specific task, such as baking cookies. The cardinal feature of the concept is that the background program can interrupt the foreground program at any time to ensure that critical needs are met. While still in the developmental stages, miniaturization to a fully portable unit may help microcomputer orthosis become a powerful concept in the management of cognitive deficits.

The use of microcomputers as tools of rehabilitation is a new concept, and advancing at an overwhelming pace. Hardware, peripheral devices, and software changes appear weekly. This rapidity of technological change has revealed the limitations of textbooks and professional journals as traditional methods of information exchange. It remains difficult to determine the answers to our clinical application questions before the information is out of date. There is a need for rapid dissemination of information so that appropriate and immediate clinical decisions can be made.

Therapeutic automata used in the treatment of aphasia and head injury have advanced tremendously since the "Electric Board" appeared 17 years ago. In the coming years we will experience additional clinically important technological advances. Developments resulting in clinically usable speaker-independent speech recognition and applied artificial intelligence capabilities will fundamentally alter the way we train for, practice, and view our profession. If we as a profession can learn to effectively utilize this technology with our patients, then it will reap numerous clinical benefits including many which we may not yet foresee.

REFERENCES

Ben-Yishay, Y. (Ed.) *Rehabilitation Monograph No. 64: Working Approaches to Remediation of Cognitive Deficits in Brain Damaged Persons*. New York: New York University Medical Center, 1982.

Bracy, O. L. Computer based cognitive rehabilitation. *Cognitive Rehabilitation* 1:1, 1983.

Darley, F. A. Retrospective view of aphasia. *J. Speech Hear. Disord.* 42:161–169, 1977.

Gianutsos, R., and Klitzner, C. Computer programs for cognitive rehabilitation. In *IEEE Proceedings of Johns Hopkins First National Search for Applications of Personal Computing to Aid the Handicapped*. Los Angeles: IEEE Computer Society, 1981.

Katz, R. C. Using microcomputers in the diagnosis and treatment of chronic aphasic adults. *Semin. Speech Lang.* 5:11–22, 1984.

Katz, R. C., and Nagy, V. T. A computerized treatment system for chronic aphasic patients. In R. H. Brookshire (Ed.), *Clinical Aphasiology: Conference Proceedings 1982*. Minneapolis: BRK Publishers, 1982.

Kearns, K. P. The application of phonological process analysis to adult neuropathologies. In R. H. Brookshire (Ed.), *Clinical Aphasiology: Conference Proceedings, 1980*. Minneapolis: BRK Publishers, 1980.

Keith, R. L., and Darley, F. L. The use of a specific electric board in rehabilitation of the aphasic patient. *J. Speech Hear. Disord.* 32:2, 1967.

Kertesz, A. *Aphasia and Associated Disorders: Taxonomy, Localization and Recovery*. New York: Grune & Stratton, 1979.

Kirsh, N. L., and Levine, S. P. A compensatory microcomputer intervention for patients with cognitive limitations. Paper presented to the Conference on Models and Techniques in Cognitive Rehabilitation—IV. Indianapolis, March 30–April 4, 1984.

Lynch, W. J. Cognitive retraining using microcomputer games and commercially available software. *Cognitive Rehabilitation* 1:1, 1983.

McDonald, E. T. *A Deep Test of Articulation*. Pittsburg: Stanwix House, 1964.

Miller, J. F., and Chapman, R. S. SALT: Systematic Analysis of Language Transcripts. A computer program developed on the Harris/5 computer, The Research Computing Facility, Waisman Center on Mental Retardation and Human Development, University of Wisconsin at Madison, 1982.

Mills, R. H. Microcomputerized auditory comprehension training. In R. H. Brookshire (Ed.), *Clinical Aphasiology, Conference Proceedings, 1982*. Minneapolis: BRK Publishers, 1982.

Mills, R. H., and Thomas, R. P. Microcomputerized language therapy for the aphasic patient. In *IEEE Proceedings of the Johns Hopkins First National Search for Applications of Personal Computing to Aid the Handicapped*. Los Angeles: IEEE Computer Society, 1981.

Porch, B.E. *Porch Index of Communicative Ability*. Palo Alto: Consulting Psychologists Press, 1967.

Rahimi, M. Prosthetic communication devices that learn and teach. In *IEEE Proceedings on Application of Personal Computing to Aid the Handicapped*. Long Beach: IEEE Computer Society, 1980.

Seron, X., Deloche, G., Moulard, G., and Rousselle, M. A computer-based therapy for the treatment of aphasic subjects with writing disorders. *Brain Lang.* 45:45–58, 1980.

Telage, K. M. A computer place-manner distinctive feature program for articulation analyses. *J. Speech Hear. Disord.* 45:481–494, 1980.

Willis, J., and Miller, M. *Computers for Everybody* (3rd ed.). Beaverton, Oregon: Dilithium Press, 1984.

Wilson, P. B. Software selection and use in language and cognitive retraining. *Cognitive Rehabilitation* 1:1, 1983.

8

Microcomputer Language Assessment, Intervention, and Enhancement

Mary Sweig Wilson and Bernard J. Fox

The microcomputer revolution has just begun to impact on the field of communication disorders. During the next decade, software that can deliver clinical services will become increasingly available. The task at hand is to determine how best to use microcomputers to provide language assessment and intervention. There is also a need to determine how best to use computers for the enhancement of oral and written communication. The intelligent use of microcomputer software requires careful analysis of every approach to the treatment of communication disorders. We must be prepared to rethink, and change, if necessary, the roles that speech-language pathologists will play in the future.

Evans' prophetic book, *The Micro Millennium* (1979), describes developments leading up to the computer revolution. Three phases are identified: the pioneering stage, the medium-term future, and the final phase. Evans predicted that the pioneering phase of the computer revolution would come to an end by 1982, and we would move into a phase of rapid consumer growth. During the final phase of the revolution, which Evans predicted will begin in 1991, the industrial era will come to an end, and society will change radically.

In terms of timing, his "guess-timate" of when the first phase would end was fairly accurate. It must be remembered that he made these predictions before personal computers were even being sold. By the beginning of 1984, most analysts and commentators agreed that we had moved into the second, or mass market, phase of the microcomputer revolution. During this second phase Evans predicted the decline of professions. Information and services currently provided by professionals could, according to Evans, be cheaply disseminated to the general public via computer. This is beginning to happen in communication disorders with the introduction of talking programs that provide language assessment, intervention, and enhancement (Fox and Wilson, 1983; Geiger, 1983; Mills, 1983; Wilson and Fox, 1982, 1983a, 1984). However, we do not believe that using microcomputers to deliver clinical services will cause our profession to decline; in fact, our profession will improve if we are willing to change our roles.

Developing effective software for language assessment and intervention is an important professional goal, but not an easy task. In addition, the education of people in the use of computer software is not inherently difficult. However, in a passage on educational philosophy Evans (1979) points out, ". . . no one, not even the most experienced and eminent teacher, the most knowledgeable educator or the most perceptive psychologist, has the faintest idea what the best methods of teaching are. We do not even know how human learning takes place, or what ensures that one thing is learned rather than another."

Today most educators would agree with Evans that there is still some mystery involved in teaching and learning. Had Evans made this statement in 1960, most educators would have violently disagreed. By the late 1950s most educators were feeling confident that they knew what to teach and how to teach it. The teaching machine and programmed texts exemplified this belief.

Neither the microcomputer revolution nor our current approaches to language intervention developed in a vacuum. Twenty-five years of educational software development on mainframe computers preceded the microcomputer revolution. Similarly, twenty-five years of revolutionary advances in linguistics and psycholinguistics undergird our current approaches to language intervention. We will trace developments in linguistics and psycholinguistics over the past quarter century before discussing the convergence of these two revolutions.

THE LINGUISTIC REVOLUTION

By the mid-1950s, American structuralism was the dominant linguistic theory, and behaviorism was dominant in psychology (Newmeyer, 1980). Structuralists prided themselves on being close to an accurate and complete description of language. Similarly, psychologists believed they could explain how we learn. Structuralists based their description on recordings of the sounds of a language. Phonetic analysis provided the basis for the description of the three rule levels: *phonology, morphology*, and *syntax*. Linguists at that time were in general agreement as to what one learned in acquiring a language—sounds, words, and then strings of words. Psychologists (Skinner, 1957; Staats and Staats, 1963) felt confident that behavioral principles could account for the learning of language. They described how parents, through reinforcement of successive approximations, trained children to talk.

Within the field of language disorders, approaches to remediation have relied on linguistics to determine *what* to teach and psychology to reveal *how* to teach. In the 1950s language delays were frequently characterized as speech delays (Van Riper, 1954), since both linguists and psychologists emphasized the importance of sounds. Approaches to intervention emphasized the importance of shaping as well as reinforcement.

Chomsky's proposal of a transformational, generative, grammatical approach to linguistic theory (1957) totally transformed the fields of linguistics, psycholinguistics, and, ultimately, communication disorders. Unlike the structuralists, syntax was viewed as central in transformational grammar. By the time Chomsky's second book, *Aspects of the Theory of Syntax* (1965), was published, structural approaches to linguistic analysis had fallen by the wayside. In the late 1960s and early 1970s, generative semantics emerged to challenge the tenets of standard-theory generative grammar, or, as it is now known, interpretive semantics. By 1980, Newmeyer (1980, p. 133), speaking of the fundamental hypotheses of generative semantics, said, "Today many of these hypotheses have no public adherents at all, and the term 'generative semantics' itself evokes nostalgia rather than partisan fervor."

The debates among psychologists were as heated as those among linguists. As was the case with structuralism in the field of linguistics, strict behavioral accounts of language acquisition were quickly laid to rest. Chomsky's critical review (1959) of Skinner's *Verbal Behavior* (1957) was never countered by an acceptable rebuttal. In 1965, Chomsky introduced the concepts of language competence and performance, the former being one's knowledge of the rules of language, and the latter being one's use of the rules in speaking and listening. Chomsky proposed that what a child had to acquire was a generative grammar that had both deep and surface structures. Linguistic universals, which are both species-specific and task-specific, guide language acquisition.

After strictly empirical accounts of language acquisition were dismissed, the emphasis in debates about language acquisition shifted. Behavioral challenges to Chomsky's account were replaced by those from cognitive psychologists who accepted Piaget's general account of language acquisition. The basic difference between these two approaches is that the cognitive, or Piagetian, position holds that the child brings species-specific information to the task of language acquisition, but nothing task-specific. The Chomskian position is that both cognitive and specifically linguistic universals are necessary to explain language acquisition.

A welcome proliferation of studies on the normal development of language accompanied the debates in linguistics and psycholinguistics. Simplistic behavioral explanations that described language as being learned through shaping and reinforcement were clearly insufficient to account for the acquisition of a generative grammar. This new research was important to the development of new approaches to treating language disorders (Crystal, Fletcher, and Garman, 1976; Hubbell, 1981; Leonard, 1984; Wiig and Semel, 1980; Wilson, 1977).

Our approach to the development of microcomputer courseware is based on our conception of how language is used for communication. Figure 8-1 depicts the components important to using language for communication. Language requires cognition: the speaker must have something to say (content), a way to say it (structure), and an appropriate context in which to deliver the message (function). The processes of perception and integration are also critical to the normal acquisition and use of language.

The structural component of language consists of rules governing the expression of meaning (semantics), choice of words (lexicon), ordering of elements (syntax), linguistic context (discourse), and finally sound production of a message (phonology). Whereas the rules of syntax govern the construction of sentences, the rules of discourse apply across sentences. For example, if someone asks, "Where are you going?" one could reply, "Home," or "I'm going home," but not, "I go home." A query in the present progressive requires a response in that mode if a verb is included in the reply. Similarly, if asked, "Where do you go after work?" one could correctly respond, "Home," or "I go home," but not, "I'm going home." Children with language disorders typically have problems in this area concomitant with problems with syntactic rules. These problems must be distinguished from those in the pragmatic realm.

Normally developing children in an adequate linguistic environment will induce the structures of the language. They will use them in pragmatically acceptable ways to extract and exchange content with other persons. Both linguistic and cognitive universals guide this induction. If the acquisition process is partially genetically determined, can we ever

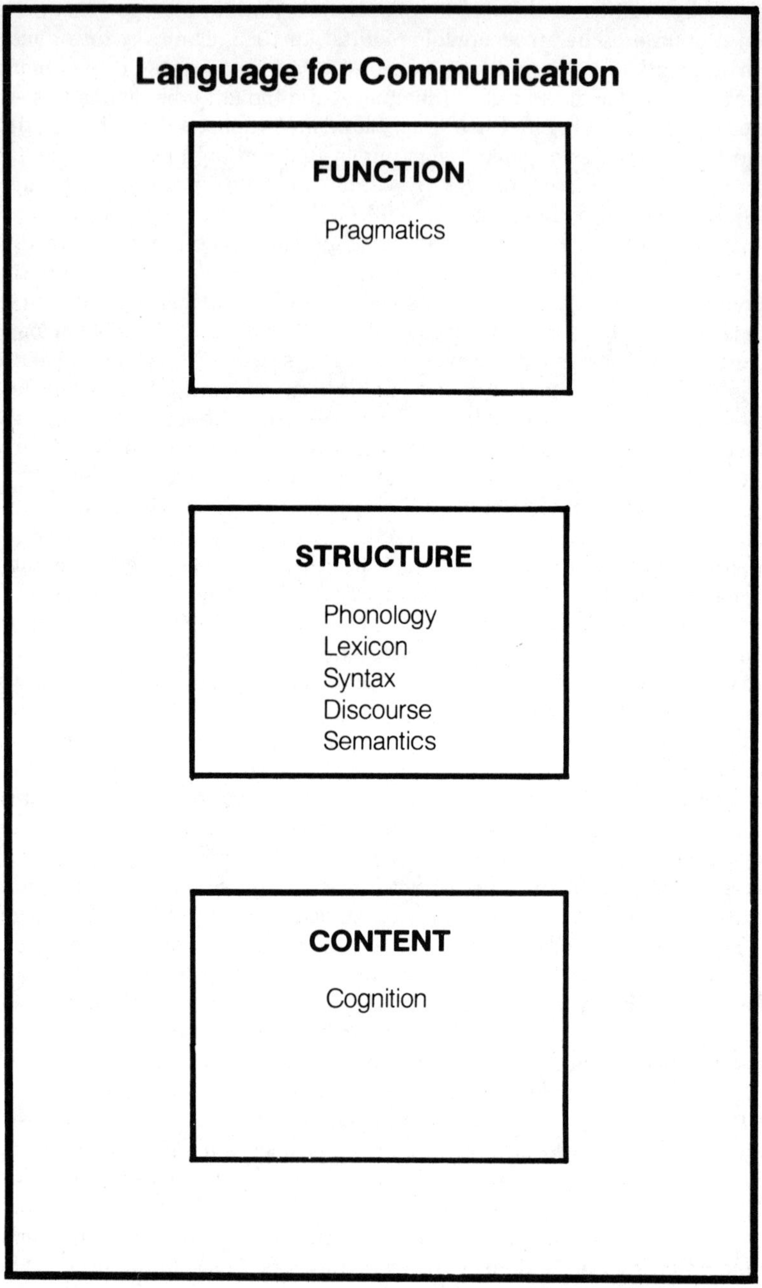

Fig. 8-1. The relationship between language function, structure, and content.

"teach" language to language-impaired children? If *teach* means systematically training a transformational grammar through successive approximation and reinforcement, then the answer is *no*. If, however, *teach* means to arrange the environment and the input to the child in such a way that the child is able to induce the concept, then the answer is *yes*.

APPLICATIONS OF MICROCOMPUTER TECHNOLOGY

Microcomputer technology can be applied in all areas of language assessment, intervention, and enhancement with children. Currently a significant amount of clinician time is spent in direct clinical-therapy service. This service area is the logical place for the microcomputer to augment effectiveness. As clinicians and authors of clinical materials begin seeing the microcomputer as a means through which to deliver services, a proliferation of alternative approaches to language assessment and instruction will begin. Just as clinicians now choose from a variety of print-media tests and intervention programs, clinicians will soon have these choices in microcomputer software programs.

The current inexpensive speech-generation units can produce speech of a quality that is adequate for receptive language assessment and intervention (Cater, 1983; Munro, 1982; Stoughton, 1983). To date we have developed, tested, and published language testing and training programs in both the lexical (Wilson and Fox, 1982) and syntactic (Wilson and Fox, 1980, 1983b, 1984) areas. We have also developed a program in the area of categorization (Wilson and Fox, 1983b) that cuts across lexical, semantic, and cognitive areas. Concepts, words, syntactic structures, and elements of discourse all lend themselves to computer applications given the current technology. In the future, better speech-recognition units will give us the capability to provide expressive language intervention.

One way of looking at the microcomputer in language assessment and intervention is as a trained clinical aide. This perception has been the usual response to our receptive software (Wilson, 1984). Certainly microcomputer software is providing the kind of receptive language testing and instruction that has typically been provided by humans with the assistance of print media (Semel, 1982; Wiig and Semel, 1980; Wilson, 1972, 1976). The microcomputer fulfills the role of a tireless clinical aide. However, the microcomputer can do much more than take over necessary repetitive tasks, as it can provide a different, yet complementary, aid to our own clinical services.

Children find microcomputers to be nonjudgmental and, hence, nonthreatening (Hagen, 1984). The children benefit from increased attention span, greater average time on task, improved sense of self-esteem, improved emotional response to learning, and an increased sense of accomplishment (Jenkins, 1983). Those who fear that children might become isolated quickly change their minds when they observe language-learning disabled youngsters proudly teaching peers how to operate a computer program. There are also cognitive and social advantages to having children work in pairs on computer programs (Dickson and Vareen, 1983). Playing cooperative and turn-taking games together at a microcomputer provides a setting in which the speech-language pathologist can easily work on pragmatic skills.

MICROCOMPUTER-ADMINISTERED ASSESSMENT

Computers have been used for both test construction and test administration. Schmidt, Urry, and Gugel (1978) reported that their adult subjects preferred computer-administered testing to live testing. In our first study, we found that both young and handicapped children preferred microcomputer to live testing (Fox, 1980; Fox and Wilson, 1981). This response was ascertained by having the children choose either live or microcomputerized testing following exposure to both methods.

Apparently, computer testing has a greater "comfort factor" than live testing. Anyone who has given a test on which the child reached "the guessing level" before making enough errors to terminate testing has a vivid appreciation of the discomfort experienced by both child and clinician in this situation. With older language-learning disabled children, we tell them the nature of the test so they will understand why we continue to press on past the point where both parties in the dyad know that the child is guessing. All dyadic communication expectations are removed in computer testing, and hence the entire procedure is less threatening.

Assessment is the first step in the remediation process. As more sophisticated microcomputer programs become available, the area of clinical assessment will be enriched. Many procedures that are deemed useful, such as free speech and linguistic and phonologic analysis, are not routinely done in school programs because they are too time-consuming. Today, programs such as *Lingquest 1* (Mordecai, Palin, and Palmer, 1982) and *Systematic Analysis of Language Transcriptions* (SALT) can be used to provide a linguistic analysis of a language sample entered through the microcomputer keyboard.

As voice-entry systems are improved, we will see the development of data collection combined with real-time analysis. This combination will radically change linguistic-analysis tasks. With real-time analysis and computerized data reporting, assessment strategies can be changed immediately. A report of inconsistencies in the area of verb usage, for example, could be followed by the introduction of certain tasks designed to target verbs. This can be done in a number of ways, for example, the child responds to computer-presented stimuli in various naming and description tasks. The computer could also analyze the child's utterances while he or she interacts with the clinician. This analysis would provide the clinician with immediate information on the child's use of language structure for communication. Very complex linguistic and pragmatic assessments would be possible in the same amount of time currently utilized to administer some diagnostic test battery.

Today, the main stumbling block to the development of sophisticated diagnostic tools is the lack of devices that recognize free speech. Instruments are currently available that can recognize voices and a small vocabulary from a number of different speakers. Tools are also available that can be trained to recognize unlimited sets of vocabulary items from an individual speaker who has gone through a training sequence. However, we do not have a computer that can interpret what a speaker has said.

Problems in developing free-speech analysis center around our limited understanding of language comprehension. We do not simply take an acoustic signal and analyze it to extract communicative content. Our processing of acoustic data in speech is a linguistic process that includes analysis using various rule levels. Limited speech analysis is a reality, although the better systems are still quite expensive. With today's technology, however, one could design a battery of diagnostic tests of expressive language wherein the computer presents pictures and sentences to which the child responds. The current microcomputer can be instructed to deal with the individual child's phonologic system before having to analyze responses to vocabulary, concept, and syntax testing.

LANGUAGE INTERVENTION WITH MICROCOMPUTERS

We have been using audible software with language-impaired children and adults since 1980. Delivery of receptive language instruction via computer has numerous advantages over live instruction. Some of these advantages are due to the machine's superiority in the rapid handling of numbers. For example, in the delivery of picture stimuli, randomization is easy for the computer. The computer can also collect data "invisibly" so the clinician no longer has to sneak out a pencil to record checks and minuses. Watching another human being record your cumulative failures is not a pleasant experience. Data collection has been something clinicians have accepted as part of instruction, but as human beings there is no easy way to do it on the spot without causing some client discomfort. Moreover, most clinicians have neither the time nor the facilities for data collection via the analysis of video tapes.

Other related advantages of computer instruction include consistency and focus on relevant stimuli (Lesgold, 1983). Learners can be aided by having the cuing standardized. In the human tutorial dyad, the instructor is, in many ways, a distraction. The clinician moves, makes sounds, dresses differently from day to day, and presents nonvocal feedback that can distract the learner from the task. The presence of a human instructor may lengthen the time the child spends figuring out to what to attend.

If receptive microcomputer software can do a more effective job of instructing in content areas, will clinicians be out of work when computers can listen as well as talk? The answer to that question depends on how professionals incorporate microcomputer technology into clinical service programs. There are many roles the computer cannot play in the lives of language-impaired children. Fortunately, it is these roles that most clinicians find challenging and exciting. Computers cannot advocate on behalf of language-learning disabled children. The school speech-language pathologist can aid a child with language-processing problems significantly by instructing regular educators and advocating on the child's behalf when behaviors are misunderstood. The speech-language pathologist can also play a significant role in helping the language-learning disabled cope with stressful pragmatic situations. This kind of personalized instruction provided to children, parents, and others is not likely, in the near future, to be assumed by computer software.

Microcomputer software is ideal for offering the extended number of stimulus presentations necessary for children with language disorders to induce a concept. For example, numerous studies have documented syntactic deficits in populations with mental retardation (Goda and Griffith, 1962; Graham and Graham, 1971; Lozar, Wepman, and Hass, 1972; Lyon, 1975). Whereas studies have shown lexicons to be commensurate with mental ages, this has not been the case with syntax. It remains to be proved whether this relationship is a special characteristic of the mentally retarded population or is related to the lack of continued training on syntactic rule induction.

Simulation software for modeling real-life situations aids efforts in rehabilitation. Children have the opportunity to practice their shopping skills, for example, before they go to the supermarket. A wide range of simulation activities can be created on the computer, and children can be provided with experiences they might not otherwise have. Software can be created that allows the child to "fly" over the United States, learning states, directions, and experiencing a sense of controlling "the ship."

LANGUAGE ENHANCEMENT WITH MICROCOMPUTERS

Microcomputers are capable not only of augmenting or increasing the power of communication, but also of contributing to qualitative enhancements or improvements. The most powerful written enhancement tools today are word-processor programs. During the past six years we have been using word-processing software with children who have language-learning disabilities. Word-processing software aids these children in producing good-quality written documents. For example, a teen-aged learning-disabled youngster announced for the first time that he wanted to put his written work up on the bulletin board. Using a pencil or pen, the child must encode each letter without cues. While this aspect of writing is not of concern to the accomplished writer, the learning-disabled child frequently experiences difficulty.

In addition to regular word processing with these youngsters, we have used audible software to generate written work (Fox and Wilson, 1983). This provides the children with a multisensory feedback and monitoring system. Children with severe writing disabilities find this especially useful. A fourth-grade girl with language-learning disabilities and motoric impairments delighted in using the audible program to write a sentence independently. At first she wrote, "Today I am going to work with a computer." She then expanded it to, "Today I am going to go to work with a computer." Finally she produced, "Today I am going to go to work with a people computer." When queried why it was a "people computer," she responded, "Because it talks." Her mother commented that that was the longest sentence she had ever seen her daughter generate!

The particular program the child used facilitated the production of her sentence partly because she could have the sentence spoken as she built it. Probably more important, however, was that she built this sentence not by typing the words letter by letter, but rather by choosing words by number from a dictionary listing displayed on the screen. She would first specify the beginning letter of the word she wanted and subsequently choose from the alphabetical listing on the screen. This process of generating written work is dramatically different from the total encoding process involved in using a pen or pencil.

The speech-language pathologist can be the advocate for language-learning disabled students to have access to word-processing software for alternative written output. These students should start benefiting as soon as possible from the use of word processing. The speech-language pathologist can also use this technology as the focus for language-experience approaches to reading that incorporate work on oral language. School-aged language-learning disabled children benefit from a coordinated approach to listening, speaking, reading, and writing.

Another augmentative use of the microcomputer is as an oral-communication device. The rehabilitation engineering approach to the development of augmentative communication devices was to design a machine that would perform certain functions and then build it. Devices developed in this manner are costly to manufacture and market because of the relatively small number of nonvocal clients who benefit from any particular device. With the advent of microcomputers, however, software programs can be developed that can be easily modified before committing to hardware design. In the future this approach will help bring down the cost of such dedicated devices.

Today's challenge to those committed to improvement of communication aids for nonvocal persons is to figure out how best to arrange linguistic data to increase speed and offer maximal spontaneity to the nonvocal person. As with speech recognition, these are nontrivial problems. No longer can we claim to be limited in the linguistic design of programs because of the media. When restricted to a direct-select board that has to fit on a wheelchair, communication designs are limited. Conceptually, memory size is no longer a consideration in linguistic design; the challenge is organizing and accessing the data base in the most effective and efficient manner.

One of our original designs for an augmentative communication system used a number of ways to speed the generation of a spontaneous sentence (Wilson and Fox, 1980). The program was designed to be operated by a single-switch user. Sentences were constructed by having the user first choose a word from the noun column. Depending on which noun was specified, only certain verbs were presented. Similarly, the noun phrase and the verb phrase were constrained to grammatically possible combinations. The program defaulted to the definite determiner, thus eliminating the necessity for choosing it. After the base sentence was generated, the user could specify the single-based transformation to be applied with the program defaulting to present the declarative form. The elements of this initial design were incorporated in two different software programs (Fox and Wilson, 1981; Hillinger, Fox, and Wilson, 1981.)

In 1980, when we began designing microcomputer-based augmentative communication systems, we used Mountain Computer *Supertalker*. This is a digitization or waveform-encoding unit. The human voice is sampled and stored in digitized form. This technique preserves the quality of human speech but uses up a lot of computer memory and takes more room to store on diskette. The highest digitization rate (4KB) produces the best speech quality. At this rate, however, only about 25 seconds of running speech can be stored on a single diskette.

We stopped using the *Supertalker* to develop the audible component for our software in 1981, when Street Electronics came out with the *Echo II* speech synthesizer. It uses a Texas Instruments speech processor chip. Since then the chip has been updated a number of times. The chip can produce different modes of speech. For the audible courseware used in language assessment and intervention we use custom-encoded speech. In this mode, a custom set of words and phrases are digitized and then encoded for a program. The process of data compression uses linear predictive coding (LPC). The LPC process compresses the data, thereby allowing it to be stored using less memory. Formulas are used to code data for storage and subsequently re-encode it for production. This mode of speech generation preserves vocal quality, but one is restricted to the encoded base. In the phoneme mode allophones are concatenated. This mode offers both flexibility and small memory demands. For comparison, the *Supertalker* at the highest digitization rate can use 3000 to 4000 bytes of memory per word, whereas the phoneme mode of the *Echo II* uses between 2 and 40 bytes per word (Munro, 1982).

Using inexpensive speech-generation units, speech-language pathologists can begin working on the design of augmentative communication systems.

We developed *Speak Up* (Fox and Wilson, 1983) for augmentative communication purposes. The program can be used to create words and phrases that subsequently can be included in an individually designed software program. Alternatively, the speech-language pathologist who does not program and does not have access to a programmer can use it in conjunction with the *Fast Access Scan Talker* (Fox and Wilson, 1985). FAST is a "shell program" in the sense that the data can be changed for a specific user. The program gives a single-switch user access to a maximum of 20 different individualized phrase files in memory. Each file can have 40 phrases, which are shown on the screen by two columns of words representing the phrases. The word and phrase editor on *Speak Up* can be used to build any phrase. An index builder is used to assign a word to represent the phrase. By building phrase files in forty-phrase units, the user has access to a large pre-established sentence base. The phrase generator on *Speak Up* can be used to generate spontaneous utterances. The user chooses from a dictionary either by specifying word number or choosing from an alphabetical listing on the screen.

Accessing pregenerated phrases as just described is relatively fast in terms of the units of information communicated in a minute. The limitation, of course, is lack of spontaneity. Spontaneous communication demands the ability to encode content using sentence structures with access to one's lexicon. A dictionary of 40,000 words can be stored on a hard disk, but how can the nonvocal person access this lexical data? Prediction formulas can be used after both letter selection and word selection, but no system yet devised comes close to the speed and flexibility of oral language. Today the barriers to the development of portable, flexible communication devices are no longer technical. Our challenge is to apply our knowledge to the design, development, and use of effective software.

REFERENCES

Cater, J. *Electronically Speaking: Computer Speech Generation.* Indianapolis: Sams, 1983.

Chomsky, N. *Syntactic Structures.* The Hague: Mouton, 1957.

Chomsky, N. Review of B. F. Skinner, verbal behavior. *Language* 35:26–57, 1959.

Chomsky, N. *Aspects of the Theory of Syntax.* Cambridge, Mass.: MIT Press, 1965.

Crystal, D., Fletcher, P., and Garman, M. *The Grammatical Analysis of Language Disability.* New York: Elsevier, 1976.

Dickson, W. P., and Vereen, M. A. Two students at one microcomputer. *Theory Into Practice* 22:296–300, 1983.

Evans, C. *The Micro Millennium.* New York: Viking, 1979.

Fox B. A study comparing live and computer-assisted receptive syntax items testing the prepositions in, on and under. University of Vermont Master's Thesis, 1980.

Fox, B., and Wilson, M. *Speak Up.* Burlington, Vt.: Laureate Learning Systems, 1983.

Fox, B., and Wilson, M. Microcomputer administered receptive language testing: A new alternative. Unpublished manuscript, 1981a.

Fox, B., and Wilson, M. Augmentative communication demonstration. Presented to the American Association on Mental Deficiency, Region 10 Convention, Montreal, Canada, 1981b.

Fox, B., and Wilson, M. *Fast Access Scan Talker.* Burlington, Vt.: Laureate Learning Systems, 1985.

Geiger, C. *Say It.* Syracuse: Schneier Communication Unit, Cerebral Palsy Center, 1983.

Goda, S. and Griffith, B. Spoken language of adolescent retardates and its relation to intelligence, age and anxiety. *Child Dev.* 33:489–498, 1962.

Graham, J., and Graham, L. Language behavior of the mentally retarded: Syntactic characteristics. *Am. J. Ment. Defic.* 75:623–629, 1971.

Hagan, D. *Microcomputer Resource Book for Special Education.* Reston, Va.: Reston Publishing Co., 1984.

Hillinger, M., Fox, B., and Wilson, M. Computer-enhanced communication systems for the Apple II. In *Proceedings of the Johns Hopkins First National Search for Applications of Personal Computing to Aid the Handicapped.* New York: IEEE Computer Society, 1981.

Hubbell, R. D. *Children's Language Disorders.* Englewood Cliffs, N.J.: Prentice-Hall, 1981.

Jenkins, Providing CAI for the mentally retarded. *Closing The Gap* 2:10, 1983.

Leonard, Normal language acquisition: Some recent findings and clinical implications. *Language Disorders in Children.* San Diego: College-Hill Press, 1984. Pp. 1–36.

Lesgold, A. M. When can computers make a difference? *Theory Into Practice* 22:247–252, 1983.

Lozar, B., Wepman, J., and Hass, W. Syntactic indices of language use of mentally retarded and normal children. *Lang. Speech* 16:1972.

Lyon, S. G. Transformational mastery and expressive vocabulary levels in mentally retarded children. University of Vermont Master's Thesis, 1975.

Mills, R. Microcomputerized Language Therapy Program, 1983.

Mordecai, C., Palin, M., and Palmer, C. *Lingquest 1: Language Sample Analysis*. Napa, Ca.: Lingquest Software, 1982.

Munro, A. An overview of speech synthesizers. *Softalk* May 1982.

Newmeyer, F. *Linguistic Theory in America*. New York: Academic Press, 1980.

Schmidt, F., Urry, V., and Gugel, J. Computer assisted tailored testing: Examines reactions and evaluations. *Educational and Psychological Measurement* 38:265–273, 1978.

Semel, E. *Language Intervention Activities*. Columbus: Charles E. Merrill Publishing Co., 1982.

Semel, E., and Wiig, E. *Clinical Language Intervention Programs*. Columbus: Charles E. Merrill, 1982.

Skinner, B. *Verbal Behavior*. New York: Appleton-Century-Crofts, 1957.

Staats, A., and Staats, C. *Complex Human Behavior*. New York: Holt, Rinehart and Winston, 1963.

Stoughton, A. M. Personal computers deliver speech aids to the handicapped. *Speech Technol.* 1:80–88, 1983.

Van Riper, C. *Speech Correction*. Englewood Cliffs, N.J.: Prentice-Hall, 1954.

Wiig, E., and Semel, E. *Language Assessment and Intervention*. Columbus: Charles E. Merrill, 1980.

Wilson, M. *Wilson Initial Syntax Program*. Cambridge, Mass.: Educators Publishing Service, 1972.

Wilson, M. *Wilson Expanded Syntax Program*. Cambridge Mass.: Educators Publishing Service, 1976.

Wilson, M. *Syntax Remediation*. Cambridge, Mass.: Educators Publishing Service, 1977.

Wilson, M. Microcomputers in communication disorders. Presented at the Annual Meeting of the South Carolina Speech-Language-Hearing Association, Hilton Head, S.C., 1984.

Wilson, M., and Fox, B. Computer managed language diagnosis and treatment. Scientific Exhibit, ASHA Convention, Detroit, 1980.

Wilson, M., and Fox, B. *First Words*. Burlington, Vt.: Laureate Learning Systems, 1982.

Wilson, M., and Fox, B. Microcomputers: A Clinical Aid. In H. Winitz (Ed.), *Treating Language Disorders*. Baltimore, Md.: University Park, 1983a. Pp. 235–248.

Wilson, M., and Fox, B. *First Categories*. Burlington, Vt.: Laureate Learning Systems, 1983b.

Wilson, M., and Fox, B. *Microcomputer Language Assessment and Development System*. Burlington, Vt.: Laureate Learning Systems, 1984.

9

Microcomputer Applications in Audiology

Brad A. Stach and James F. Jerger

For the past several years at the Neurosensory Center of the Baylor College of Medicine and The Methodist Hospital, Houston, Texas, we have been applying microcomputer technology to our audiology research laboratory and clinical service. Our applications range in scope from administrative tasks, such as report writing, to electrophysiologic and electroacoustic data collection, such as an acoustic reflex-averaging system. As we have begun to appreciate the immense power of this new technology and the extent to which it has increased our efficiency and productivity, we have also begun to understand the need to guard against the "technological imperative" approach to its application. That is, because the use of microcomputers has profoundly increased efficiency and productivity, there is a tendency to want to automate those tasks in the laboratory and clinic that either can be done as easily without a computer or should not be done by a computer at all. Certain aspects of patient testing and data collection are enhanced by microcomputer use, whereas other aspects are much more appropriately carried out by the audiologist.

NEW SURGE OF INTEREST IN COMPUTERS

Because microcomputers gained popularity so quickly, there is a tendency to think that audiologic applications are equally novel. Actually, little of what is being done with microcomputers today is new. Indeed, many of our current applications have been carried out with mini- and main-frame computers for years. For example, evoked-potential data collection was done with a computer in the late 1950s (Geisler, Frishkopf, and Rosenblith, 1958). Large computers were used for statistical analysis even earlier. Keeping patient records on computer has been suggested for over a decade (Elliot, Vegely, and Falvey, 1971). Almost since the birth of the programmable computer, researchers have tried to automate the testing of auditory thresholds (Brogan, 1956; Weiss, 1961). For the past several years, acoustic reflexes have been subjected to computer averaging (Jerger, Mauldin, and Lewis, 1977). Computers have also been used for speech audiometry for many years (Wittich, Wood, and Mahaffey, 1971). Clearly, the use of computers in audiology is not new. Why, then, has there been a sudden surge of interest in the application of microcomputers to audiology?

The most obvious reason for a resurgence of interest in computers is a financial one. Truly, this is a phenomenon that needs little explanation. A minicomputer system that costs $25,000 ten years ago has been scaled down to a microcomputer that costs one tenth the price. Perhaps equally important, however, is that the systems that can be bought today are so sophisticated that they are simple to program and use. Indeed, computer power costing one tenth of what it would have cost 10 years ago is also far more flexible and easier to use. The simple fact of affordability has created a situation wherein many facilities now have microcomputers that are in search of applications.

A less obvious reason for the new interest is that, because microcomputers are easy to use, many professionals with a background in programming secondary to an expertise in audiology are becoming involved in the development of microcomputer programs. The result is that programmers with a perspective on audiologic applications are designing and building systems. Some will argue that such a trend is leading to a decline in program elegance. While this is quite likely to be the case, what is traded for the price of this decline is the availability of programs that address real audiologic needs and that carefully blend appropriate use of automation with continued reliance on clinical judgment. Professional programmers have a tendency to see only the need to automate. They tend not to allow the user to bring to the process the experience and knowledge that are uniquely human and that contribute so much to the clinical evaluation of patients.

ADVANTAGES OF MICROCOMPUTER USE

In the research laboratory there are at least three major advantages to the use of microcomputers. First, since computers have storage capability, data can be collected on more patients. That is, storage of behavioral or electrophysiologic data during a measurement procedure results in less patient-contact time and allows more patients to be seen during the workday. Offline data analysis and printing of results can be done later, when time constraints are minimal. A second advantage to computer use is that data analysis is much more refined. For example, quantification of acoustic reflex waveform characteristics such as amplitude and latency can be made with much greater resolution by computer analysis than by analysis with a ruler and pencil. Refinement such as this leads, almost inexorably, to the discovery of subtle changes resulting from pathologic conditions that would otherwise remain unnoticed. Third, the number of parameters that can be evaluated efficiently has increased. For example, the spectral components of an evoked response, such as the 40-Hz potential, can be measured objectively, providing amplitude and phase information about a particular frequency component. The phase measurement, which is difficult to make with a visual detection technique, can be made very easily with a microcomputer. Use of microcomputer technology in the clinical audiology laboratory, then, results in more data being collected and analyzed in more ways with more refinement than ever before.

Benefits from the clinical use of microcomputers are also numerous. First, more patients can be seen in a given amount of time. This has the effect of either increasing patient case load or increasing noncontact time during the workday. A second benefit is that less professional time and effort are spent on clerical matters such as report writing and file maintenance. Automating the report-writing process and using a data-base management system reduce the amount of time necessary for such tasks. Additionally, the accuracy with which information is reported is increased by this process. Third, psychophysical paradigms and electrophysiologic measures previously considered too complex for routine clinical application can be automated to an extent that makes their administration clinically feasible. Thus, the number of procedures included in a battery of tests can be increased to include more sophisticated measurements. Finally, results can be subjected to complex analyses to determine their relationship to what might be expected from a patient in a given population—for example, a particular age and hearing-loss group. In this manner, the decision-making power of the professional is increased. Microcomputers in the clinic, then, can aid the audiologist by refining the nature of the tests used and by allowing more professional time for meeting patient-care needs.

PURE-TONE AUDIOMETRY

Early in the history of the programmable computer, researchers saw the potential for automating the psychophysical paradigms used for the measurement of auditory sensitivity (Brogan, 1956; Weiss, 1961). Since that time, on computers ranging from main-frame to micro, numerous attempts have been made to evaluate the efficacy of various computerized psychophysical procedures (Almqvist and Aursnes, 1978; Campbell, 1974; Cook and Creech, 1983; D. A. Harris, 1979a, 1979b; J. D. Harris, 1978, 1979, 1980; Hashimoto et al., 1977; Jerivall, Dryselius, and Arlinger, 1983; Mahaffey, 1975; Sakabe et al., 1975, 1978; Sparks, 1972; Wood, 1971; Wood et al., 1971, 1973a, 1973b). Today, such procedures are successfully applied for screening purposes in industrial and educational settings.

The use of microcomputers for mass screening is an excellent example of an appropriate computer application. It is certainly not that the typical "down-10, up-5" threshold-searching technique is so complex that it requires computer control. Rather, keeping records of large amounts of data and screening more than one person at a time are tasks that a computer can do especially well. As long as careful control over response inconsistency is maintained, the microcomputer is a very useful tool for screening purposes.

In contrast, the use of automated threshold measurement for routine clinical use is probably not an appropriate application. The computer still cannot perform pure-tone audiometry as efficiently and effectively as a human. Whereas the audiologist has developed judgment based on training and experience, the computer has only a finite set of structured rules on which to base its decision. Should all possible contingencies on which a response is judged as present or absent be truly definable, their inclusion in a computer program would probably render the program too slow to be useful. The same finely tuned judgment that allows the audiologist to obtain a reliable audiogram on a young adult with normal hearing in less time than a computer could also allows the audiologist to evaluate certain members of the geriatric population whose responses are delayed or inconsistent enough to be rejected by a structured, inflexible set of rules. Considering the differences between an industrial screening population and a typical clinical population, success with computerized techniques in the former case is hardly evidence for probable success in the latter.

One other area of interest related to pure-tone audiometry is the application of microcomputers to the problems of masking. Masking of the nontest ear during threshold-seeking procedures has been successfully programmed (Sparks, 1972; Wood, Wittich, and Mahaffey, 1973b). Perhaps a more appropriate use of the microcomputer in terms of masking is to aid the tester, on request, by determining an appropriate starting level for the masking procedure (Lehnhardt, Battmer, and Becker, 1980). Still more appropriate, however, is to use a microcomputer to teach students of audiology how to make such determinations for themselves (Hood and Zimmerman, 1981). In short, conventional pure-tone audiometry is still done better by a well-trained human than by computer.

THE AUDIOMETER

The audiometer has undergone significant change over the past few years as a result of microprocessor technology. One useful addition to the audiometer is the ability to communicate (interface) with a microcomputer. In many instances, the computer can receive information from the audiometer and can send information to the audiometer. An example of audiometer-to-computer communication is the automatic transfer of pure-tone threshold data from the audiometer to a data-base management system in the microcomputer. The values may be plotted on an audiogram by the computer and saved in an electronic file. Computer-to-audiometer communication may consist of a computer-controlled adaptive psychophysical procedure, whereby the computer changes the audiometer signal attenuation in a specified manner depending on the patient's response. This capability of audiometer-computer communication results in the potential for automating the audiology laboratory and clinic (e.g., Lehnhardt, Battmer, and Becker, 1980).

The audiometer-microcomputer paradigm is one approach to microcomputer use in the audiology clinic. The most important advantage of this approach is that it is maximally flexible. Appropriate manual testing can be carried out without alteration of existing hardware. The computer can be called on as needed for the tasks it does best—data storage, manipulation, and control of complex psychophysical rules.

There is, however, an alternative approach to microcomputer use in an audiology clinic. Instead of using a microcomputer as a supplement to a stand-alone hardware instrument, the microcomputer can become the audiometer (e.g., Sakabe et al., 1975). The computer in this case is used to generate signals (e.g., Polich, Fischer, and Starr, 1983; Wolf and Bilger, 1977), as well as attenuate, amplify, and direct them to the proper earphone. Testing is done either automatically or by manual control through the computer keyboard. Data are automatically stored in a data base and printed out in a report format. Although such an approach is quite possible and relatively inexpensive, it can be inflexible and difficult to use.

One can hope, however, that the future audiometer will appear as neither of the present alternatives, but as a combination of both. Evoked-potential instruments have changed over the years from totally hardware to mostly software systems. But the inflexibility of the all-software approach has become so glaringly apparent that many of the newest systems are returning to hardware switching or keyboard override capabilities. We can only hope that audiometer development will avoid this intermediate step. Instead, the new audiometer should not only use a microcomputer to its fullest potential for data acquisition, analysis, and storage, but also be designed with appropriate hardware switches and dials to allow the audiologist the flexibility necessary to meet patient needs adequately, appropriately, and efficiently, while measuring hearing.

OTHER PSYCHOPHYSICAL APPLICATIONS

Computers have also been used to automate other psychophysical procedures. These other uses fall into two categories: (1) those that represent refinements in existing clinical procedures, and (2) those that are not routine clinical procedures, but, because of their ease once automated, may become routine in the future. At least two traditional clinical procedures have been computer-automated. They are the alternate binaural loudness balance (ABLB) test (Fritze, 1978) and the tone-decay test (Sakabe, Hirai, and Itami, 1978). In the case of ABLB, the author concluded that the sensitivity of the measure could be increased by refining the analysis of the response with a computer technique. In addition to these refinements, other procedures that are not commonly used clinically have been automated with the computer and hold promise for future use. These include adaptive psychophysical procedures for measurement of various auditory phenomena (e.g., Levitt, 1978, 1980; Tyler, 1979, 1982), reaction-time measurement (Tyler, 1982; Wood, Goshorn, and Peters, 1974), and sound localization measurement (Gilman, Dirks, and Hunt, 1979; Thompson and Cortez, 1983). All these procedures have been shown to be quite useful in the laboratory but have failed to be adopted clinically. With the addition of microcomputers to the clinic, the feasibility of using these procedures routinely will increase substantially.

SPEECH AUDIOMETRY

Early application of microcomputers to speech audiometry involved simple control over signal presentation levels (Wittich, Wood, and Mahaffey, 1971; Wood, Wittich, and Mahaffey, 1971). With these early exceptions, little has been done with computers in this area. This is not surprising since the presentation and scoring of all speech audiometry procedures in routine use are simple enough to preclude any need for computer assistance. The area of speech audiometry, however, is on the verge of major changes in terms of microcomputer applications.

One major change is the application of adaptive psychophysical paradigms to speech audiometry (Dirks, Morgan, and Dubno, 1982; Stach and Jerger, 1982; Tecca and Binnie, 1982). An example of an adaptive speech audiometric algorithm is illustrated in Figure 9-1. For the particular procedure shown here, the patient is listening to PB (target) words in the presence of single-talker competition presented to the same ear. Presentation level of the PB-words is constant, and presentation level of the competition is varied depending on the patient's response. If, for example, the patient responds correctly to the target word *hot*, the level of competition is raised to make the task more difficult, and another word is presented. If that word is repeated correctly, the competition is raised again. If not,

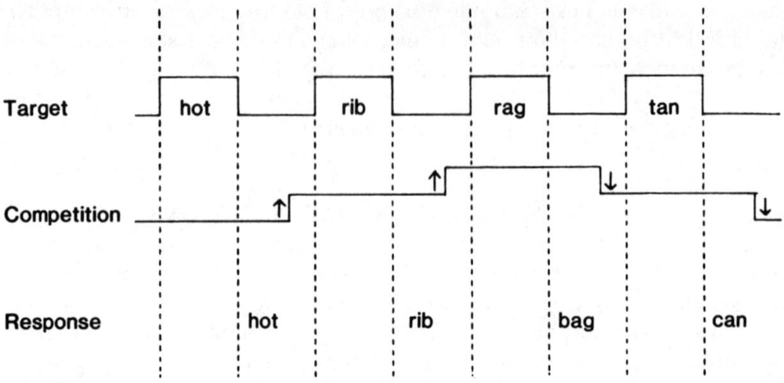

Fig. 9-1. An adaptive speech audiometry paradigm. PB (target) words are presented at a constant intensity level, and the single-talker competition level is increased after a correct response and decreased after an incorrect response.

then the presentation level of the competition is lowered to make the task easier. This procedure is continued until some specified criterion is met. For example, if a criterion of 50% is used, the competition level is varied up and down until a determination of the message-to-competition ratio (MCR) at which 50% of the words were repeated correctly is met. A sample of a search for this level is shown in Figure 9-2. Competition is increased after a correct response and decreased after an incorrect response. A *reversal* is specified as the level at which a correct response occurs following an incorrect response. The points of reversal are shown by the arrows in Figure 9-2. Testing is terminated after three reversals. In this example, the first two reversals occurred at −5 MCR (message at 70 and competition at 75 dB sound pressure level [SPL]), and the third reversal occurred at 0 MCR (message and competition at 70 dB SPL). The mean MCR, therefore, was −3.3 dB. This value is called the MCR 50, or the MCR at which the 50% criterion is reached, and can be plotted as a function of target SPL.

Figure 9-3 shows right- and left-ear functions for PB words from a 34-year-old patient with left acoustic neuroma. The shaded area represents normal limits. This patient had normal auditory thresholds and conventional PBmax scores of 100% for the right ear and 90% for the left ear. With an adaptive procedure, speech understanding was within the normal range for the right ear and grossly abnormal for the left. In addition to being sensitive to eighth-nerve disorder, the adaptive technique also appears to be more sensitive to the effects of cochlear hearing loss than traditional measures (Stach and Jerger, 1982).

The important point to be made about adaptive speech audiometry is that it lends itself well to microcomputer control. Although it can be done without computer assistance, it is tedious to control, simultaneously, signal presentation, competition attenuation, and response scoring. We have developed a microcomputer-based system for adaptive speech audiometry in which the level of the competition is controlled by a custom-built programmable attenuator, which is under software control. The tester sim-

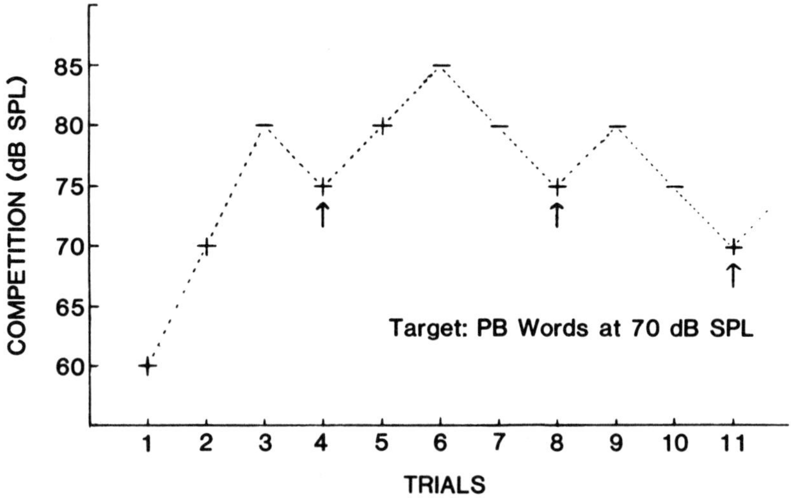

Fig. 9-2. An adaptive speech audiometry search procedure. PB words are presented at 70 dB sound pressure level. Single-talker competition is increased after a correct response (+) and decreased after an incorrect response (−). Arrow indicates a point of reversal, or the level at which a correct response occurs after an incorrect response. The procedure is terminated after three reversals.

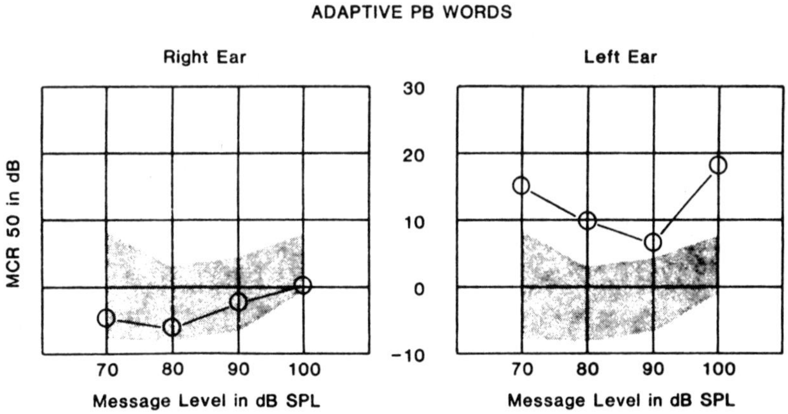

Fig. 9-3. Adaptive performance-intensity function from a 34-year-old patient with left acoustic neuroma. MCR 50 is an estimate of the level at which 50% of PB words are repeated correctly. Performance is inversely related to the MCR 50 decibel value. Shaded area represents normal limits.

ply decides if a response is correct or incorrect and the computer makes the decision about increasing or decreasing attenuation depending on a specified set of criteria. The MCR at which criterion is met is determined automatically. Such an automated procedure makes clinically feasible a complex psychophysical speech audiometry technique that had previously been restricted to the laboratory.

The other major change in the area of speech audiometry is that the tape recorder is being replaced by computer-synthesized or digitized speech (for an excellent discussion of this concept see Kamm et al., 1980; and Chapter 12). Many speech-synthesis devices are commercially available and are used for purposes ranging from cash registers that inform a customer of the outrageous price of eggs to devices designed specifically for augmentative communication. Many devices use different speech-synthesis algorithms, and the intelligibility of the speech produced by each can vary considerably (Chial, 1984).

For the past several years, we have been investigating the application of this technology to speech audiometry procedures. We find that there is a very clear trade-off involved in the decision regarding what type of computer-generated speech to use. On one hand, the microcomputer can be used as a digital tape recorder. That is, by means of an analog-to-digital (AD) converter, the analog voltage transduced by a microphone is converted to digital form and stored in memory in the computer. Then, by digital-to-analog (DA) conversion, the numbers stored in memory are translated to voltage, which can then be applied to an earphone or loudspeaker. Fidelity of the speech (and consequently intelligibility) depends on two factors: (1) the amplitude resolution of the AD and DA converters, and (2) the rate at which the AD and DA conversions are made. Assuming that an appropriate converter resolution is used, speech intelligibility will depend almost entirely on the digitization rate of the system. If, for example, speech was sampled at a rate of 16,000 per second, fidelity of the signal would be far greater than if it were sampled at 4000 per second. What this means is that using the digital tape-recorder approach requires a large amount of memory. If, for example, a sentence required three seconds of time and the digitization rate was 12,000 per second, then 36,000 bytes of memory would be required for one sentence. The digital tape-recorder approach, then, provides excellent computer-generated speech but at a considerable cost in memory.

The other approach is to use some type of synthesized speech. While not nearly as much memory is required, intelligibility of the speech produced is not so good. And, although synthesized speech is improving rapidly, it is still quite expensive to create a customized vocabulary. In the not-too-distant future, most of these trade-off problems will be solved. Synthesized speech will be highly intelligible and more affordable. Also, with bigger and better microprocessors conveniently available, memory will not be a concern, and the digital tape-recorder approach will be more practical.

There is one other approach that might be taken that would allow microcomputer control of speech presentation. Instead of computer-generated speech, the tape recorder may be replaced by the compact digital audio disk system that is rapidly gaining on the traditional "LP" audio market. This system is essentially a digitized approach to recording, except that the music or speech is saved on small disks and reproduced with a laser beam. Speech recorded in this way could be accessed by the computer, with proper computer-to-disk-system interface, in a programmed manner similar to computer-generated speech. The great advantage of this type of system is that it would require no computer memory to operate, yet it could be controlled by the computer to present speech segments in any order.

In our applications of the microcomputer to speech audiometry, we have developed a microcomputer-based system that uses the digitized speech approach. Speech is converted from AD and DA with an 8-bit converter at a rate of 12,500 per second. The PB words or sentences are saved on a rapid-access, 6-megabyte disk drive. We see the following as advantages to the use of computer-generated speech for speech audiometry purposes: (1) Control over stimulus presentation and interstimulus interval is simple and can easily be manual or automatic. (2) Repeating the presentation of a word or sentence is immeasurably easier by computer than by tape recorder. (3) Randomization of stimulus presentation is simplified by computer use. For example, the ten sentences of the Synthetic Sentence Identification test (SSI) need to be saved in memory only once. All scramblings can be generated randomly by the computer. (4) Speech in digital form can easily be altered in sophisticated ways. For example, speech materials can be time-compressed by the computer. (5) Use of computer-generated speech will (we hope) solve the problems associated with interlaboratory inconsistency of speech materials.

Clearly, microcomputers and speech audiometry are quite compatible. Not only are computers replacing tape recorders, but the methods of speech audiometry are expanding under computer control.

ACOUSTIC REFLEX MEASUREMENT

Immittance measurement devices, like audiometers, are currently based on the microprocessor. While perhaps more reliable and certainly more cosmetic technologically, their capabilities are quite similar in scope to their analog predecessors. Perhaps the most useful advance has been the addition of a serial interface that allows the device to communicate with a microcomputer for data storage or test-parameter manipulation.

For a number of years, our laboratory has been actively involved in computerized acoustic reflex averaging (e.g., Jerger and Hayes, 1983; Jerger, Mauldin, and Lewis, 1977; Stach, Jerger, and Jenkins, 1984). The initial work was carried out using a PDP-8 minicomputer. The procedure has since been adapted for microcomputer use (see Stach and Jerger, 1984, for a complete description). Briefly, an immittance probe is placed in each ear canal of a patient. The computer has been programmed to alternate signal presentation between the ipsilateral transducer of each probe. After the computer turns on a switch to present a signal to the left ear, it simultaneously measures immittance change from the probes in both ears. The signal is then presented to the right ear, and, again, immittance change from both ears is measured. The process is repeated eight times, and the reflex responses are signal-averaged. The result of this procedure is that all four possible reflexes—the right uncrossed, right crossed, left uncrossed, and left crossed—are averaged and stored in separate memory lo-

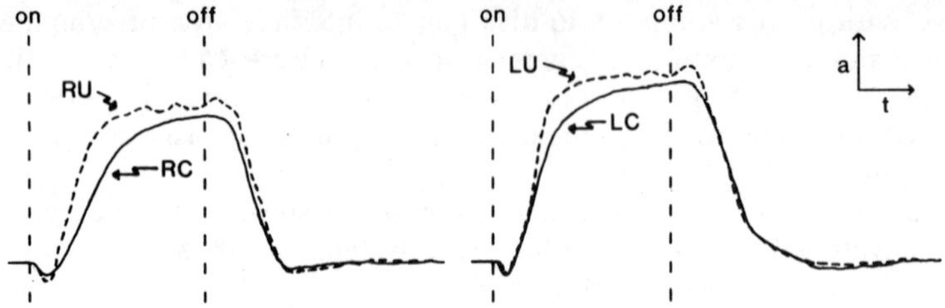

	Signal to Right Ear			Signal to Left Ear		
			Amplitude in dB			
Crossed		1.29			1.41	
Uncrossed		1.35			1.48	
			Latency in msec			
	20%	50%	80%	20%	50%	80%
Crossed Onset	100	144	226	86	134	194
Crossed Offset	840	738	666	862	758	642
Uncrossed Offset	886	752	672	860	756	650

Fig. 9-4. Signal-averaged acoustic reflexes from a subject with normal hearing. Signal averaging and measurement of amplitude and latency are controlled by an Apple microcomputer. Latency is expressed as time, in milliseconds, required to reach a percentage (20, 50, and 80) of reflex amplitude. Vertical dashed lines represent signal boundaries. Signal duration was 500 msec. Signal was a 2000-Hz sinusoid presented at 100 dB SPL. RU = right uncrossed; RC = right crossed; LU = left uncrossed; LC = left crossed; a = amplitude; t = time.

cations. These reflexes are then stored on disk for later analysis. Reflex waveform analysis is also computer controlled and consists of measures of amplitude and latency. Figure 9-4 is an example of normal reflexes, latency, and amplitude values obtained with this procedure.

Along with others (Bruschini et al., 1984; Gorga and Stelmachowicz, 1983; Hall, 1982; Yamane and Nomura, 1984), we have found computer averaging and suprathreshold reflex measurements to provide additional diagnostic information that would not have been obtainable by conventional methods. Quite aside from the diagnostic benefits, however, are advantages that a microcomputer brings to the entire process of reflex measurement. First, by using the computer to average signals, the amount of probe-tone filtering necessary for noise reduction is reduced. This allows the analysis of undistorted temporal characteristics of the reflex. Also, averaging reduces the equipment noise floor to such a degree that threshold detection is enhanced. Second, by using the computer for data storage, less actual testing time is required. It has been our experience that the time a patient must spend being evaluated by the reflex procedure has been reduced by half due to storing data on disk rather than printing or plotting results immediately after they have been collected. Third, by computer analysis of reflex results, the precision of analysis has increased. With this technique, latency resolution is 2 msec, and amplitude can be resolved to a hundredth of a decibel. Also, analysis can be done much more quickly and thoroughly by the computer.

By using a microcomputer for acoustic reflex measurement in the laboratory, we have been able to collect more data on a larger number of patients in less time and analyze those data in more ways with greater refinement than ever before. It seems reasonable to believe that microcomputer use for this purpose in a clinical setting would result in similar benefits.

EVOKED POTENTIALS

Use of an averaging computer for measuring auditory evoked potentials has a history dating back almost three decades. The first commercial evoked-potential units were available in the early 1960s. Like the audiometer, instruments for measuring evoked potentials have undergone great changes over the years. Today, most units take one of two forms: (1) a hardware averaging device to which a microcomputer is interfaced, or (2) a microcomputer-based averaging system with various degrees of external control of equipment parameters (e.g., Raviv et al., 1982).

There are several advantages to attaching a microcomputer to a signal averager.[1] Perhaps the single most useful application of microcomputers in this regard is for storage of averaged waveforms. Storage of results on disk for later analysis significantly reduces patient-contact time. Such time reduction is often critical when testing of sedated children is being carried out. Waveforms do not need to be plotted during testing. Instead, they can be saved on disk and printed out later when time constraints are minimal. And, of course, a reduction in patient-contact time allows for services to be provided to more patients in a given time period. Another benefit of adding a microcomputer to a stand-alone evoked-potential unit is that specialized data analysis, not available on the hardware unit, can be added easily. For example, spectral analysis of the high-rate, driven response (the so-called 40-Hz ERP) can be determined objectively with a fast Fourier transform (FFT) technique programmed to be used on a microcomputer. So, in addition to speeding up clinical testing, the microcomputer can also be used for sophisticated data analysis. One other advantage of such an arrangement is that all of the benefits accruing from the addition of a microcomputer to the system are achieved with no loss of flexibility inherent in a hardware averager. That is, the averager, with all of the externally controlled signal and measurement parameters that provide excellent flexibility for clinical use, remains essentially unaltered by the addition of a microcomputer.

The second type of system, the microcomputer-based averager, covers quite a range of hardware-software configurations. Our initial experience with microcomputer-based systems encompassed the range. On one end was a software averaging program written for a commercially available personal computer.[2] This program uses the microcomputer for signal

[1] We have interfaced a Nicolet 1170 averager to a Crommemco Z-2D microcomputer and a Nicolet CA-1000 to an Apple II.

[2] This program can be purchased from Dr. Glenn Thompson, Department of Otorhinolaryngology, Baylor College of Medicine, One Baylor Plaza, Houston, TX 77030. The program is written for the Apple II.

averaging, control of averaging epoch, number of sweeps, and for data storage, retrieval, and printing. All signal generation and control of physiologic amplifiers are external. Such an arrangement permits adequate flexibility while allowing appropriate use of the computer for rapid data acquisition, storage, and analysis. Because of limitations of microcomputer speed and power, however, the system does not permit more than single-channel recording or measurement at high stimulus rates. Still, for simple applications, it is quite adequate and is available at a substantially lower cost than most dedicated systems.

At the other end of the range are commercially available units that might best be described as dedicated evoked-response systems. The entire apparatus is under microcomputer control. Selection of earphone, stimulus rise-time, duration, intensity, and all other parameters is made from menus built into the software programs. Amplifier gain is set automatically, as is a delay to eliminate signal artifact. All scaling of results plotted on the cathode-ray tube (CRT) and subsequently printed is done automatically. Such systems represent perhaps the ultimate in automation of evoked-potential measurement. They are also among the most difficult and least flexible systems to use in the clinical situation.

Our experience with evoked-potential systems has greatly clarified, for us, the role of microcomputers in audiology and has confirmed our thoughts about the need for systems that blend the talents of the audiologist with the power of the computer. Certain aspects of evoked-potential systems seem to defy automation. Amplifier gain may be one. Scaling of the y axis of a plot on the CRT is another. Also, flexibility for efficient clinical use is enhanced by resisting the temptation to make all signal parameters menu-driven. There needs to be a blend of hardware dials and knobs with software switches and menus. Automation for the sole purpose of automation takes no account of the fact that one black box is not testing another. Purposeful inclusion of external parameter controls permits maximal use of those aspects of patient testing that require flexibility on the part of the audiologist. Fortunately, some manufacturers of evoked-potential systems have become aware of such criticism and have begun to move in the direction of balancing automated versus manual and hardware versus software considerations.

COCHLEAR IMPLANTS

Cochlear implants are gaining rapidly in sophistication and complexity. We have used a multichannel system that requires independent control of as many as 21 different electrodes.[3] The level of current necessary to reach the threshold of audibility and the maximum comfort level can be set independently for each electrode. A map of the current levels for the electrode array is created from these determinations and programmed into the implant processor. Table 9-1 is an example of the threshold and comfort current levels for each electrode in a typical map. Table 9-2 shows the minimum and maximum comfort levels for electrodes in another map.

[3]Implant and speech processor are manufactured by Nucleus Limited. A Sanyo microcomputer is used for interfacing.

Table 9-1. Electrical-current step levels necessary to reach threshold and comfort level for each of 20 electrodes in a cochlear-implant map.

Current	Electrode						
	1	2	3	4	5	6	7
Threshold	112	99	126	131	130	122	127
Comfort	147	157	175	159	190	167	200
	8	9	10	11	12	13	14
Threshold	131	127	127	125	122	124	120
Comfort	172	195	167	175	165	200	167
	15	16	17	18	19	20	
Threshold	121	99	113	113	109	121	
Comfort	185	165	165	165	159	195	

Table 9-2. Electrical-current step levels necessary to reach minimum and maximum comfort level (C.L.), and frequency range assigned to each electrode in a cochlear-implant map.

Electrode No.	Minimum C.L.	Maximum C.L.	f_2 Frequency Range (Hz)
20	122	152	0– 924
18	115	165	925–1066
16	101	165	1067–1238
14	122	167	1239–1442
12	124	165	1443–1662
10	129	167	1663–1928
8	133	172	1929–2226
6	124	167	2227–2572
4	132	159	2573–2979
2	101	157	2980–3450
1	113	147	3451–4000

f_2 = second formant.

Also shown are second-format (f_2) frequency ranges that are programmed to correspond to the various electrodes. When f_2 of an acoustic event falls within a certain range, the corresponding electrode will be stimulated.

The microcomputer has been invaluable for this multichannel implant application. It is especially useful for keeping records of the values contained in an implant map. Creating a map or changing a map can be done efficiently and accurately. Map values can be saved on disk and used as necessary. In addition to this important data-management role, the microcomputer can also be programmed to carry out complex psychophysical procedures for the evaluation of implant function. For example, a two-alternative, forced-choice paradigm has been programmed to measure the patients' ability to pitch-rank the electrodes.

The microcomputer has made clinical control of sophisticated multichannel cochlear implants feasible. Function of the implant can be as-

REPORT WORKSHEET

Date: 11/18/84 Exam: ___BA X DA ___PA ___HAC ___HAE

Name: Smith, Bob Age: 27 Sex: M

Address: 210 Cherry St. Phone: 666-2233

Referred by: J. Jones (on file) Tested by: Sallie Adams

Hospital File # 84736

RESULTS

Right Ear: N2, ARTABN, SPPBROL, ABRABN

Left Ear: N2, IMPNORM, ABRNORM

Comments and Recommendations: SITEVIII - right

A

Fig. 9-5. Sample report worksheet (A) and corresponding word-processed report (B). A label on the report worksheet is the name of a stock paragraph that is stored on disk and loaded into the report format. For example, ARTABN is the

sessed easily, and any necessary change can be made. Complex diagnostic and therapeutic paradigms can be controlled accurately. Instrument parameters and results from psychophysical procedures can be stored and analyzed efficiently. It seems likely that, as the technology of conventional hearing-aid systems increases, the microcomputer applications used so effectively with cochlear implants will extend into the realm of more traditional amplification.

November 18, 1984

J. J. Jones, M.D.
6565 Woodlawn Blvd
Suite 1222
Houston, Texas 77030

REPORT OF AUDIOMETRIC EVALUATION

NAME: Smith, Bob
ADDRESS: 210 Cherry Street
Houston, Texas 77025

AGE: 27
FILE#: 84736

Dear Dr. Jones:

We evaluated your patient, Bob Smith, on November 17, 1984. Audiometric results were as follows:

RIGHT EAR

*Normal sensitivity.
*The tympanogram is normal, but acoustic reflex thresholds are abnormally elevated.
*Speech audiometric results show significant rollover of the PI-PB function.
*Auditory brainstem response (ABR) audiometry shows abnormal responses to click stimuli. Both the absolute latency of Wave V and the I-V interwave interval are significantly prolonged.

LEFT EAR

*Normal sensitivity.
*Acoustic immittance measures indicate normal middle ear function.
*Auditory brainstem response (ABR) audiometry shows well-formed responses to click stimuli at normal absolute and interwave latencies over a stimulus rate range of 20 to 70 clicks per second and to both high intensity (80 dBnHL) and low intensity (60 dBnHL) click stimuli.

The overall pattern of results is most consistent with Eighth Nerve site on the right side.

Sincerely,

James F. Jerger, Ph.D.
Director of Audiology

Sallie Adams, M.S.
Audiologist

B

Fig. 9-5. (continued) name of the stored file that describes abnormal acoustic-reflex thresholds for the right ear in the final report.

REPORT WRITING

For several years we have taken advantage of the power of word-processing software and microcomputers by automating the report-writing task. We realized that nearly 95% of all reports written to referral sources by audiologists in our service comprised summary information and recommendations that could be contained in a relatively small number of stock paragraphs. That is, a small, finite number of descriptions of hearing sensitivity, speech audiometry, immittance measures, auditory brain-stem response results, and recommendations made up nearly all of the reports being written to referral sources. The advent of sophisticated word-processing software made it possible to store the descriptive paragraphs and recall them to an appropriate location in a standard report format.

Figure 9-5 shows an example of the form an audiologist fills out and the resultant report that is processed. The audiologist needs to note only the label for each test result and each recommendation. A stock sentence or paragraph, stored on disk under a short name, can then be loaded quickly and placed appropriately into the report. Commonly used referral-source names and addresses are also saved on disk and loaded into the report at the proper location within the format.

We have found several advantages to using microcomputers for report writing in this manner. First, the amount of professional time and effort spent on clerical matters has decreased substantially. Second, the turn-around time necessary for reporting results has also decreased because of the increased simplicity of the clerical task. Third, the overall quality and accuracy of the report-writing process has improved dramatically. Of course, there are still instances when the format will not be appropriate for a particular report. In that case, the report will need to be processed in a conventional manner. It has been our experience, however, that the flexibility of this approach minimizes such instances.

HEARING AID INVENTORY

Another administrative application of the microcomputer that we have found to be valuable in the clinical setting is the use of a data-base management system for hearing aid inventory. When the dispensing of hearing aids was initiated at our facility, there was little need for a sophisticated electronic file system to keep track of the small number of hearing aids dispensed. However, as the service grew, the number of hearing aids in stock, on loan, on order, and dispensed increased to a level where a simple paper filing system was no longer adequate. The application of data-base management software to inventory control of the hearing aid stock has increased the efficiency of the entire process.

Table 9-3 is a sample of the data kept on file for each hearing aid. All information deemed relevant for a particular aid is thus kept as one page in electronic storage. If the clinician wishes to know the disposition of a particular aid, information on the aid can be called up from the data base by model and serial number. If the clinician wishes to know the type of aid dispensed to a certain patient, the patient's name can be called up from the data base. The efficiency of such a technique becomes very obvious as the number of hearing aids increases.

One other important aspect of electronic inventory control is the simplicity with which administrative questions can be answered. For example, suppose that an administrator wanted to know the distribution of the various makes of hearing aids dispensed in a given year. A simple sorting and counting procedure can be carried out by the computer within minutes. The computer can even be instructed to plot and print the distribution. It is quite a simple matter to know how many of a certain type of hearing aid were dispensed, to know how many monaural or binaural fit-

Table 9-3. Sample of one "page" of an electronic filing system used for hearing-aid inventory.

Make model	Supertone A55
Make serial no.	Supertone AX1938722
Invoice no.	53491
Date rec.	05/23/84
Disposition	Sold 06/12/84
Case manager	Sallie Adams
Patient name	John Jones
Patient file no.	184-1234
Fitting	MON BTE UO/EM
Settings	G/10 VC3/4 MPO/120 FE/N CMP2/3
Warranty	06/12/84 to 06/12/85
Insurance	06/12/84 to 06/12/86
Repairs	Replaced gain control: 10/02/84

tings were recommended, or to get a breakdown of the ratio of aids tried to aids dispensed for a particular model. This type of sorting, which is quite tedious to do manually, is inherently easy to do with a microcomputer. The administrative efficiency and accuracy of such a system makes it well suited for a large hearing aid data base.

DECISION MAKING

One final application of the microcomputer is its use as an instrument to aid in the decision-making process. The microcomputer is excellent at remembering, comparing, sorting, and categorizing numbers. In the clinical setting, the clinician is often asked to do similar tasks with test results. In many instances these tasks are quite simple and require no microcomputer assistance. Placing a test result into a normal or abnormal category often requires no more than deciding whether it is larger or smaller than a well-known criterion. Using a microcomputer in such a case is unnecessary. There are instances, however, when the decision of normal or abnormal is based on a more complex interaction of test results that need to be compared to criteria that vary over age, across gender, or over signal intensity or frequency. In such a case, the computer's proficiency with numbers makes a cumbersome decision-making task much more efficient.

We have developed a computer algorithm for the determination of auditory brain-stem response (ABR) normality. This development was motivated by the desire to answer rationally such evasive questions as, "Is a wave I-V interval of 4.5 abnormal?" Table 9-4 shows the criteria used to categorize ABR latencies. Four latency measures are used: I-V interval, I-V ear difference, absolute wave V latency, and absolute wave V ear difference. The interpretation can fall into one of three categories: normal, questionable, or abnormal. The probability levels (0.05 and 0.01) are based on empirically determined means and standard deviations. The absolute wave V latency means are adjusted for peripheral sensitivity loss.

All comparisons and categorizations are automated. The clinician needs to supply the computer with only the wave V and wave I-V interval latency values. If wave I cannot be measured, interpretation will be made

Table 9-4. Auditory brain-stem response interpretation.

Measure	*Normal*			*Questionable*						*Abnormal*					
I-V interval	>0.05	CNE	<0.05		CNE	CNE	<0.01		<0.05		<0.05	<0.05	CNE	CNE	CNE
I-V ear difference	>0.05	CNE		<0.05	CNE	CNE		<0.01	<0.05	<0.05		<0.05	CNE	CNE	CNE
V latency	NA	>0.05			<0.05				<0.05	<0.05	<0.05		<0.01		<0.05
V ear difference	NA	>0.05				<0.05				<0.05	<0.05	<0.05		<0.01	<0.05

NA = not applicable; CNE = could not evaluate.

on the basis of wave V alone. Currently, the program evaluates results obtained only at a high stimulus level with no account taken of patient gender or age. The addition of these other factors, if found to be necessary for valid interpretation, could be added quite simply once appropriate means and standard deviations were determined.

To validate the interpretation paradigm, ABR latency values from 34 patients with confirmed acoustic neuromas and from 34 patients with cochlear hearing loss were evaluated. Of the patients with tumors, 2 (6%) were categorized as normal and 13 (38%) as abnormal. The remaining patients had no measurable wave V on the affected side and thus were considered abnormal with no interpretation necessary. Of the cochlear hearing-loss patients, 31 (91%) were classified as normal and 3 (9%) as questionable. From these results, we conclude that the interpretation paradigm used is a valid one for separating cochlear and retrocochlear hearing-loss groups.

The ABR interpretation program is just one example of the manner in which microcomputers can be used to aid in the decision-making process. The advantage of using a microcomputer for this application is not that it can interpret more accurately than a human, but that it can compare and classify results more efficiently on the basis of specified criteria that might change with patient or procedural variables. Quite simply, it can make a cumbersome interpretation task much easier.

FUTURE DIRECTIONS

The future of microcomputers in audiology is bright. Just as the vacuum tube made practical the reliable delivery of sounds to earphones, the microcomputer is making practical the rapid and complex manipulation of large amounts of information. It seems important to point out that neither the vacuum tube nor the microcomputer was, or is, inherently audiologic. That is, there is nothing about a microcomputer that has anything to do with audiology. It is the application of this microcomputer technology to audiologic problems that is of interest. And it is toward this end that we see microcomputers helping the audiologist to be more efficient and effective.

We envision the audiology test room to look different in the near future. At center stage will be a microcomputer, perhaps an off-the-shelf personal computer. Each room will have one, and each computer will be in a network that is linked to a common mass-storage device. Attached to each computer will be several modules. One will be what was formerly known as an audiometer, and, via computer keyboard command, will perform similar functions. The audiometer module will, of course, have appropriate knobs and dials used in combination with software switches. In one of the computer's expansion slots will be a board that contains all the PB word lists and synthetic sentences. The computer will be able to access these speech materials rapidly and in any order. Another module will contain the hardware for immittance measurements, including acoustic reflex averaging. Still another module will be used for evoked potentials. The audiologist will direct the functions of these modules as necessary. All results will be incorporated into a data base and saved in electronic storage. Reports will be processed immediately and will be waiting to be signed at the printer station. Much of the free time that will result from this increased efficiency will be used for meeting patient-care needs and, perhaps, reading professional journals.

Microcomputers will impact audiology in several important ways. They will permit more complex procedures to be used routinely. They will refine the measurement procedures in current use. They will aid the audiologist in the decision-making process. Most important, microcomputers will increase efficiency and thus increase time for patient care and professional growth.

REFERENCES

Almqvist, B., and Aursnes, J. Computerized pure tone audiometry. *Scand. Audiol.* [*Suppl.*] 8:193–196, 1978.

Brogan, F. S. An automatic audiometer for Air Force Classification Centers. *Noise Control* 2:58–59, 1956.

Bruschini, P., Sellari-Franceschini, S., Bartalena, L., Aghini-Lombardi, F., Mazzeo, S., and Martino, E. Acoustic reflex characteristics in hypo- and hyperthyroid patients. *Audiology* 23:38–45, 1984.

Campbell, R. A. Computer audiometry. *J. Speech Hear. Res.* 17:134–140, 1974.

Chial, M. R. Comparison of commercial speech synthesis systems for micros. Presented at the American Speech-Language-Hearing Foundation Conference, The Personal Computer as a Professional Tool. Las Vegas, February 1984.

Cook, G., and Creech, H. B. Reliability and validity of computer hearing tests. *Hearing Instruments* 34:10–13, 39, 1983.

Dirks, D. D., Morgan, D. E., and Dubno, J. R. A procedure for quantifying the effects of noise on speech recognition. *J. Speech Hear. Dis.* 47:114–123, 1982.

Elliot, L. L., Vegely, A. B., and Falvey, N. J. Description of a computer-oriented record-keeping system. *J. Am. Speech Hear. Assoc.* 13:435–443, 1971.

Fritze, W. A computer-controlled binaural balance test. *Acta Otolaryngol.* 86:89–92, 1978.

Geisler, C. D., Frishkopf, L. S., and Rosenblith, W. A. Extracranial responses to acoustic clicks in man. *Science* 128:1210–1211, 1958.

Gilman, S., Dirks, D. D., and Hunt, S. Measurement of head movement during auditory localization. *Behav. Res. Methods Instr.* 11:37–41, 1979.

Gorga, M. P., and Stelmachowicz, P. G. Temporal characteristics of the acoustic reflex. *Audiology* 22:120–127, 1983.

Hall, J. W. Quantification of the relationship between crossed and uncrossed acoustic reflex amplitudes. *Ear Hear.* 3:296–300, 1982.

Harris, D. A. Microprocessor versus self-recording audiometer in industry. *J. Audiol. Res.* 19:137–149, 1979a.

Harris, D. A. Microprocessor, self-recording and manual audiometry. *J. Audiol. Res.* 19:159–166, 1979b.

Harris, J. D. Proem to a quantum leap in audiometric data collection and management. *J. Audiol. Res.* 18:1–29, 1978.

Harris, J. D. Optimum threshold crossings and time-window validation in threshold pure-tone computerized audiometry. *J. Acoust. Soc. Am.* 66:1545–1547, 1979.

Harris, J. D. A comparison of computerized audiometry by ANSI, Bekesy fixed-frequency, and modified ISO procedures in an industrial hearing conservation program. *J. Audiol. Res.* 20:143–167, 1980.

Hashimoto, T., Murata, K., Minami, S., Taniguchi, I., and Katayama Y. Computer-aided group audiometry. *J. Audiol. Res.* 17:59–76, 1977.

Hood, R., and Zimmerman, H. Computerized audiometric programmable simulator. *Hear. Aid J.* 34:6, 20, 1981.

Jerger, J., and Hayes, D. Latency of the acoustic reflex. *Arch. Otolaryngol.* 109:1–5, 1983.

Jerger, J., Mauldin, L., and Lewis, N. Temporal summation of the acoustic reflex. *Audiology* 16:177–200, 1977.

Jerivall, L., Dryselius, H., and Arlinger, S. Comparison of manual and computer-controlled audiometry using identical procedures. *Scand. Audiol.* 12:209–213, 1983.

Kamm, C., Carterette, E. C., Morgan, D. E., and Dirks, D. D. Use of digitized speech materials in audiological research. *J. Speech Hear. Res.* 23:709–721, 1980.

Lehnhardt, E., Battmer, R. D., and Becker, D. Storage of audiometric data—online—with a small computer. *Arch. Otorhinolaryngol.* 226:199–206, 1980.

Levitt, H. Computer applications in audiology and rehabilitation of the hearing impaired. *J. Commun. Dis.* 13:471–481, 1980.

Mahaffey, R. B. The Measurement of Hearing by Computer. In S. Singh (Ed.), *Measurement Procedures in Speech, Hearing, and Language.* Baltimore: University Park Press, 1975.

Polich, J., Fischer, A., and Starr, A. A programmable multiple-tone generator. *Behav. Res. Methods Instr.* 15:39–41, 1983.

Raviv, G., Raviv, G., Weingarten, C. Z., and Lapin, G. D. A multipurpose microcomputer system in the physician's office. *J. Med. Systems* 6:329–334, 1982.

Sakabe, N., Hirai, Y., and Itami, E. Modification and application of the computerized automatic audiometer. *Scand. Audiol.* 7:105–109, 1978.

Sakabe, N., Ooki, T., Terai, E., Shinozaki, K., and Itami, E. A computerized automatic audiometer. *Scand. Audiol.* 4:75–81, 1975.

Sparks, D. W. The feasibility of computerized audiometry. *J. Audiol. Res.* 12:62–66, 1972.

Stach, B. A., and Jerger, J. F. Clinical experience with adaptive speech audiometry techniques. Presented at the Annual Convention of the American Speech-Language-Hearing Association. Toronto, November 1982.

Stach, B. A., and Jerger, J. F. Acoustic reflex averaging. *Ear Hear.* 5:289–293, 1984.

Stach, B. A., Jerger, J. F., and Jenkins, H. A. The human acoustic tensor tympani reflex: A case report. *Scand. Audiol.* In press, 1985.

Tecca, J. E., and Binnie, C. A. The application of an adaptive procedure to the California consonant test for hearing aid evaluation. *Ear Hear.* 3:72–76, 1982.

Thompson, G. C., and Cortez, A. M. The inability of squirrel monkey to localize sound after unilateral ablation of auditory cortex. *Behav. Brain Res.* 8:211–216, 1983.

Tyler, R. S. Measuring hearing loss in the future. *Br. J. Audiol.* 13:29–40, 1979.

Tyler, R. S. Minicomputers and the Assessment of Hearing Loss and Tinnitus. In J. Raviv (Ed.), *Uses of Computers in Aiding the Disabled.* Amsterdam: North-Holland Publishing Company, 1982.

Weiss, E. A Computing Automatic Audiometer for Testing Hearing Loss. In P. L. Frommer (Ed.), *Digest of 1961 International Conference on Medical Electronics.* New York: Institute of Electrical and Electronic Engineers, 1961.

Wittich, W. W., Wood, T. J., and Mahaffey, R. B. Computerized speech audiometric procedures. *J. Audiol. Res.* 11:335–344, 1971.

Wolf, R. V., and Bilger, R. C. A digital noise and sine-wave generator. *Behav. Res. Methods Instr.* 9:345–348, 1977.

Wood, T. J. A computerized audiometric system for the fail-detect monitoring and self calibration of frequency and hearing level. *J. Audiol. Res.* 11:325–334, 1971.

Wood, T. J., Goshorn, E., and Peters, R. W. Auditory reaction times as an index of functional hearing loss (abstract). *J. Acoust. Soc. Am.* 55:40, 1974.

Wood, T. J., Mahaffey, R. B., and Peters, R. W. A six-man computerized audiometer (abstract). *J. Acoust. Soc. Am.* 54:338, 1973a.

Wood, T. J., Wittich, W. W., and Mahaffey, R. B. An application of digital computer logic to pure-tone and speech audiometric procedures (abstract). *J. Acoust. Soc. Am.* 49:131, 1971.

Wood, T. J., Wittich, W. W., and Mahaffey, R. B. Computerized pure-tone audiometric procedures. *J. Speech Hear. Res.* 16:676–684, 1973b.

Yamane, M., and Nomura, Y. Analysis of stapedial reflex in neuromuscular disease. *ORL* 46:84–96, 1984.

10

Computer Technology in Hearing-Conservation Programs: Schools and Industry

David M. Lipscomb and Russell J. Fankhouser

Over a decade ago, a number of consulting firms and school systems had computerized at least some of their activities and records. There are two major reasons for the proliferation of interest in computer applications for industrial and school hearing-conservation programs. (1) Microchip technology has provided affordable and manageable computers for the relatively unsophisticated user engaged in hearing-conservation activities. (2) Individuals involved in this area are being forced into some form of mass data storage and analysis simply because of the sheer quantity of numbers with which they deal. Thus, the practitioner engaged in hearing conservation, either in the schools or in industry, is moving increasingly toward various computer applications to increase work efficiency and to provide requisite record keeping and documentation.

It may seem strange to see this topic combined for both industry and schools. Nevertheless, few elements in hearing-conservation programs differ for these two seemingly disparate settings. Both settings require identification of hearing-hazardous areas and conditions, both utilize alterations in processes and environments that are deemed hazardous, and both undertake identification audiometry for purposes of recognizing those persons with hearing conditions that exceed normal limits.

TYPES OF COMPUTERS

It will suffice in this chapter to discuss only a few types of computer. In fact, just three categories apply to this chapter, since the assumption is made that most readers will be interested in microcomputers rather than

The authors gratefully acknowledge the support and encouragement of Dr. W. T. Mathes, Dr. Arthur Harris, and Dr. James F. Wood, owners of Watauga Hearing Conservation, Inc.

Figures 10-3, 10-4, and 10-5 were printed using a Commodore 64 computer system linked to an Okidata 92 printer. This system was selected to demonstrate the versatility and applicability of even small systems.

A CPT 8525 was used to generate the materials shown in Figures 10-6, 10-7, 10-8, and 10-9.

The example form in Figure 10-3 was designed using the *Codewriter* software distributed by Dynatech Microsoftware, Inc., Niles, Ill. These figures were designed with the assistance of Ms. Deborah Arthur.

Spread-sheet software used to develop Figures 10-4 and 10-5 was *Omnicalc*, distributed by Human Engineered Software, Brisbane, Calif.

The hearing-protector selection program shown in Figure 10-9 was developed in association with Michael Seilo, Ph.D.

main-frame computers or minicomputers. The three categories are dedicated computers, restricted computers, and general-purpose computers.

Dedicated Computers

These devices are produced with a very restricted purpose in mind and, therefore, are unable to perform outside the limited range of functions for which they were designed. A digital watch is an example of a dedicated computer. In recent years, hearing conservationists have seen numerous dedicated computers enter their hardware armamentarium. Many digital sound-level meters are microchip-based units with the advantages of computerization, but with limitations in their range of capabilities and programmability.

One such meter is illustrated in Figure 10-1. This device is capable of measuring steady-state and impulse sound. Moreover, it contains microchip circuitry to integrate sound levels by sampling the sound pressure four times per second, combining each measure with those preceding. In 60 seconds, a time-weighted energy average is obtained. Such detailed and rapid integrative functions depend on computer technology.

Devices that measure and analyze sound are being integrated with more complex computer systems in order to expand and facilitate use of the inherent capabilities of the units. With the combination of ultraminiaturization and microchip technology, some very sophisticated but compact devices have been developed. The unit in Figure 10-1 easily fits into one's back pocket, even though a decade ago a device with the same capability would have required a van to move it about.

The introduction of digital devices into the field of sound measurement has been one of the truly remarkable recent improvements. With the use of some of these devices, one can take more sound measurements and conduct more thorough analyses in one day than all the people who have taken sound measures by hand during the entire history of sound measurement.

Another important dedicated computer now available to hearing conservationists is the microchip-based audiometer, as shown in Figure 10-2. Regarded as an "automatic audiometer" in a truer sense than the self-recording (Bekesy-type) audiometers of times past, microchip-based hearing-test apparatus is often programmed to conduct threshold audiometric measures and to recognize any of several subject-response problems and conditions. Some of these devices are capable of reporting hearing-test results to a central computer for additional analysis and printout. The range of abilities of these devices is quite large, but, at this writing, perfection in this realm is still a gleam in the eyes of equipment designers. Future units will indeed be both utilitarian and lower in cost than is currently the case.

Restricted Computers

Restricted computers are limited in their range of applications. Some small calculators are programmable, but they cannot accept preprogrammed software. Although some small calculators and so-called pocket computers do accept predeveloped software, their range of function, size of available memory, and input/output peripherals are so limited that they are inadequate for most purposes set forth in this chapter.

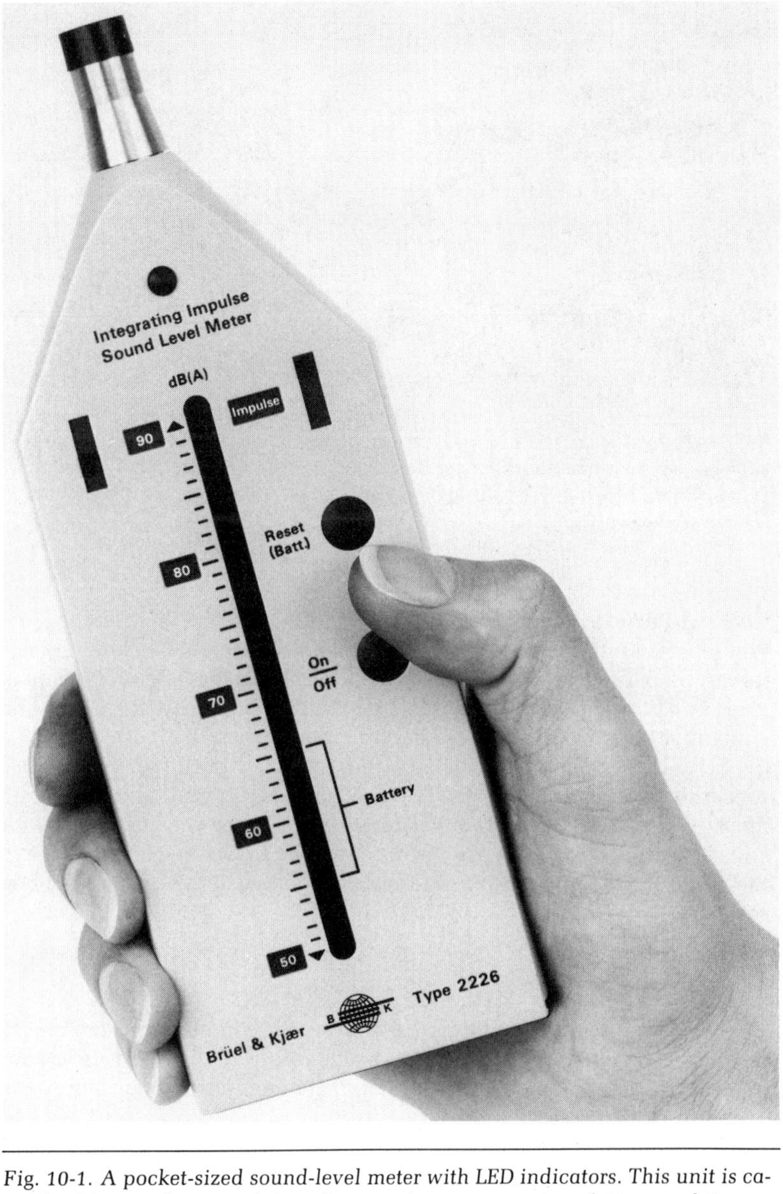

Fig. 10-1. A pocket-sized sound-level meter with LED indicators. This unit is capable of fast or slow speed, impulse sound measurement, and 60-second time-weighted energy-average determinations. Leq (60s). (Photograph courtesy of Brüel & Kjaer.)

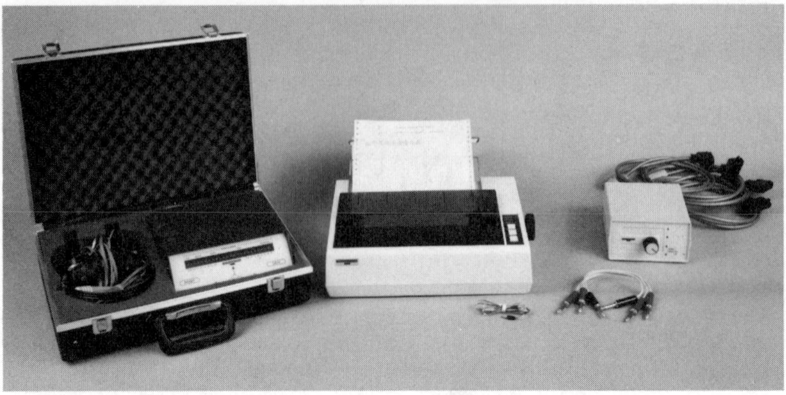

Fig. 10-2. Microchip technology has been applied to audiometric equipment such as this automatic audiometer. Nearly all adjustments commonly used in the conventional hearing-test paradigm are available in these devices. In essence, the audiometer tests the subject itself, leaving the operator free to take care of other duties during testing. (Photograph courtesy of Tracoustics, Inc.)

General-Purpose Computers

When a computer can be programmed, has considerable memory, is well served by peripheral input/output devices, and makes use of large quantities and types of software, it offers the type of flexibility that is most desirable for the purposes of this chapter. Some general-purpose computers are actually expanded dedicated computers. For example, some word-processing systems are convertible to data processing, but the efficiency is not always good. A true general-purpose computer can use both word- and data-processing software for the procedures we cite. Therefore, it is the general-purpose computers that are used in industrial and school settings.

TYPES OF LANGUAGES

The speed of program performance and ease of computer use are closely related to the level of computer language used. The three levels of computer languages are: machine, assembler, and high-level languages.

Machine Language

Because this language is in binary code, the computer can operate directly on the instructions issued. Nevertheless, humans find binary code (a series of ones and zeros) difficult to read and write (see Chap. 3).

Assembler Language

This system is based on a series of abbreviated instructions and commands (mnemonics) that can be used to program the unit. Again, the coding of these commands is complex and is used only by highly skilled programmers. This language requires some interpretation before the computer can act on it. The assembler language must be converted to binary for the computer to take action. Therefore, computer action based on assembler language instructions is slower than the same action based on binary instructions.

High-Level Languages

Such programming systems as BASIC (Beginners All-purpose Symbolic Instruction Code) provide much more easily understood commands for program preparation, but run slowly on the computer. These languages are even more distant in structure from binary and require two levels of interpretation: high-level language to assembler language, and then assembler language to binary. After computer action has taken place, the interpretation process must be repeated in order for the computer to communicate with the operator.

It is beyond the scope of this effort to discuss the many high-level languages currently available. However, mention will be made of a small number that are particularly useful in hearing-conservation programming applications.

BASIC

Far and away the most commonly used high-level language, BASIC offers relatively simple commands and understandable structure (often termed *syntax*). All or most of one's custom-written programs can be written effectively in BASIC.

LOGO

LOGO was developed by scientists at the Massachusetts Institute of Technology to meet the growing need for a structured approach to the introduction of programming techniques to children. It soon became obvious that the language was extremely powerful and was by no means to be restricted to children and early beginners. *Structured language* means that the parts of a program are developed in patches or modules. In fact, in LOGO, there are a very limited number of commands. The programmer actually constructs custom commands as a composite of the LOGO commands available. Integral with the LOGO language is a useful graphics mode called *turtle graphics*. (The name derives from the use of a "turtle," or indicator, which is directed around the screen by the programmer.) Very complex designs and illustrations are possible with this component of LOGO. For example, one can construct a command called *square* by combining those LOGO commands required to move the turtle in a path that outlines a square. Thereafter, the only command required to produce a square is the *square* command itself. This application of structured language offers considerable power and flexibility. LOGO is particularly useful when graphics are needed for a computer application.

PILOT

PILOT is a very simple, but limited, language developed for the preparation of instructional interactive programs. Thus, for certain teaching and informative functions, PILOT may be deemed useful. It is mentioned here for its possible use in interactive programs.

```
        ^XYZ MANUFACTURING COMPANY^

STS'DATA FOR .............................

      ^BASELINE^ ^LAST TEST^^DIFFERENCE^
      ^--------^ ^----------^^----------^

DATE   ../../.. DATE ../../..

^R^
^I^    2K ..#        2K ..#         2K ..#
^G^    3K ..#        3K ..#         3K ..#
^H^    4K ..#        4K ..#         4K ..#
^T^

^L^
^E^    2K ..#        2K ..#         2K ..#
^F^    3K ..#        3K ..#         3K ..#
^T^    4K ..#        4K ..#         4K ..#

   AVERAGE SHIFT = RIGHT ..#    LEFT ..#

PRINT FOR HARDCOPY : EXIT  P
```

A

MANIPULATION OF HEARING-TEST DATA

The number-crunching capabilities of computers are of great benefit in industrial and school hearing-conservation programs involving large numbers of personnel. This is particularly true when each data file contains complex matrices of information, such as data on serial audiometric tests. Computer programs are generally receptive to procedural changes, data interpretation and reinterpretation, and format modifications. Computers also provide rapid restructuring of file-keeping systems and facilitate the introduction of changes that might otherwise be rejected because of the turmoil involved in adapting to the changes. Corrections and modifications in computer formats are often effected with either overstrikes or reorganization of the instruction set. Essentially, the computer does not care about reorganization so long as its instructions agree with the format and syntax required by its construction and design.

Three general computer functions apply to the organization of hearing-conservation programs.

1. Massive amounts of data can be handled with microcomputers. There is no more need for volumes of forms, file drawers filled with individual health records, crowded offices overrun with charts, carbon paper, etc. Organization of data banks using computer capabilities is becoming the rule.

```
            XYZ MANUFACTURING COMPANY

 STS'DATA FOR SAMPLE'-'YURI'''''''''''''''

          BASELINE    LAST TEST   DIFFERENCE
          --------    ---------   ----------

 DATE  08/04/83 DATE 09/01/84

  R
  I      2K 15'       2K 20'         2K    5
  G      3K 25'       3K 40'         3K   15
  H      4K 40'       4K 55'         4K   15
  T

  L
  E      2K 10'       2K 15'         2K    5
  F      3K 20'       3K 35'         3K   15
  T      4K 35'       4K 45'         4K   10

   AVERAGE SHIFT = RIGHT 11.    LEFT  10

 PRINTING...
```

B

```
READY.

1 REM *PROGRAM NAME IS STS/T*
2 CLR:DF$="STS0/D":REM DATA FILE NAME
3 HF$="STS/X":REM HASH FILE
4 MS= 50 :REM *NUMBER OF RECORDS
5 KF= 1 :RS= 74
8 SF$="STS/S":REM SCREEN FILE
10 POKE808,237:GOSUB52210:GOSUB 33000
20 Y$=""
21 SS$="":FORI=1TO80:SS$=SS$+CHR$(160):NEXTI
22 SP$="":FORI=1TO39:SP$=SP$+CHR$(32):NEXT I
25 DT$="":FORI=1TO39:DT$=DT$+CHR$(46):NEXT I
30 PRINTCHR$(14)
35 REM
37 DIM F$(NF),G$(NF),DT%(12),GS%(NF+NC)
52 FOR I=1TO12:DT%(I)=31:NEXTI
54 DT%(2)=29:DT%(4)=30:DT%(6)=30:DT%(9)=30:DT%(11)=30
55 TT$="FINISHED WITH ENTRY? (RETURN=NO)"
70 OPEN2,8,2,"0:"+HF$+",L,"+CHR$(5)
71 INPUT#2,NR$:NR=VAL(NR$):INPUT#2.NXR$:INPUT#2.XFS$:INPUT#2,XFS$:CLOSE2
72 PO=1:IF ASC(NR$)=255 THEN PO=0
80 DIM CS%(NC):FORI=1TONC:READCS%(I):NEXTI
82 DATA 0.0.0.0.0.0,0.0
```

C

Fig. 10-3. An example form generated for record-keeping purposes. (A) The form was laid out on the terminal screen using a program-writing software system. (B) A printout of the form after data input. (C) A portion of the software-generated program listing.

2. Computerized information can help managers analyze effects of changes in procedures. Temporal alterations of program components—for example, conducting hearing tests during the spring rather than the fall season—can be assessed according to planning schedules and staff availability. This knowledge can be gained from studying computer data regarding the availability of staff, facilities, and equipment.
3. Policies can be updated by utilizing various forms of trend analysis currently available through computer-based programming. The spread sheet, for example, with its "what if?" application can be used to create numerous hypothetical conditions in order to evaluate effects of policy changes prior to their initiation.

HEARING-CONSERVATION BUSINESS SOFTWARE

A growing number of software packages are useful for the business side of hearing-conservation activity. Reviews of these software programs are available in many of the popular computing magazines.

Accounting Software

Such items as general ledger, accounts receivable, accounts payable, payroll, and tax preparation programs should not be disregarded if one is active in the hearing-conservation consulting and service business.

Word Processing

Word processing has become extremely popular for business applications. This facility is now found in many homes. It is an indispensable aid for correspondence, formatting forms, or preparing newsletters and reports.

Custom Programs

A recent advancement in software that has dramatic promise in hearing conservation allows one to lay out the format of a record form and, with appropriate instructions to the program, activate the unit to write a BASIC program that uses the new format. Formerly, a programmer had to write and develop a custom program to achieve the desired function. This new system uses software to generate other software. Figure 10-3 presents an illustration of a customized record form generated by *Codewriter*. By indicating those portions (fields) of the form to be input from the keyboard, those to be calculated by the program, and those to be global (accumulated from one form to another), a vast amount of flexibility in customizing business and data records is now available without the need to retain computer specialty personnel.

USE OF SPREAD SHEETS

Another important application allows one to construct complex tabular files called spread sheets. The spread sheet is organized in rows and columns with each coordinate point being called a cell. Cells contain either data or descriptions. All numerical data can be calculated according to standard arithmetic means, or data can be manipulated by custom equations. The strengths of such capabilities are evident. Most business-application software makes use of some form of spread sheet for con-

PUBLIC SCHOOL HEARING CONSERVATION RECORD --1985--

SCREENING RESULTS

SYSTEM: SCHOOL: TEACHER: GRADE: ROOM:

STUDENT NAME:	PURE TONE SCREENING 1000*		2000*		4000*		NUMBER OF FREQUENCIES FAILED		TYMPANOMETRY SCREENING*		FOLLOWUP CODE
	RIGHT	LEFT	RIGHT	LEFT	RIGHT	LEFT	RIGHT	LEFT	RIGHT	LEFT	
	Ø	Ø	Ø	Ø	Ø	Ø	Ø	Ø	Ø	Ø	
	Ø	Ø	Ø	Ø	Ø	Ø	Ø	Ø	Ø	Ø	
	Ø	Ø	Ø	Ø	Ø	Ø	Ø	Ø	Ø	Ø	
	Ø	Ø	Ø	Ø	Ø	Ø	Ø	Ø	Ø	Ø	
	Ø	Ø	Ø	Ø	Ø	Ø	Ø	Ø	Ø	Ø	
	Ø	Ø	Ø	Ø	Ø	Ø	Ø	Ø	Ø	Ø	
	Ø	Ø	Ø	Ø	Ø	Ø	Ø	Ø	Ø	Ø	
	Ø	Ø	Ø	Ø	Ø	Ø	Ø	Ø	Ø	Ø	
	Ø	Ø	Ø	Ø	Ø	Ø	Ø	Ø	Ø	Ø	
	Ø	Ø	Ø	Ø	Ø	Ø	Ø	Ø	Ø	Ø	
	Ø	Ø	Ø	Ø	Ø	Ø	Ø	Ø	Ø	Ø	
	Ø	Ø	Ø	Ø	Ø	Ø	Ø	Ø	Ø	Ø	
	Ø	Ø	Ø	Ø	Ø	Ø	Ø	Ø	Ø	Ø	
	Ø	Ø	Ø	Ø	Ø	Ø	Ø	Ø	Ø	Ø	
	Ø	Ø	Ø	Ø	Ø	Ø	Ø	Ø	Ø	Ø	
	Ø	Ø	Ø	Ø	Ø	Ø	Ø	Ø	Ø	Ø	
	Ø	Ø	Ø	Ø	Ø	Ø	Ø	Ø	Ø	Ø	
	Ø	Ø	Ø	Ø	Ø	Ø	Ø	Ø	Ø	Ø	
	Ø	Ø	Ø	Ø	Ø	Ø	Ø	Ø	Ø	Ø	
	Ø	Ø	Ø	Ø	Ø	Ø	Ø	Ø	Ø	Ø	
	Ø	Ø	Ø	Ø	Ø	Ø	Ø	Ø	Ø	Ø	
	Ø	Ø	Ø	Ø	Ø	Ø	Ø	Ø	Ø	Ø	
	Ø	Ø	Ø	Ø	Ø	Ø	Ø	Ø	Ø	Ø	
	Ø	Ø	Ø	Ø	Ø	Ø	Ø	Ø	Ø	Ø	
	Ø	Ø	Ø	Ø	Ø	Ø	Ø	Ø	Ø	Ø	
	Ø	Ø	Ø	Ø	Ø	Ø	Ø	Ø	Ø	Ø	
	Ø	Ø	Ø	Ø	Ø	Ø	Ø	Ø	Ø	Ø	
	Ø	Ø	Ø	Ø	Ø	Ø	Ø	Ø	Ø	Ø	
TOTALS:											

* Ø = PASSED TEST FREQUENCY
1 = FAILED TEST FREQUENCY

FOLLOWUP CODES:

A = AUDIOMETRIC REFERRAL
AC = AUDIOLOGY CONSULT
MD = MEDICAL REFERRAL
R3 = RETEST AFTER 3 MONTHS (TYMPANOMETRY)
RT = RETEST TYMPANOMETRY IN 1Ø-14 DAYS
SP = SPEECH PATH REFERRAL
O = OTHER

Fig. 10-4. Spread-sheet application for school hearing-conservation programs.

structing tabular summaries. Numerous spread-sheet programs are currently available. They can often be identified by the letters *calc* somewhere in the name of the program (e.g., *Visicalc, Supercalc, Omnicalc, Easycalc*).

Perhaps the greatest power provided by the spread sheet is the so-called *what if* function. In addition to holding real data, spread sheets can be injected with hypothetical figures in order to note the effect such numbers might have on the total of certain parts of the spread sheet. Thus, spread sheets allow hypothetical outcomes to be manipulated by specific data variations.

For the most part, the use of spread sheets in hearing conservation provides a useful means of displaying the results of some aspect of the program. The recording and analysis of expenses is one area that lends itself well to the spread-sheet approach. For example, by constructing a

SYSTEM: SCHOOL: TEACHER: GRADE:

	PURE TONE THRESHOLDS (HZ.)									
	250		500		1000		2000		3000	
STUDENT NAME:	RIGHT	LEFT	RIGHT	LEFT	RIGHT	LEFT	RIGHT	LEFT	RIGHT	LEFT
	0	0	0	0	0	0	0	0	0	0
	0	0	0	0	0	0	0	0	0	0
	0	0	0	0	0	0	0	0	0	0
	0	0	0	0	0	0	0	0	0	0
	0	0	0	0	0	0	0	0	0	0
	0	0	0	0	0	0	0	0	0	0
	0	0	0	0	0	0	0	0	0	0
	0	0	0	0	0	0	0	0	0	0
	0	0	0	0	0	0	0	0	0	0
	0	0	0	0	0	0	0	0	0	0
	0	0	0	0	0	0	0	0	0	0
	0	0	0	0	0	0	0	0	0	0
	0	0	0	0	0	0	0	0	0	0
	0	0	0	0	0	0	0	0	0	0
	0	0	0	0	0	0	0	0	0	0
	0	0	0	0	0	0	0	0	0	0
	0	0	0	0	0	0	0	0	0	0
	0	0	0	0	0	0	0	0	0	0
	0	0	0	0	0	0	0	0	0	0
	0	0	0	0	0	0	0	0	0	0

FOLLOWUP CODES:

A = AUDIOMETRIC REFERRAL
AC = AUDIOLOGY CONSULT
MD = MEDICAL REFERRAL
R3 = RETEST AFTER 3 MONTHS (TYMPANOMETRY)
RT = RETEST TYMPANOMETRY IN 10-14 DAYS
SP = SPEECH PATH REFERRAL
O = OTHER

Fig. 10-5. A spread sheet designed to provide follow-up information in a school screening program.

format that allows space for information on travel—such as date, destination, purpose, distance, and expenses such as meals, lodging, car, fares, tolls, and entertainment—one can generate detailed travel-expense information for tax purposes and for other financial analyses. Other useful applications of the spread sheet are the production of income summaries, activity plans, trend analysis, and data compilation. It is safe to say that one is limited only by the strength of one's imagination in the use of the spread sheet.

Figures 10-4 and 10-5 show examples of spread sheets. These figures illustrate two possible compilations of data for a school hearing-conservation program. Figure 10-4 shows a spread-sheet layout for the results of hearing-screening tests organized by classroom. A statistical aid is provided by the spread sheet in that the column totals are calculated automatically, so the number of failures is shown by ear and frequency or frequencies failed. A spread-sheet format for follow-up information, including hearing retest results and referral information, is shown in Figure 10-5. In both illustrations the cells contain zeros. This is to facilitate the insertion of data. Each cell must be defined as to the type of information

ROOM:

4000		6000		8000		3 FREQ. AVERAGE		4 FREQ. AVERAGE		
RIGHT	LEFT	RIGHT	LEFT	RIGHT	LEFT	RIGHT	LEFT	RIGHT	LEFT	FOLLOWUP CODE
0	0	0	0	0	0	0	0	0	0	
0	0	0	0	0	0	0	0	0	0	
0	0	0	0	0	0	0	0	0	0	
0	0	0	0	0	0	0	0	0	0	
0	0	0	0	0	0	0	0	0	0	
0	0	0	0	0	0	0	0	0	0	
0	0	0	0	0	0	0	0	0	0	
0	0	0	0	0	0	0	0	0	0	
0	0	0	0	0	0	0	0	0	0	
0	0	0	0	0	0	0	0	0	0	
0	0	0	0	0	0	0	0	0	0	
0	0	0	0	0	0	0	0	0	0	
0	0	0	0	0	0	0	0	0	0	
0	0	0	0	0	0	0	0	0	0	
0	0	0	0	0	0	0	0	0	0	
0	0	0	0	0	0	0	0	0	0	
0	0	0	0	0	0	0	0	0	0	
0	0	0	0	0	0	0	0	0	0	
0	0	0	0	0	0	0	0	0	0	
0	0	0	0	0	0	0	0	0	0	

to be inserted. Rather than having data input impeded by repetitive cell definition, the procedure can be done in the spread-sheet format. The software system automatically inserts zeros in cells that will eventually contain numerical data. These sample formats can be modified to suit the needs of each individual program, another indication of the value and versatility of spread sheets.

DATA-BASE MANAGEMENT

Nearly all information files can be called data bases. The concept is as old as the first filing cabinet—perhaps older, if one includes ancient demographics etched in stone. In general, a data base is simply systematized information, as explained in Chapter 4. Computer data-base management systems access stored information for any of several purposes. One common application is the organization and utilization of mailing lists. Mailings can be sent to different combinations of addresses, depending on the material contained in the data base and the sorting instructions used by the manager. For example, mailings can be organized according to zip code, state, city, name, or any other characteristic found in the data being accessed.

Data-base management systems are being produced by software-development firms in increasing numbers. Many of these programs have the letter *d* or the word *manager* in the name (e.g., *dBaseII* and *Knowledge Manager*). Some software packages now combine data-base management and spread sheets. This combination is useful because data can be accessed from, or inserted into, the spread-sheet format. With the advent of this capability, hearing-conservation records can be readily handled by data-base software.

The major limitation to data-base management has been restrictions in text use. Word-processing programs are now being integrated into data-base systems to provide the aggregate power of word processing, spread sheeting, and data-base management. Thus, hearing-test records can be stored along with appropriate demographic information on the student or worker. These data can be accessed, organized, manipulated, tabulated, and reported according to pre-established format instructions. For industrial applications, calculations required by the Occupational Health and Safety Administration (OSHA) are also possible. Ultimately, the display (report) processed by the data-base manager provides all pertinent data and calculations. It can summarize in written form those points cogent to the hearing condition of the student or worker.

The "search" capability of data-base programs is especially useful for hearing-conservation programs. Once the data have been stored and reports on individuals generated, data can be accessed again to provide statistical information. For example, data-base managers are capable of responding to inquiries for lists of persons whose hearing thresholds exceed a certain level (in decibels), lists of industrial personnel who were found to have a standard threshold shift, or lists of those whose noise exposure exceeded a certain level (in dBA). Thus, with the recently expanded power of data-base management, data on both individuals and groups can be readily obtained and displayed.

RECORD KEEPING BY COMPUTER

Not many people relish the opportunity to be directly involved in the voluminous record-keeping chores associated with school and industrial hearing-conservation programs. It is in this area that the computer shines, because, when properly organized and programmed, it essentially eliminates the mundane tasks of keeping records, thereby freeing professionals to discharge duties more fitting to their training and preparation. It must be clear that the approaches discussed previously derive from our experiences and do not constitute the only way to keep adequate records. The methods cited represent useful steps in reducing the load of paperwork for school and industrial programs.

Broad-Based Statistical Reports

Here, records are handled and reported in groups. The computer printout lists all workers in various areas of a plant or all students in a classroom. The listing includes pertinent information regarding hearing-test results, date of test, identification of the hearing-test technician, and equipment used. An obvious advantage of such data manipulation is the "single-glance" identification of the relative hearing conditions of persons cited in the report. Another notable advantage is the availability of summary statistics, such as the number of persons tested, proportion of the group whose hearing fell into various categories, and totals of those for whom there were specific recommendations for follow-up activities.

Individualized Reports

Figure 10-6 shows a sample printout for an industrial worker. Perhaps the greatest positive feature of this program is that a history of hearing-test data is available in a single place. Each year, the printout updates the hearing-test history so refiling of each hearing test is rendered unnecessary. Hearing-test printouts for all program participants can be organized in a binder as a single volume. Some hearing-conservation programs discard the old printouts when new annual tests are completed because the data are updated. Others retain the bound volumes of printouts labeled for each test year. From a programming standpoint, the computation of standard threshold shift (STS) is more easily accomplished by this method because data files generated for each individual are readily accessed by the program. Moreover, other information can be included on the printout to facilitate counseling and follow-up. An obvious drawback to this type of record keeping is that summary data for the group are more difficult to generate.

Both of the above record-keeping approaches have their strengths. We opted for the latter format because it summarizes individual data and because it allows a convenient means for providing a letter to each individual tested (Fig. 10-7). In the industrial setting, this form of communication is required for those found to have defective hearing. However, when letters are sent to all workers, there is less of a "singling-out" phenomenon that can influence worker morale. Moreover, individualized letters inform workers of their hearing-test results efficiently, and thus save considerable time for the personnel administering the hearing-conservation program. With appropriate modifications, a similar printout can be used for a school-based program.

The computerized hearing-test report form we developed consists of two parts. (1) The first page contains information for the program administrator. Although it is considered a confidential form only for the use of hearing-conservation program managers, it is available to the worker or student under the Freedom of Information Act. Therefore, care is exercised in the wording of notes on the printout. (2) Page two of the printout is a personalized letter outlining to the individual the results of the test in noninflammatory language. It also makes recommendations specific to test results.

Generally, a hearing-health history is taken for each participant in a hearing-conservation program. The question is whether to include those facts in the computer printout. If the program utilizes group-summary printouts, the decision will be made automatically by the printout format to exclude detailed information from individual histories. For the individualized printout, however, information from the history can be included. We prefer to keep the history information separate because it takes up a great deal of space on the printout, it consumes huge amounts of memory, the computer program is increased in size and complexity, and the time required to input data from the history raises the cost of providing com-

WATAUGA HEARING CONSERVATION, INC.
REPORT OF HEARING TEST INTERPRETATIONS

NAME: Sample, Ima IDENTIFICATION NUMBER: 000-00-0000 BIRTHDATE: 8/9/57

	RIGHT EAR							LEFT EAR						
	.5K	1K	2K	3K	4K	6K	8K	.5K	1K	2K	3K	4K	6K	8K
DATE: 9/3/80	5	10	10	5	15	15	10	5	10	10	5	10	15	20
DATE: 9/7/81	10	15	15	15	20	25	20	10	10	15	10	20	25	20
DATE: 9/5/82	10	20	20	25	25	25	20	10	15	15	25	25	30	20
SHIFT:	5	10	10	20	10	10	10	5	5	5	20	15	15	0

BRIEF SUMMARY OF THE MOST RECENT TEST:

A STANDARD THRESHOLD SHIFT HAS BEEN NOTED FOR THE RIGHT EAR.

A STANDARD THRESHOLD SHIFT HAS BEEN NOTED FOR THE LEFT EAR.

PERCENTAGE HEARING IMPAIRMENT:
RIGHT EAR: 0 % -- LEFT EAR 0 % -- BINAURAL: 0 %

INTERPRETATION OF MOST RECENT HEARING TEST

There is a mild high frequency hearing impairment.
The use of hearing protection is strongly advised.
NOTE -- There has been a shift from the baseline test of an average of 10 dB or more. If this is the first time a shift of this magnitude has been noted, be sure to concentrate on this worker. Whether the shift is due to work related noise or other causes, steps for prevention are advisable.

ADDITIONAL COMMENTS:

DATA REVIEWED BY:

Code 2
Code 4

Fig. 10-6. Computer printout of the hearing-test history of a hypothetical industrial worker. (See explanation in text.)

puterized readouts. Although we are not de-emphasizing the value of the history, we recommend that those records be kept separately and be updated as necessary.

The example printout in Figure 10-6 includes a number of features that provide worthwhile information to administrators of hearing-conservation programs. One apparent omission is that the printout does not contain

---

TO: Ima Sample

EMPLOYEE I.D. NUMBER : 000-00-0000

The hearing test you received is part of our comprehensive hearing conservation program. The purpose of this effort is to monitor your hearing from year to year and to recognize if there is any change. In the case of hearing disorders, as with many other physical problems, early identification is important.

For your most recent hearing test, the results can be summarized as follows:

The hearing test shows you have some reduction in hearing sensitivity. Use of hearing protection is mandatory while you are working in high noise areas. Although we have no control over your activities off the job, we strongly urge that you avoid excessive noise exposure then and use hearing protection if the noise cannot be avoided.

We have noted that your hearing has changed since your baseline hearing test. Since there are many causes resulting in hearing decrease, we suggest that if you haven't done so recently, you should consult an ear specialist (Otolaryngologist) to determine if there is a medical reason for the change.

We urge that you comply with these recommendations. If you have questions regarding this information, feel free to contact the Personnel Office.

Fig. 10-7. Continuation of the form shown in Fig. 10-6 illustrating an example letter to the worker after computerized analysis of the hearing evaluation.

any record of the audiometric equipment used or its calibration. This information, although necessary for compliance with federal guidelines, is redundant when placed on each printout form. Therefore, industries should keep information on audiometer calibration and use on file so each printout can be traced back to the equipment with which the test was conducted.

The Printout

Major components of the printout include the following:

HEARING-TEST HISTORY

By noting sequential (serial) hearing-test results, it is possible to spot trends in hearing-condition changes. The three annual hearing tests shown in the sample (Fig. 10-6) reveal the development of a progressively greater hearing impairment.

THRESHOLD SHIFT

Negative numbers indicate an improvement in the most recent test as compared to the base-line test. This information gives a valuable indication about the direction of changes in hearing. It is not uncommon to note with newly established hearing-conservation programs that the first annual retest results show many persons with "improved" hearing. In all likelihood, the hearing has not changed; rather, the contaminating influence of temporary threshold shift (TTS) has been reduced or eliminated. Moreover, it can be determined at a glance the extent to which a person's hearing has worsened and the frequency range in which the downward trend is taking place.

NOTIFICATION OF STANDARD THRESHOLD SHIFT

If the most recent hearing-test results show hearing has worsened by an average of 10 dB or more for the frequencies 2, 3, and 4 kHz, a statement will appear under the audiometric test results indicating that STS was noted for the ear(s) involved.

PERCENTAGE OF HEARING IMPAIRMENT

The percentage of hearing impairment is added to the printout to indicate to the administrator of an industrial program the degree to which there is possible culpability. The method of calculation we have chosen is that recommended by the American Academy of Ophthalmology and Otolaryngology (1979).

STATEMENT OF HEARING-TEST INTERPRETATION

In the program we use, there are 11 possible types and magnitudes of hearing impairment plus a rating of normal. Although it was difficult to program the computer to make those determinations, the effort has proved to be worthwhile.

IDENTIFICATION OF REVIEWER

Each printout should be reviewed by a competent audiologist or physician. That person is identified, and space is provided for the reviewer to make additional comments.

EMPLOYEE-NOTICE CODES

Since the letter sent to the employee is not available in the file and since it would require excess paperwork to make copies of each letter, codes are used to indicate the contents of each letter. The program providing the printout in Figure 10-6 has four possible codes: code 1, normal hearing; code 2, some hearing impairment; code 3, medical referral; code 4, STS.

Although the example in Figure 10-6 illustrates hearing-test data and interpretations for an industrial hearing-conservation program, slight modifications make the printout appropriate for school programs as well, and the letter can be altered to be appropriate for notification of parents.

NOTIFICATION LETTER

Based on the data reviewed by the computer program, a letter is written to the employee (or parents of the student). Note that the example in Figure 10-7 uses general terminology to avoid upsetting the person, but is sufficiently specific to make appropriate recommendations.

EQUIPMENT RECORDS

Depending on the availability of programming assistance, since no software currently exists for this purpose, one may wish to computerize all equipment maintenance and calibration records. The federal guidelines for hearing-conservation programs in industry require annual checks of electronic audiometer calibration. Yearly calibration of sound-measuring equipment is also mandated in order to trace the equipment to the National Bureau of Standards. Regardless of the environment for hearing-conservation activity, it is good practice to have the equipment checked each year. A form for recording the pertinent information on the calibration can be generated using the *CodeWriter* program mentioned earlier.

REPORTING SOUND-MEASUREMENT RESULTS

Word processing offers assistance in generating reports of sound measurement and analysis. If the word-processing program has even limited graphic capability, data sheets can be enhanced by diagrams showing the floor plans of areas being assessed for noise level. One such diagram is shown in Figure 10-8. In subsequent years, repeated measures can be obtained using the diagram as a guide. Since it is already on the disk, the sketch does not need to be redrawn. It can be duplicated by the word-processing program. A blank version of the form in Figure 10-8 is stored in the computer system and is simply filled out each time data are entered into a report.

The body of sound-measurement reports contains numerous paragraphs that are either identical or quite similar from one report to another, since all follow the standardized method of reporting cited in ANSI S1.13-1976. Word processing avoids the need to type these sections repeatedly by allowing the automatic insertion of recurring passages, thus speeding up preparation time and reducing the possibility of errors.

FOLLOW-UP RECORDS

The use of spread sheets offers the potential for generating systematized accounts of follow-up activities. Often, recommendations are made for medical intervention, rehabilitative procedures, hearing-aid consideration, periodic retest, etc. Unfortunately, many such recommendations are not filed systematically. Thus, program directors do not have a convenient means of following up on recommendations. As shown earlier in Figure 10-5, recommendations can be cited in code on a spread sheet, and columns can be added for recording when appropriate follow-up action has been taken.

HEARING-PROTECTOR SELECTION

It has always been worthwhile to document the selection of hearing-protection devices used in hearing-conservation programs. More often than not, however, protectors are chosen on the basis of cost, availability, suggestion by sales personnel, impressions made in exhibit halls during a convention, or other spurious reasons. A number of methods have been advanced to quantify the match between hearing-protection devices and the environments in which they are being used. Of these, the noise reduction rating (NRR) has enjoyed considerable popularity of late. Conventional use of the NRR calls for subtracting 7 dB from the NRR rating when

Watauga Hearing Conservation, Inc. Page 10

Attachment 1 OCTAVE-BAND SOUND SURVEY FORM

Date: February 15, 1984

Instrument(s):
B & K 2209/1613/2226
M/Sonics db 301/306/352

Location: Main Building
Rear Shop/Finish Whse

By: R. Fankhouser

Notes:

* = personal dosimetry

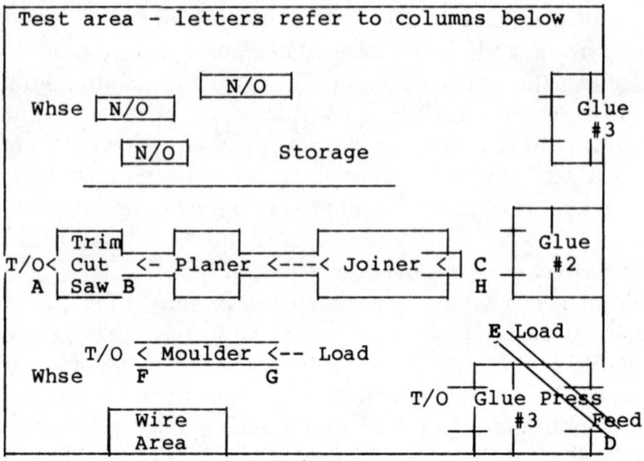

MEASURES TAKEN (in dB):

Center Frequency (hz)	A	B	C	D	E	F	G	H*	I	J	K
63	78	80	86	80	80	84	___	___	___	___	___
125	79	82	88	83	83	86	___	___	___	___	___
250	94	95	108	92	90	99	___	___	___	___	___
500	86	94	94	80	83	102	___	___	___	___	___
1000	80	87	87	86	76	100	___	___	___	___	___
2000	76/83	80	84/8	87	75	101	___	___	___	___	___
4000	76/82	80	82	72	72	93	___	___	___	___	___
8000	77	76	80	66/8	65	84	___	___	___	___	___
Lin	95	100	109	94.5	93	104	___	___	___	___	___
dBA	88	96	100	86	87	106	___	97/8	___	___	___
Leq(60)	90.5	96	101.4	___	___	104.6	___	___	___	___	___
L(osha)	90	96	101	86	88	105	87	98	___	___	___
L(max)	95	94	103	98	93	114	___	101	___	___	___
Impulse	___	97	104	___	___	116	92	___	___	___	___
Sample Time Min/Sec	14:30	5:40	19:25	12:14	7:22	8:30	10:01	18:29	___	___	___

Fig. 10-8. Data for use in reporting the results of sound measures taken in specific areas of an industrial plant.

matching a protective device to an environment whose measurement was in A-weighted dB values (dBA=NRR−7). This 7-dB adjustment was inserted in an effort to compensate for the fact that real-world hearing-protector performance does not equal the laboratory test data on which the NRR for each protector is based. At this writing, the U. S. Department of Labor is contemplating a policy of reducing NRR values by 50% across the board, further negating any value of the descriptor.

It is our belief that single-number attempts to determine the appropriateness of hearing-protection devices, though convenient, leave much to be desired in adequacy of selection. Now that computers are abundantly available, we advocate using their speed and versatility for this application. A program has been written to select hearing protectors appropriate to a given noise environment using a more defensible protocol than NRR. In Figure 10-9, a printout from the program lists those hearing-protection devices projected to allow no more than 80 dB in any octave band on the back side of the protector. The program takes into consideration specifications for a total of 30 protective devices. For each device, it adjusts the mean attenuation by two standard deviations (to increase the estimated success of the protector to nearly all personnel, 97.5%), then subtracts that "effective-attenuation" value from each appropriate octave band level. It then compares the estimated level at the ear with an 80-dB criterion. If any of the comparisons predict that the attenuated sound level will exceed 80 dB, the device is rejected, and the next device is evaluated by the program. When a hearing protector meets the criterion, its name is typed on the form.

This program offers two major advantages. (1) There is documentation that the protectors selected, if worn and used correctly, will be adequate for the environment into which they will be introduced. (2) There is documentation for purchasing agents that these protectors must be selected in order to achieve the purpose of the devices.

COMPUTER-ASSISTED INSTRUCTION

Training of Hearing-Test Technicians

The interactive abilities of computers fit nicely with the educational and training materials used for hearing-conservation purposes. Computerized resource, reference, and drill materials are useful as adjuncts in the training of industrial hearing-test technicians. It is anticipated that such training programs will soon be able to augment lectures and laboratory experiences with computer-assisted instruction techniques.

Actually, computer technology has been employed in audiometry training programs for several years. Hearing-impairment simulators allow an instructor to program an electronic device to respond during simulated testing as if it were a person with a predetermined hearing impairment. Use of these simulators is convenient, because hearing-test practice laboratories usually have students test each other. Most often, all the students have normal hearing, and no experience is gained in testing persons with hearing impairments. Granted, simulator use is not identical to testing a real person, but the recently improved quality of simulators and a wider

WATAUGA HEARING CONSERVATION, INC.

HEARING PROTECTOR SELECTION PROGRAM

This hearing protector use analysis was prepared specially for XYZ MANUFACTURING

Date of analysis: 2/19/84

Work location under consideration: MOULDER "F" LEVEL: 106 dBA

Octave-band levels at the work location:

FREQUENCY BAND:	125Hz	250Hz	500Hz	1000Hz	2000Hz	4000Hz	8000Hz
	86	99	102	100	101	93	84

The following named hearing protective devices have been found to allow no more than 80 dB at the ear. The procedure used in this analysis was to reduce the specified attenuation (noise reduction) for each protector by two standard deviations. This insures that the protector(s) named below can be expected to provide adequate protection for 97.5% of the workers in the area for which the octave-band levels were listed above. This assumes, of course, that the hearing protective device has been appropriately fitted to each ear and that it is worn properly.

AMERICAN OPTICAL 1720 EARMUFFS
BILSOM SOFT EAR PLUGS
BILSOM PER-FIT EAR PLUGS
BILSOM VIKING EARMUFFS
CESCO El-2 EAR INSERTS
DAVID CLARKE 10A EARMUFFS
E-A-R PLUGS
MINE SAFETY APPLIANCES MARK II EARMUFFS
MINE SAFETY APPLIANCES MARK IV EARMUFFS
MINE SAFETY APPLIANCES MARK V EARMUFFS
NORTON SILENT PARTNER
NORTON 4540 INDUSTRIAL EARMUFFS
NORTON 4530 SOUND-OFF EARMUFFS
NORTON COMFIT EAR PLUGS

There are 14 hearing protectors suitable for this work location:

The listed protectors are available from:

SAFECO - Kingsport, TN (246-4164)
- or -
Safety Equipment Distributing Co. - Knoxville, TN (584-8663)

Fig. 10-9. Example printout of a hearing-protector selection program. (See text for description.)

variety of programmable test-response parameters gives a real-world feel to the testing situation.

One of the requirements set forth by the Council on the Accreditation of Occupational Hearing Conservationists is that the instructional period be terminated by written and practical examinations. A written examination can easily be computerized to take advantage of the interactive and graphic features of microcomputers. Moreover, test results can be calculated and combined for statistical purposes.

Employee Education

A weakness in nearly all hearing-conservation programs is in the area of employee education. Various resources have been brought to this phase of some programs, including lectures, instructional films, video tapes, and demonstrations. Unfortunately, employee attention is often directed to other activities, such as dozing, flirting, or reading other materials.

An interactive educational program that uses graphics to hold the attention of workers while it instructs them is past due. With the proliferation of inexpensive microcomputers, this approach is both possible and economically feasible. The format of such a program can be structured according to the programmed learning paradigm. Instructive statements are followed by questions. When answers are incorrect, the passage is repeated with its significant part highlighted in order to clarify the concept being transmitted. At the end of the exercise, a printout can be provided to signify that the worker has successfully completed the instructional program, and a copy can be kept in the worker's file.

Although this approach has its limitations, it offers several advantages. (1) It provides a type of individual instruction. (2) It requires participation by the employee. (3) It documents that the program has been completed and thus satisfies the OSHA requirement for employee instruction. The topic areas of instructional programs can be varied each year so that the instructional activities will expand worker understanding of the hearing-conservation program.

School hearing-conservation programs can utilize similar programming techniques with appropriate modifications.

REFERENCES

American National Standards Institute. *American National Standard Methods for the Measurement of Sound Pressure Levels.* ANSI S1.13-1971 (Revised 1976).

American Academy of Otolaryngology Committee on Hearing and Equilibrium and American Council of Otolaryngology Committee on the Medical Aspects of Noise. Guide for the evaluation of hearing handicap. *J.A.M.A.* 241:2055–2059, 1979.

11

Computer-Assisted Instruction for the Hearing Impaired

Donald G. Sims and
E. William Clymer

Computer-based education (CBE) is the term used to describe the many educational applications in which the computer is directly or indirectly involved in the creation, delivery, evaluation, and management of instructional activities. Educators who specialize in CBE generally agree that there are two separate components, computer-assisted instruction (CAI) and computer-managed instruction (CMI). The difference between them is that CAI refers to the delivery of specific instructional content by a computer, whereas CMI refers to the application in which the computer is used to monitor and manage administrative aspects of an academic or clinical program.

COMPUTER-MANAGED INSTRUCTION

Software packages for CMI are specially designed data-base systems used for monitoring and controlling instructional and therapeutic activities. Most CMI systems provide a means of storing and retrieving information about student demographics and test data, and monitor progress toward specific instructional objectives. Microcomputer-based versions of mainframe-type CMI programs are being introduced so that smaller schools and agencies will be able to manage their programs better.

COMPUTER-ASSISTED INSTRUCTION

Computer-assisted instruction can be defined as an instructional system in which the computer is the primary means of delivering instruction, and in which the learner is an active participant in the learning process. Typically, the learner is required to make overt responses to statements, questions, and problems posed by the computer. Most CAI programs are able to evaluate a learner's response and alter the sequence of the instructional presentation accordingly.

Attributes of CAI

INDIVIDUALIZED INSTRUCTION

Computer-assisted instruction is individualized because it is intended to be used by one learner at a time, and the user controls the rate of presentation. The individualized nature of CAI is appealing to teachers because hearing-impaired students need an instructional system that is patient yet alert to the needs of the learner and can present information at an appropriate rate (Newell, Sims, and Clymer, 1984).

FEEDBACK AND BRANCHING

Good CAI provides feedback and adaptive instruction in a way that is not possible in a typical classroom setting. When feedback is used appropriately, each student (1) receives instant confirmation of performance (feedback), (2) is allowed to try alternative instructional paths for remedial or accelerated learning activities (branching), and (3) is coached in alternative problem-solving strategies if unsuccessful.

STUDENT RECORDS

A CAI lesson can be designed to keep an exact record of student responses to selected questions throughout the program. This permits detailed analysis of the effectiveness of a lesson and provides the instructor with information regarding the performance of an individual student or the entire class.

GRAPHICS

Programming languages and authoring systems give the CAI lesson designer the ability to produce high-quality visual displays that can bring about understanding that would not otherwise be feasible. The computer is capable of using color, graphics, animation, and alternative character sets to display information on the monitor. For example, at the National Technical Institute for the Deaf, special character sets have been developed to incorporate Webster's diacritical markings and selected phonetic symbols in communication lessons.

EXTERNAL DEVICES

A CAI lesson can also control external audiovisual devices. By controlling an audiocassette, videotape, or videodisk, it is possible to merge the power of CAI (feedback, branching, record keeping) with prerecorded communication events. This is particularly significant for communication training, as it would not otherwise be possible with computers.

Types of CAI Lesson Designs

DRILL AND PRACTICE

Drill and practice exercises are the most common type of CAI lesson. Generally, teachers use drill and practice to supplement classroom instruction for the habituation of some newly acquired skill. Drill and practice programs can randomize presentation of items and can control the degree of difficulty of the problems.

TUTORIAL LESSONS

Tutorial CAI designs are complete instructional modules that serve as the primary mode of instruction. Tutorial lessons provide the learner with all the elements of instruction—the objectives, the presentation of concepts, the drill and practice, and the subsequent analysis of performance.

GAMES

The tremendous popularity of videogames can be used to instructional advantage in the form of CAI lessons. According to Driskell and Dwyer (1984), videogames thoroughly engage the user because (1) they provide a quick-action activity that is competitive, challenging, and interesting to the player, (2) the players receive immediate feedback regarding performance, and (3) they involve fantasy. Examples of game-type CAI software can be found in commercially available math and language drill and practice lessons.

SIMULATIONS

Computerized simulations are an excellent way for learners to integrate new concepts and skills by applying them to life-like situations without penalty for exploration of a wide range of alternative responses. Simulation is used when the real-life situation is too costly or dangerous, too difficult to replicate repeatedly, or too sensitive an issue psychologically. The simulation develops a scenario that requires the learner to make a decision, enter it into the computer, and then witness the consequences of the decision.

Very effective simulations can be created by using external audiovisual devices, such as videotapes or videodisks. By using the presentation capabilities of the computer, it is possible to provide learners with very realistic simulations of communication situations (Sims, Scott, and Myers, 1982).

REVIEW OF CBE FOR THE HEARING IMPAIRED

Watson (1979) traced the history of CAI for the handicapped and the hearing impaired starting with several large mainframe-computer projects at Stanford, the National Technical Institute for the Deaf, Gallaudet College, the California School for the Deaf at Riverside, and other institutions funded by universities and private organizations. A common trait of each of these projects is that the subject matter of the CAI lessons was typically mathematics or English. Little, if any, of the specialized software developed for these mainframe projects has been adapted for use on microcomputers.

More recently, two conferences—The Conference of Educational Administrators Serving the Deaf and The Convention of American Instructors of the Deaf—were devoted to the use of microcomputers with the hearing impaired. The proceedings of these seminars are reported in the September 1982 and 1983 issues of the *American Annals of the Deaf*. These issues are a very useful resource for detailed descriptions from practitioners regarding their use of microcomputers with the hearing impaired.

The following review of CBE for the hearing-impaired learner is limited to instruction for communication training and does not include academic subjects or language.

Computer-Managed Instruction

SPEECH-LANGUAGE PATHOLOGY

Parrish and De Bold (1982) have used the *DB Master* data-base management software package to generate reports summarizing test results, instructional goals, and skills requiring carry-over activities. Similarly, Stoker (1983) devised a learning-management system that provides (1) a listing of current speech skills in profile form, and (2) a listing of the antecedent skills and proper order of instruction for the six most relevant speech subskills not currently being produced by the student.

SIGN LANGUAGE

Grossman, Siders, and Garraway (1983) developed a system for applying precision teaching principles to sign-language instruction. They input student speed and accuracy of expression and reception for a series of one-minute computer-managed tests. The computer provides the student with updated performance standards (for motion, placement, hand shape, and linguistic content), advises the student on study strategies, and completes a class profile for the instructor.

Computer-Assisted Instruction

SPEECH-LANGUAGE PATHOLOGY

Most CAI development for speech-language applications has centered on the application of various computer- or microprocessor-based visual or tactile sensory aids to replace the auditory feedback channel necessary for the development of speech. Rudimentary drill and practice exercises have been coupled with *mainframe* computers, which performed real-time signal analysis of speech. Parameters such as pitch and intensity over time or spectrogram-like displays of the teacher's and the student's speech have been used (Boothroyd et al., 1975; Nickerson and Stevens, 1980).

The English scientists Fallside, Guilian, Hinds, and Keiller (1983) reported using a *microcomputer* as a visible speech and timing aid for correct production of fricatives and the voicing distinction over a 6-month training period.

Nickerson et al. (1983) and Braeges and Houde (1982) state that more information is needed regarding the relationship between the physical measures of speech and intelligible speech so that training objectives can be set. In this regard, Osberger et al. (1981) recommended that computer-assisted speech training not concentrate initially on prosodic aspects of production, as this may *not* improve intelligibility.

From their considerable experience, Nickerson et al. (1983) suggest the following functional capabilities for visible sensory-aid speech-training devices of the future: (1) Continuous real-time and freeze-frame capture of 2 seconds of speech should be displayed as (a) an amplitude envelope, (b) format frequencies, (c) nasalization, or (d) a spectrogram. (2) Display options should be measurable with cursors. (3) Digital record, playback, and editing should be done easily at the student's station. Prerecorded segments of natural speech should also be available for target comparisons.

In a different approach, Osberger et al. (1981) found qualified success with digitizing and storing a deaf child's personal best utterance of vowel targets. She used this as a template for the computer to judge subsequent productions by the child as appropriate. Preliminary results with this system resulted in a greatly increased number of target phoneme productions by the client during the therapy sessions and an apparent improvement in the average proportion of intelligible vowel productions from 73% to 93%.

REHABILITATIVE AUDIOLOGY

CAI for auditory training could conceivably be accomplished with low-cost speech-synthesis equipment for microcomputers. In theory, the courseware could generate an infinite variety of artificial speech stimuli for evaluation and training. However, speech synthesis has not yet found widespread use for clinical activities with hearing-impaired persons.

Mills and Thomas (1983) report a five-program set designed for evaluation/treatment of auditory comprehension/memory impairments in language-impaired adults and children. Color graphic representations of objects and color chips are coupled with speech synthesizer output for drill and practice sequences. There is extensive control of the stimulus presentation parameters and the collection of response data, including reaction time.

With regard to lipreading, Hight (1982) designed a software package that converts typed sentences into graphic, animated mouth movements. His *Lip-Reader Trainer* package uses idealized and stylized mouth shapes that represent each of 18 visually identifiable phonemes. Easy-to-use programs were developed for the teacher to generate lipreading exercises and obtain records of student responses. Students control the speed of animation and select answers from a multiple-choice answer format. Software control of a Votrax speech synthesizer is an option. No data have been reported to date as to the accuracy and naturalness of the graphic representations, or whether training results in improved lipreading skills.

Saunders, Hill, and Easley (1979) initiated the development of a computer-assisted speech-perception training program for profoundly deaf children. They used a prototype 20-channel electrotactile sensory aid and the *PLATO* mainframe time-share CAI system. The natural speech stimuli for training were prerecorded on a random-access magnetic disk and then converted to touch patterns by the "tickle belt" tactile display worn on the child's abdomen. The CAI lessons required students to listen to single words while viewing a graphic image depicting the word. Students touched the screen in one of two places to hear the item again or to continue. A two-item choice was then presented in a similar way. Then previously learned words were embedded in short sentences and students used a four-choice response format to select the target word used in the sentence. Ten hours of training were needed to discriminate basic phonemic features. Common words, consisting of a few dozen items presented in isolation, were learned in a comparable period of time (Saunders, Hill, and Easley, 1979). However, Saunders et al. also say "the process . . . of learning fluent comprehension of ongoing speech is much more difficult and is . . . equivalent to the learning of a new language."

TELECOMMUNICATION

Glaser (1982) and Pflaum (1982) report successful interfacing of microcomputers to teletype devices for the deaf (TDD) such that the hearing-impaired person can use a personal computer for communication with the Baudot code TDDs or the American Standard Code for Information Interchange code to access online computer information services and electronic mail. This type of computer-assisted communication has been used successfully between deaf students to improve written-language skills.

SOFTWARE: PURCHASE OR DEVELOPMENT

Before the decision is made to create or to purchase any CAI materials, it is wise to analyze the instructional problem being encountered and to formulate specific educational goals.

Instructional Development

An academic specialty known as instructional development (ID) (Dick and Carey, 1978; Diamond, 1975; Mager, 1979) offers educators systematic development procedures for the acquisition or creation of instructional materials. Kearsley (1978) and Fletcher (1974) describe how instructional development techniques can be used to manage the development of CAI specifically for the hearing impaired.

The first step in any ID process must be to gather information about the learners and the information and skills they are to acquire.

Student Characteristics

Student demographic information should be obtained, such as grade level, handicapping condition, age, social and intellectual development, and attitudinal characteristics. By combining this information with the likes and dislikes of students, it is possible to obtain a "picture" of the typical student that can be very useful in the creation of instructional materials.

For example, Harding and Tidball (1982), in a national survey of microcomputer hardware and software used in schools for the hearing impaired, found that respondents expressed the need for adaptation of existing CAI software to the needs of the deaf student. Because of restricted English reading and writing skills, the hearing-impaired student's CAI lessons must be carefully written to avoid complex grammatical structures and unfamiliar vocabulary. (See Shulman and Decker, 1980, for a description of adaptation methods.)

Objectives

Well-thought-out instructional objectives take the mystery out of the entire instructional development process because they indicate exactly what is to be learned and how the learner will demonstrate competency after finishing the instruction.

Media Selection

By considering the characteristics of learners and by carefully determining precisely what the learner should be able to do after completing instruction, it is possible to decide what medium is best able to deliver instruction.

Mager (1979) indicates that media selection should depend on two criteria.

1. *Learning.* The medium should be appropriate for the content presented. "It should demonstrate the desired performance, prepare the student to practice, and provide both feedback and practice."
2. *Administrative.* The medium selected should be the "simplest, cheapest, readily available that will get the job done."

Gagne, Wager, and Rojas (1981) caution that CAI may be appropriate only for certain categories of learning outcomes. They believe that CAI may be useful for verbal information, concrete and defined concepts, rules, and problem-solving outcomes. These types of learning outcomes are frequently found in communication-training activities.

When it is determined that CAI is an appropriate instructional medium for a particular situation, it is wise to review existing commercial software to determine whether it is appropriate for the established objectives. It is very expensive to create software when just a few hours of searching for existing software can result in a tremendous savings. Lathrap and Goodson (1983) describe procedures for searching for, acquiring, and storing educational software.

Hagan (1984) lists over 200 distributors and producers of software for special-education applications. She reviews specific software packages for use with specific handicaps, such as deafness and blindness, describes more than 20 different authoring systems for use with microcomputers, and lists several sources of special input/output microcomputer devices for the handicapped. Hagan also offers several rules for acquiring software for use with special-education students. One rule that is particularly pertinent for the hearing impaired states that software does not have to say "handicapped" (deaf) on the label to be useful in special education. In other words, the teacher should judge the applicability of software packages for hearing-impaired students against specific objectives, and not rely on the advertising claims for the packages. LINC (1983) also lists software packages for use with disabled persons. The list is organized by handicapping condition.

Software packages should be purchased with the agreement that the buyer can return materials that are not appropriate for the target population. This is especially true for materials not originally designed for use with the deaf.

DEVELOPING CAI MATERIALS

In order to create CAI lessons, the nonprofessional CAI developer must acquire or compensate for two essential skills—computer programming and CAI lesson design.

Computer Programming

Several different levels of programming languages can be used to develop CAI lessons. Traditional programming languages such as BASIC or PASCAL are fairly sophisticated languages that can be intimidating for novice programmers. A disadvantage of using languages like BASIC is that they are primarily intended to manipulate numeric and mathematical information, and CAI lessons for the hearing impaired are generally language-oriented and do not require mathematical sophistication. They require instead a conversational dialogue between the user and the program. Authoring languages, such as Apple's Super PILOT (Huntington, 1983) offer an easier approach to writing CAI lessons. Authoring languages are simplified versions of programming languages containing predetermined programming routines that simplify the writing of text and the judging of responses, feedback, and branching. Using an authoring language facilitates the development of lessons; however, the trade-off for the ease of development is a reduction in flexibility. Zemke (1984) and Data Training (1983) describe the features of many of the available authoring languages for use with various microcomputers.

Authoring systems are even simpler to use than authoring languages because they are actually software programs in which entire structures of lessons are already programmed. The teacher simply inserts the content to be presented to the student. Typically, these systems are used for more routine drill and practice applications, primarily for math and language.

Slovick (1982) and Irwin (1982) created the *BLOCKS 82* authoring systems, which are designed to be used for CAI lesson development by teachers of the hearing impaired. In order to increase the utilization of visual aids in lessons, hundreds of different stock computer graphic images are included with the software system.

CAI Lesson Design

Gagne and Briggs (1974) and Alesandrini (1983) describe nine events that can be used in the development of individualized instruction. These nine instructional events are useful references when writing CAI lessons and are also a good checklist when evaluating existing software.

1. *Gain attention.* In order for a learner to be ready for the instruction, he or she must be aware that the lesson is about to begin and must attend to the display on the computer. Frequently, clever graphics that appeal to the learner's interests are used to gain attention. The attention-getting format should relate directly to the content to follow. However, attention-getting devices can become tedious after repeated viewings.
2. *Inform learner of objectives.* Frequently, teachers carefully compose instructional objectives that they never reveal to the learners. The primary reason for writing objectives is to provide students with knowledge of what they will be learning and how they will be evaluated. Objectives should be worded so that the learner understands exactly what is expected. To clarify an objective further, one might show a representative sample question before starting the lesson. In this way, the learner is better prepared for the content.
3. *Activate prior knowledge.* By starting instruction at a point where the student recalls past rules or examples from previous work, the stage is set for a smoother transition to content that is a continuation of past work. The most direct means of activating prior knowledge is to pose a recall question to the learner. When a learner cannot recall past information, a remedial lesson should be used rather than continuing instruction based on concepts not yet mastered.
4. *Present information.* The sequence and timing of the content presentation should follow the order in which learners are expected to perform newly acquired skills. Information should be presented with the characteristics of the learner in mind. For example, images and words should be used that are meaningful to the hearing-impaired population at a specific age level.
5. *Guide learning.* By recognizing common errors, it is possible to coach the student by prompts or hints when he or she makes anticipated errors or when the response time is excessively long. This form of communication makes the CAI lesson more self-sufficient.
6. *Elicit responses.* Once the concepts have been presented to the learner, it is important to provide an opportunity for practice that permits a demonstration of new competencies. The practice activities should relate to stated instructional objectives.

7. *Provide feedback.* Feedback should be given so that the learner understands how well he or she performed during the practice segments of a lesson. Ideally, feedback should communicate to the learner specific information about the degree of correctness of the answer. It helps the learner if the feedback is displayed while the question and answer are still on the screen.
8. *Assess performance.* Testing the learner's ability to demonstrate the skills called for in the objective is the primary means of determining the success of a CAI lesson. The key to successful assessment hinges on the reliability and validity of the test.
9. *Promote transfer.* The ability of the learner to recall newly acquired information can be enhanced by including review activities in subsequent related lessons. Future lessons should incorporate a capsulization of key aspects of past lessons. This promotes a better understanding of the linking of information and reinforces central concepts. It helps to ensure generalization of the concepts.

EVALUATION

Instructional Quality

Hunka (1982), Cohen (1983), and Zemke (1984) provide practical and detailed guidelines for evaluating the quality of CAI programs. Hunka's checklist includes five items that should be used in high-quality CAI:

1. The use of microlearning strategies such as advanced organizers, schedules, and transfer-of-learning support techniques, which are thought to improve comprehension and retention (McCann, 1981; Tobias, 1980).
2. The use of macroinstructional strategies such as drill and practice, tutorial sequences, simulations, fixed formats, and discovery approaches. The use of game-like formats for increased motivation through the challenge, fantasy, and mastery aspects of successful video games (Driskell and Dwyer, 1984).
3. The use of learner intervention into the instructional sequences. A great degree of learner control is desirable at one extreme, whereas no student control is desired at the other.
4. The use of alternate pathways associated with major portions of the lesson. This capability indicates the degree to which the student is recycled through the same material even though it may not have resulted in learning during the first pass.
5. The use of specific student-response techniques to enhance cognitive involvement such as constructed (open set) responses or associations (Jay, 1983). The use of multiple modes of response—that is, not only multiple-choice responses, but also flexibility for phrase and sentence input.

Student Performance

During the development of a CAI lesson, it is important to establish that the software is accomplishing its intended instructional purposes. This process is called formative evaluation (Dick, 1977; Gokes, 1983). Formative evaluations are used as a means of fine-tuning software by closely monitoring its effectiveness with a sample from the target population.

Once a program has been de-bugged as a result of a formative evaluation, it is ready for a summative evaluation to determine whether the newly created program reliably produces improvement in student performance (Knapper, 1980). Unfortunately, formative and summative evaluations have not often been completed for courseware used with the hearing impaired. Kelly (1982) says that "a disproportionate number of 'thought' papers (are) presented versus data-based research papers (regarding effectiveness). A major emphasis should clearly be on learner characteristics and performance data.

CAI has been proved effective with normally learning elementary, secondary, and college pupils (Hartley, 1977; Visonhaler and Bass, 1972). Kulik, Kulik, and Cohen (1980) state in their meta-analysis of the effectiveness of computer-based college-level teaching that the principal beneficial effects of CAI when compared to conventional instruction are (1) improved student achievement (about 10% improvement in percentile ranking), (2) improved student attitude toward instruction, and (3) a decrease of about one third in the time necessary to complete the instruction.

Nevertheless, history has also shown that there are many subtleties in the research designs used to evaluate CAI that can result in support for the educational researcher's null hypothesis that there is little or no difference in student achievement with CAI when compared with other instructional methods. The evaluator must keep in mind that a CAI lesson will never produce more measurable learning than the live, one-on-one instruction that occurs so often in the speech and hearing remediation process. No matter how sophisticated the computer lesson is, it will not match the accumulated knowledge and flexibility of an experienced therapist who can interact with the individual student and meet educational needs spontaneously.

Principles of Evaluation

Evaluation should control confounding factors that may limit applicability and generality. However, the realities of the educational setting often preclude the use of strict experimental controls. This conflict of desire with the realities of educational practice is best resolved by evaluation with large numbers of students to improve ecological validity by averaging out many educational variables through closer approximation to the field population. Hunka (1982) suggests a study population of 100 to 200 as a rule of thumb.

POPULATION

If the educational circumstances allow only a small number of students, then careful experimental control is required for (1) learning potential, (2) motivation and anxiety level, (3) age, (4) relevant entry skills for the content of the course, (5) learning style, and (6) reading comprehension level.

For example, in our work with computer-assisted speech-reading training for college-aged deaf students we found that our lesson strategies worked well for intermediate and advanced-level speech-readers, but, almost invariably, poor speech-readers needed supplemental vocabulary training to acquaint them with the "survival" language used in the lessons.

CONTROLS

CAI evaluation should use rigorous methods for controlling experimental error (e.g., random assignment of students to the experimental and control groups) and for controlling the possible effects of different instructors assigned to the various treatment groups. Certain types of CAI courseware allow the student to control the amount and kind of instruction; therefore the instructional experiences may vary with each student. These variable treatment levels should be considered in the evaluation design and interpretation. Tobias (1980) states that when comparing instructional methods, macroprocessing (the frequency and intensity with which students cognitively process instructional input) is the most important comparative educational treatment variable. That is, if the method in question stimulates *more* student comprehension and *more* organization of what is learned with what has been learned before, it will result in higher achievement levels.

DEPENDENT VARIABLE

Pre- and post-test designs are commonly used for evaluation of student gain as a dependent variable. The utility of this approach is somewhat restricted, as CAI courseware is often designed for mastery at a high level of performance (Knapper, 1980). As a result, there is little student population variance with which to study learner characteristics as they interact with the treatment (i.e., correlations can be meaningless). However, when used as a dependent variable, student response or reaction time varies considerably according to individual learning style and difficulty level (Tatsouka and Tatsouka, 1978). Since response time is often related to the difficulty of the learning task and can be tracked throughout the lesson, it can be used as an online measure of skill acquisition without the necessity (and pitfalls) of a pre- and post-test design.

If skills improve on equally difficult items in the instructional sequence, one would expect response times to decrease to some floor level representing an individual student's current best performance. Time series statistical methods (Jones, Vaught, and Wienrott, 1977) may be used with single (within) subject designs using response time as the dependent variable. McReynolds and Kearns (1983) describe the advantages of this type of design as follows:

> A well matched control population sample is not needed because the subject serves as his own control. Performance is also continually assessed so that changing patterns of responses . . . present a complete profile of the effect of the independent variable on behavior . . . over time.

Evaluation of Affect

When evaluations of CAI and conventional instruction are compared for student achievement, the differences often only slightly favor CAI (Kulik, Kulik, and Cohen, 1980). However, teachers often report that CAI courseware creates much enthusiasm and motivation (Kelly, 1982). This motivation may be only the short-term infatuation with a new educational medium (novelty effect) or it may represent the development of an aptitude for mastering the new materials (Cronbach, 1972). Careful assessment of student affect is often meaningful. Usually self-report surveys are used for this process.

COMPUTER-ASSISTED INTERACTIVE VIDEO

The past 8 years have seen the development of an exciting new educational medium called interactive video. This medium marries instructional television with color, motion, and sound to computer-assisted instruction. It is called *interactive* because the instructional program's sequences and selection of messages are determined by the user's responses to the material (Cronin, 1979; Floyd and Floyd, 1982). Thus, the instruction has all the advantages of CAI—such as student pacing, individualization, immediate feedback, and mastery learning—in addition to having the realistic and compelling qualities of instructional television. Because interactive video requires substantially more development time than traditional CAI, it should be chosen only when what is to be learned requires *viewing* (or listening) to a sequence of movements. In the area of speech, hearing, and language, interactive video has been applied to drill and practice for receptive communication (speech reading and sign language), simulation of interpersonal communication interactions, and language instruction.

Interactive Video Hardware

The interactive video system typically consists of a microcomputer host (which provides the courseware), a videotape recorder (VTR) (or videodisk), and a television monitor. The VTR is controlled by the host computer through an interface controller that uses microprocessor technology to command the VTR's tape-handling functions and to read the tape's exact position. When the computer courseware calls for a particular video segment to be played, the controller takes over and finds the segment on the videotape.

VIDEODISK VERSUS VIDEOTAPE

Interactive video can utilize videotape or videodisk media. Videodisk requires highly technical mastering and reproduction procedures and therefore is relatively expensive. Subsequent copies are only a few dollars. The break-even point for videodisk versus videotape *reproduction* is approximately 100 copies. In addition, the high costs of creating a master predicate that the program material will not require change in the near future. An additional advantage of videotape is that it can be economically used for recording *during* the interactive lesson. For example, the student may need to compare his or her signed or spoken articulation to a model articulation. This can be done with interactive videotape by leaving a sufficient amount of blank tape available on the lesson tape and using a television camera in the instructional carrel to record the student articulation.

SEARCH AND ACCESS TIME

The videodisk has much faster access to programmed material than does videotape. This is important in a program such as a sign-language dictionary in which the sequences the user will select cannot be predicted, and rapid access is assumed and necessary. A search across 20 minutes of videodisk would take a few *seconds*, whereas a similar search on a videotape would take a few *minutes*. We have found, however, that videotape access times for communication training are not a source of complaint when the likely student trajectories are anticipated and video segments that may be sequentially accessed are recorded near each other during the initial production of the tape.

PICTURE QUALITY

Although videotape and videodisk both offer freeze-frame and slow motion, videodisk is, at this time, far superior for picture quality when operating in these modes. Neither play-back medium has enough picture resolution to allow one to read a video recording of a typewritten page of text.

Interactive Video and the Hearing Impaired

Brawley and Peterson (1983) have developed extensive English-language reading and writing exercises based on an interactive videodisk story titled *Dusty the Old Gold Miner*. A personal computer controls a laser videodisk. The software includes program-authoring and student data-management capabilities. Ten formats of instruction are used, and students are branched through activities

> . . . which require him or her to acknowledge captions appearing on the screen; sequence events, recognize correctness of grammar and syntax; respond to questions, and categorize, spell, capitalize, punctuate and construct sentences and questions. Student interaction is primarily through a light pen. Since the computer inserts captions and all printed tasks on the screen, rather than being embedded permanently on the videodiscs, a limitless number of reading levels, language concepts, and instructional objectives can be achieved through the use of the same sequence of video material.

Dillingham, Roe, and Roe (1982) used the computer with the BCD controller to construct safety programs presented on videotape at the Oklahoma School for the Deaf. They used authoring software that solicits instructor choices about the source and content of the instructional text, the answer options, and the appropriate interactive video treatment for each possible student response. At each step the instructor can choose to use the computer to present text material or a scene from the videotape. The use of authoring languages and systems can greatly simplify and speed the process of courseware development at the expense of a loss of some flexibility and detailed data collection and analysis for evaluation and research purposes.

Fulton, Larson, and Worthy (1983) developed a prototype system for investigating a variety of auditory-visual discrimination and training tasks. Their equipment includes a color computer interfaced to a videocassette recorder with a search controller, a programmable audiocassette, and a speech digitizer. They are investigating whether young hearing-impaired children indicate a "visual response preference when corresponding auditory stimuli are presented in a confusion context."

Kopra and Kopra (1984) used a videodisk system to build a speech-reading-training interactive video system. They carefully built a sequence of sentences controlled for level of speech-reading difficulty. These sentences will be used with a gradually faded audio level to force increased attention to the visual aspects of the sentences.

SPEECH-READING LESSON

Sims, Scott, and Myers (1982) developed interactive video software and authoring systems for speech-reading drill and practice called DAVID (Dynamic Audio Video Interactive Device). The speech-reading lesson uses videotaped sentences developed by Jacobs (1982). Students view a sentence being spoken, then type it verbatim into the computer. The student can request a stimulus repeat (front or side view of the speaker), a hint about the topic, and a letter or word fill-in of an incorrect response. The use of these aids is monitored by the program, and the student is coached for appropriate usage.

Pre- and post-test measures of gain in speech-reading skill and student preferences have compared favorably for CAI drill versus conventional videotape drill (Sims et al., 1979). However, another powerful aspect of CAI is the capability for analysis of learner performance in ways that would otherwise be difficult to obtain in typical clinical environments. Microcomputer systems can measure how long it takes a student to complete each response correctly. Previous research has shown that student skills improve if the time needed to respond correctly to equally difficult items decreases as the drill progresses (Restle and Davis, 1962). In the Sims, Scott, and Myers (1982) study, 12 equally difficult probe sentences were selected from a set of 175 sentences used for drill. It was known from previously collected data that the 12 probe sentences required roughly equal response times of 1 minute, 19 seconds. This average response time was also representative of the overall average response time of the entire practice set of 175 sentences. Since the probe sentences were spread throughout the lesson, the intention was to monitor whether student skills improved as a function of an apparent trend toward decreasing response time as practice accumulated.

Figure 11-1 is a plot of the time required to respond correctly to the first through the twelfth probe sentences. There is a clear trend toward decreasing response time. Since general orientation effects had been minimized by an initial practice block of sentences, it is suggested that the response time measure may be related to improvement in speech-reading skills for these 15 students. The greatest advantage of this design is that the skill improvement is measured *during* the instruction *with* the instructional materials so that there is no mismatch between what is being trained and the evaluation instrument. This consideration is important with prelingually hearing-impaired persons, since their level of English competence may interfere with performance measurements.

SIGN-LANGUAGE LESSON

Newell, Sims, and Myers (1983) describe a prototype interactive videotape lesson for improving reception of basic vocabulary. The student may choose to review individual vocabulary words or practice single-sentence reception prior to taking the paragraph-comprehension test. In addition, the program allows selection of two brief lectures regarding some of the principles of sign expression. Thus, the lesson is comprehensive in that

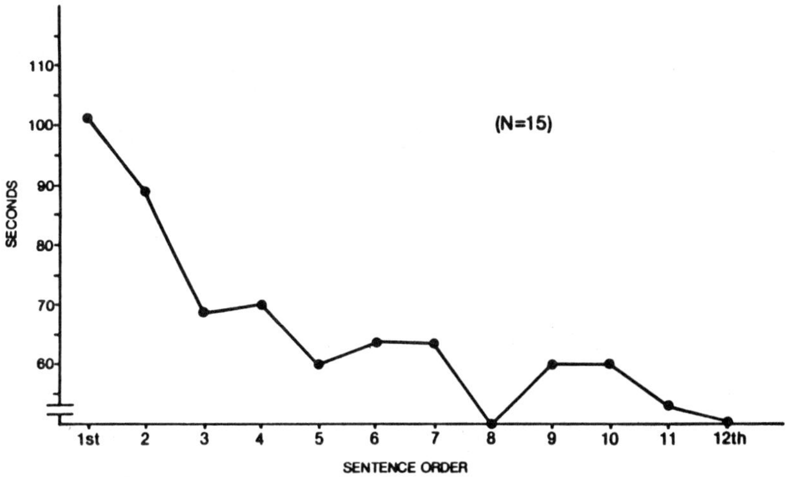

Fig. 11-1. Mean (average) time to correct response for twelve probe sentences.

the student can access practice on the word, sentence, or paragraph levels of difficulty.

COMMUNICATION SIMULATION

The most compelling use of interactive video is the simulation of dialogue. In this manner, training can focus on some of the survival strategies used when communication threatens to break down completely, or on some of the more subtle aspects of verbal and nonverbal communication in, for example, a job interview or a clinical diagnostic session. In a job interview simulation completed at the National Technical Institute for the Deaf, the student fills out an application on the computer screen and then, depending on some of the answers, various video segments are selected to test the student's reaction to problem areas that have surfaced in past real-life interviews. The student is encouraged to play the interview game several times to experience the full range of reactions from the interviewer.

THE FUTURE OF CAI

It is difficult to predict the future of CAI for the hearing impaired, but it is possible to forecast trends based on the likely direction the entire microcomputer and educational industries will take. The information that follows is based primarily on the projections of Educational Turnkey Systems of Falls Church, Va. (1983). They have surveyed industrial and special-education specialists regarding the most likely future impact of new educational technologies such as microcomputers, videodisks, and telecommunication devices.

Economics

The development and subsequent marketing of a new technology such as microcomputers is dependent on marketplace demand. The explosive

*Table 11-1. Current and proposed use of microcomputers in special education.**

	1982		1985	
	Regular Education	Special Education	Regular Education	Special Education
Instruction	100,000	15,000	400,000	125,000
Administration	25,000	10,000	100,000	25,000
Total	125,000	25,000	500,000	150,000

* From Educational Turnkey, 1983.

growth of the entire microcomputer industry is a classic example of the ability of entrepreneurs to create products to meet the needs of the market.

The special-education segment is relatively "thin" when compared with the entire microcomputer market. Major industrial research and development efforts will focus on larger segments first, and then turn to special education as a spin-off market. That is not to say that smaller organizations will not expand their development efforts for special education, only that major advances in the technology will come from firms that are attempting to exploit larger markets.

For example, it is expected that sophisticated speech-generation and recognition capabilities will be introduced as an interface mode for home appliances and military equipment. The incentive for the development of this technology is the huge market potential. The development and mass production of this technology will make it possible for handicapped individuals to have access to a tremendous communication system at a much lower cost than if it were developed only for the special-education market.

It appears that there will be a marked increase in the use of microcomputers in special education, as shown in Table 11-1. The general availability of microcomputer systems in homes and schools will grow as the price drops. Schools will acquire systems based in part on pressure from parents who want their children to have access to them. In fact, teachers and parents who own systems will become a major factor in the decision of schools to buy microcomputers.

Hardware

Microcomputers will undoubtedly become less costly and more powerful. Compatibility between systems will be less of a problem, with simpler interface systems becoming available. Telecommunications and networking applications will expand, improving the ability of the handicapped to be included in communications from various locations and through various interface systems.

Software

Educational software publishers will attempt to meet the needs of hearing-impaired learners by adapting materials from their catalogues for the general market. In addition, sophisticated authoring systems will be introduced that will permit teachers to create lessons that more closely meet the needs of their students. A reduction in unauthorized copying of software will result in the development and marketing of more and better materials for special education. It is expected that the government will provide assistance in the development of software for special education, and that telecommunication networks will be used to provide access to data bases and software on demand.

People

As both teachers and students become more sophisticated users of computers, and with continued improvement in computer-user interface, more people will use microcomputers in programs for education of the deaf. Both students and teachers will expect more than drill and practice from the computer. We hope the microcomputer will become a tool that can be used to help the hearing impaired learn and communicate, and that it will provide a means for self-expression and discovery.

REFERENCES

Alesandrini, K. L. Instructional design for CAI tutorials. *Collegiate Microcomputing* 1:207–214, 1983.

Boothroyd, A., Archambault, P., Adams, R., and Storm, R. Use of a computer-based system of speech analysis and display in a remedial speech program. *Volta Review* 77:178–193, 1975.

Braeges, J., and Houde, R. Use of Speech Training Aids. In D. Sims, G. Walter, and R. Whitehead (Eds.), *Deafness and Communication: Assessment and Training*. Baltimore: Williams & Wilkins, 1982.

Brawley, R., and Peterson, B. Interactive videodisc: An innovative instructional system. *Am. Ann. Deaf* 128:685–700, 1983.

Cohen, V. B. Criteria for the evaluation of microcomputer courseware. *Educ. Technol.* 23:9–14, 1983.

Cronbach, L. Course Improvement through Evaluation. In P. Taylor and D. Crowley (Eds.), *Readings in Curriculum Evaluation*. Dubuque, Iowa: W. C. Brown Co., 1972.

Cronin, B. The DAVID system: The development of an interactive video system at the National Technical Institute for the Deaf. *Am. Ann. Deaf* 124:616–618, 1979.

Data Training's Computer-Based Training Guide. Boston: Data Training, 1983.

Diamond, R. M. *Instructional Development for Individualized Learning in Higher Education*. Englewood Cliffs, N.J.: Educational Technology Publications, 1975.

Dick, W. Formative Evaluation. In L. J. Briggs (Ed.), *Instructional Design: Principles and Applications*. Englewood Cliffs, N.J.: Educational Technology Publications, 1977.

Dick, W., and Carey, L. *The Systematic Design of Instruction*. Glenview, Ill.: Scott, Foresman and Co., 1978.

Dillingham, L., Roe, J., and Roe, M. Selected applications of computer assisted video instruction in the education of hearing-impaired students. *Am. Ann. Deaf* 127:652–658, 1982.

Driskell, J., and Dwyer, D. Microcomputer videogame based training. *Educ. Technol.* 24:11–17, 1984.

Educational Turnkey Systems, Inc. *Microcomputers in Special Education*. Falls Church, Va.: Educational Turnkey Systems, 1983. (ERIC Document ED 231 175.)

Fallside, F., Gulian, E., Hinds, P., and Keiller, C. *Assessment and Development of a Speech Training Aid for the Deaf. A Pilot Study*. National Technical Information Service Publication PB 84-107986, 1983.

Fletcher, J. D. *Computer-Assisted Instruction for the Deaf*. Chicago: University of Illinois, 1974. (ERIC Document Reproduction No. ED 089 680.)

Floyd, S., and Floyd, B. *Handbook of Interactive Video*. White Plains, N.Y.: Knowledge Industry Publications, 1982.

Fulton, R., Larson, A., and Worthy, R. The use of microcomputer technology in assessing and training communication skills of young hearing impaired children. *Am. Ann. Deaf* 128:570–576, 1983.

Gagne, R. M., Wager, W., and Rojas, A. Planning and authoring computer-assisted instruction lessons. *Educ. Technol.* 21:17–26, 1981.

Glaser, R. Telephone communication for the deaf. *Am. Ann. Deaf* 127: 550–555, 1982.

Gokes, K. The formative evaluation of computer assisted instruction. *Educ. Technol.* 23:26–28, 1983.

Grosman, K., Siders, J., and Garraway, H. Sign teacher: A microcomputer application for the teaching of sign language. *Am. Ann. Deaf* 128: 577–584, 1983.

Hagen, R. *Microcomputer Resource Book for Special Education*. Reston, Va.: Reston Publishing Co., 1984.

Harding, R., and Tidball, L. A National microcomputer software survey of current microcomputer usage in schools for the hearing impaired. *Am. Ann. Deaf* 127:673–683, 1982.

Hartley, S. Meta-analysis of the effects of individually paced instruction in mathematics. *Diss. Abstr. Int.* 38(7-A):4003, 1977. (University Microfilms No. 77-29, 926.)

Hight, R. Lip-reader trainer: Teaching aid for the hearing impaired. *Am. Ann. Deaf* 127:564–568, 1982.

Hunka. The evaluation of CBE materials and projects. Paper presented to the University of Delaware Conference on CBE Research: Past, Present and Future. Wilmington, Del., June 1982.

Huntington, J. F. A review of SUPERPILOT. *Educ. Technol.* 23:53–55, 1983.

Irwin, M. G. CAI at CSDF: Organizational strategies. *Am. Ann. Deaf* 127:487–494, 1982.

Jacobs, M. Visual Communication (Speechreading) for the Severely and Profoundly Hearing Impaired Young Adults. In D. Sims, G. Walter, and R. Whitehead (Eds.), *Deafness and Communication: Assessment and Training*. Baltimore: Williams & Wilkins, 1982.

Jay, T. B. The cognitive approach to computer courseware design and evaluation. *Educ. Technol.* 23:22–26, 1983.

Jones, R., Vaught, R., and Weinrott, M. Time-series analysis in operant research. *J. Appl. Behav. Anal.* 10:151–166, 1977.

Kearsley, G. P. *Instructional Design Considerations of CAI for the Deaf*. Alberta, Canada: University of Alberta, 1978. (ERIC Document Reproduction Service No. ED 160 084.)

Kelly, R. Microcomputers in education: Age of romance, or age of reason. *Am. Ann. Deaf* 127:693–697, 1982.

Knapper, C. *Evaluating Instructional Technology.* New York: Wiley, 1980.

Kopra, L., and Kopra, M. Computer assisted instruction in lipreading. Paper presented at the Academy of Rehabilitative Audiology Summer Institute, Watts Bar, Tenn., June 1984.

Kulik, J., Kulik, C., and Cohen, P. Effectiveness of computer based college teaching: A meta-analysis of findings. *Rev. Educ. Res.* 50: 525–544, 1980.

Lathrop, A., and Goodson, B. *Courseware in the Classroom; Selecting, Organizing and Using Educational Software.* Menlo Park, Ca.: Addison-Wesley, 1983.

LINC Associates. *The Specialware Directory, 1983.* Columbus: LINC Associates, 1983.

Mager, R. F. *Instructional Module Development.* Los Altos Hills, Ca.: Mager Associates, 1979.

McCann, P. H. Learning strategies and computer based instruction. *Computers and Education* 5:133–140, 1981.

McReynolds, L., and Kearns, K. *Single-Subject Experimental Designs in Communicative Disorders.* Baltimore: University Park Press, 1983.

Mills, R., and Thomas, R. *Word Recognition Programs.* Ann Arbor, Mich.: Brain-Link Software, 1983.

Newell, W., Sims, D., and Clymer, W. Meet DAVID, our teacher's aid. *Perspectives* 2:15–18, 1984.

Nickerson, R., and Stevens, K. In H. Levitt and J. Pickett (Eds.), *Sensory Aids for the Hearing Impaired.* New York: Wiley, 1980.

Nickerson, R., Stevens, K., Rollins, A., and Zue, V. Computers and Speech Aids. In I. Hocberg, H. Levitt, and M. Osberger (Eds.), *Speech of the Hearing Impaired.* Baltimore: University Park Press, 1983.

Osberger, M., Moeller, M., Kroese, J., and Lippmann, R. Computer-assisted speech training for the hearing impaired. *J. Acad. Rehabil. Audiol.* 14:145–158, 1981.

Parrish, R., and De Bold, J. Computers help teachers, too. *Am. Ann. Deaf* 124:631–637, 1982.

Pflaum, M. The California connection: Interfacing the TDD and an Apple computer. *Am. Ann. Deaf* 127:573–584, 1982.

Shulman, J., and Decker, N. (Eds.). *Readable English for Hearing-Impaired Students.* Boston: The Caption Center, WGBH-TV, 1980.

Sims, D., Scott, L., and Myers, T. Past, present and future computer assisted communication training at the National Technical Institute for the Deaf. *J. Acad. Rehabil. Audiol.* 15:103–115, 1982.

Sims, D., VonFeldt, J., Dowaliby, F., Hutchinson, K., and Myers, T. A pilot experiment in computer assisted speechreading instruction utilizing the DAVID. *Am. Ann. Deaf* 124:616–623, 1979.

Slovick, L. CAI at CSDF: Microcomputer-based authoring systems. *Am. Ann. Deaf* 127:545–563, 1982.

Stoker, R. A computer-assisted diagnostic and prescriptive tool for use in teaching speech to the deaf. *Am. Ann. Deaf* 128:625–630, 1983.

Tatsouka, K., and Tatsouka, M. *Time Score Analysis in Criterion Refer-*

enced Tests, PLATO Education Group, CERL Report E-1. Champaign, Ill.: University of Illinois, Urbana, 1978.

Tobias, S. When do instructional methods make a difference? *Educ. Res.* 11:4–9, 1980.

Visonhaler, J., and Bass, R. A summary of ten major studies on CAI drill and practice. *Educ. Technol.* 12:29–32, 1972.

Watson, P. The utilization of the computer with the hearing impaired and the handicapped. *Am. Ann. Deaf* 124:670–680, 1979.

Zemke, R. Evaluating computer-assisted instruction: The good, the bad and the why. *Training* 21:22–47, 1984.

12

Speech Synthesis and Speech Recognition by Microcomputer

Conrad LaRiviere and
John Sherblom

For many years there was considerable skepticism that anyone could build a device that would produce human-like speech. This skepticism has proved largely unwarranted. Society now has "machines that speak," and we all encounter them with increasing regularity. Dialing a telephone number that has recently been changed elicits a machine's verbal response providing the updated number; a new automobile is likely to describe a malfunction verbally; video arcade games increasingly "talk" to the player; the airport shuttle announces destinations and safety reminders; "talking typewriters," allow a user to enter text at a keyboard and hear that text "spoken" by the machine. Only a few years ago, the hardware and software required to produce synthetic speech of these sorts were formidable. Now what was possible on a minicomputer can be done on a microcomputer and at surprisingly little cost. This is the beginning of an explosion of hardware and software modifications that will allow virtually any microcomputer to speak.

There is also interest in machines that "listen" and "recognize" speech. The state of the art and science of creating machines that listen is not so advanced as that for speech-synthesis devices. The principal reasons for the current interest in microcomputers that speak or listen are presented in this text.

THEORIES OF HUMAN SPEECH PRODUCTION AND PERCEPTION

Larger computers have for some time been used to answer questions about the necessary and sufficient conditions for humans to produce or recognize speech. Two general, non-mutually exclusive approaches have been used:

1. *Testing notions that have arisen from measures and manipulations of human speech.* For example, it has long been known that vowel segments in human speech are marked by a rich array of resonant or formant frequencies. The location of these frequencies appears to depend on the particular vowel segment and the gender of the speaker. A speech synthesizer could be used to ascertain which of the formant frequencies are necessary for vowel identification—the first two, three, or five?—by "building" vowels whose resonant frequencies are varied in a known way and presenting such vowels to human listeners for identification. In that way, it may be ascertained that the necessary and sufficient cues for the male vowel /*a*/ are to be found in the lowest two for-

mant frequencies, and that those frequencies need to be approximately 700 and 1100 Hz, respectively. In this application of the speech synthesizer, one has verified that not all of the acoustic information in human vowels is necessary for correct identification. In a similar vein, acoustic measures of human speech have shown that formant frequencies between adjacent speech sounds—as in the syllable /*va*/—blend into one another. The consonant /*v*/ has certain formant frequencies, the vowel /*a*/ has its own set of formants, but there is also a boundary glide in formants—known as the formant transitions—linking the consonant and vowel. How important is this transition for humans to recognize the syllable? How important are the individual characteristics of the transition—for example, its duration, its frequency range, whether it is a first formant transition, a second formant transition, and so forth? A speech synthesizer enables an investigator to generate known and highly controlled acoustic patterns. Several versions of /*va*/ can be generated and presented to listeners for identification. Transitions can be removed, lengthened, shortened, changed in frequency, and the like.

2. *Building a model from known principles that behaves like the unknown.* Computers lend themselves to a mode of inquiry called "analysis by synthesis." We try to construct (synthesize) the solution by combining constituents in the right amounts and testing the new solution for success. If it works, one has derived a working explanation (analysis) of the original solution through constructing (synthesizing) a solution that is a good model of the original. By trial and error, one can synthesize solutions from various components and in varying proportions and test them for the desired effect until one stumbles on a synthesized solution that works. Suppose someone constructed a "listening" typewriter that produced a correct, typed manuscript in response to English spoken to it by a wide range of normal English speakers. He or she would be in possession of a quite explicit theory (explanation) of human speech perception. Those principles of operation of the device—how it analyzes, categorizes, segments, and revises the incoming human speech signal—might be inferred to be the principles of operation of human speech recognition, because someone synthesized a device that behaves as a human would.

Commercial Applications

The burgeoning number of manufacturers and vendors of speech synthesis and recognition devices for microcomputers is testimony to the view that there is a potentially large market for their application as useful tools. There are a number of applications already implemented such as devices that provide verbal feedback (talking clocks), and devices that provide verbal feedback on their own performance or on the performance of the human currently using them. People whose livelihoods somehow involve sustained periods of attention on visual feedback mechanisms—for example, air-traffic controllers, computer users, employees working in most control rooms—may indeed perform more reliably and with less fatigue if they could hear their terminals and instruments talk to them. Word-processing and spread-sheet software would no doubt be less fatiguing to use if one received verbal feedback on what had been entered, rather than having to constantly glare at the monitor.

Devices for the Handicapped

A large number of individuals in our society are unable to produce intelligible speech because of congenital or adventitious handicaps. Among these handicapping conditions are severe motor disabilities secondary to cerebral palsy or acquired brain damage, severe cognitive deficits, early and profound hearing loss, and loss of organs vital for the production of speech through trauma or surgery. Although there have been many nonoral modes of communication available to such individuals—for example, communication boards containing pictures, symbols, or words; various forms of manual signaling systems; or conventional orthography—all of them have inherent limitations. These limitations have to do with portability, speed, flexibility, or the size of the population that readily comprehends and uses the symbol system. Speech-synthesis devices hold the potential for serving as effective vocal prostheses for many individuals. Electronic communication boards that allow speech output are increasingly available (see Appendix A). These devices are getting smaller, cheaper, faster, and more intelligible. In addition to such "dedicated" devices, accessories are also available for most "off-the-shelf" microcomputers that facilitate their utilization as communication prostheses. For example, most microcomputers can be attached to outboard speech synthesizers. There are also keyboard guards to help prevent unintended keyboard entries by individuals using external pointers, and, for those with severe motor deficits, keyboard emulator cards are available. These devices allow access to keyboards through virtually any external switch arrangement. The advantage of the microcomputer, of course, is that it can serve the individual in many more ways than a dedicated artificial voice. As reviewed by Shane and Bashir (1980), considerable care needs to be exercised in determining which individuals can profit from any given nonoral mode of communication. While many devices are now available that allow some handicapped individuals to "speak," there continue to be limiting factors. These concern the cognitive ability and linguistic knowledge of the user, and the speed and ready intelligibility of the speech-synthesis devices.

How successful are the speech synthesis and recognition devices currently available for microcomputers? The most stringent, widely acknowledged criterion for the extent to which a computer can model human behavior is the so-called *Turing test*, which holds that the modeling is successful if a group of judges cannot decide if the output was generated by a machine or by another human being. No available synthesis or recognition device for microcomputers can currently pass the Turing test. For most applications, the real question when evaluating success of devices should revolve around the issue of error rates—that is, the degree of intelligibility of microcomputer speech, or the "hit rate" of speech-recognition devices.

REPRESENTING SPEECH IN A MICROCOMPUTER

There exists an inherent incompatibility problem with attempting to store speech in a microcomputer. Computer memory is limited in capacity and digital in form. A microcomputer might be able to hold 128,000 bytes (128 K) of information internally. Each of these bytes comprises a number of bits (typically eight). Each of these bits has a binary digit value, which is either on or off, and represented as a one or a zero. The information stored in a byte must be represented as a digital value consisting of a pattern of these eight ones and zeros.

Speech is, of course, a continuous sound wave, an analog signal, which varies in pitch and volume. To store the speech signal in a computer the signal must be digitized (turned into a pattern of ones and zeros) and reduced to as few essential characteristics as are necessary to reproduce the original signal. An analog-to-digital (AD) converter does the conversion by taking repeated samplings of the speech waveform. This sampling must occur at a rate of 10,000 to 25,000 samples per second. If each of these sampling points is stored in one byte of the computer's memory, then only very short segments of speech can be stored in a microcomputer with 128 K of user memory (less than 12.8 seconds at the slower sampling rate, and only 5 seconds at the faster rate). In order to store longer segments of speech, techniques are used to reduce the number of samples stored and still achieve some reasonable degree of fidelity to the original analog waveform. To do this the sound is divided into frames, and a sample is taken from each frame.

Figure 12-1 shows the effects of fidelity loss caused by sampling intervals of the sound waveform. The original sound is an infinite analog waveform (Fig. 12-1*A*), which, in order to be digitized, must be sampled at various intervals (Fig. 12-1*B*). This sampling process yields a set of digital points (Fig. 12-1*C*) from which the original waveform can be roughly reproduced (Fig. 12-1*D*). The longer the interval between samples, the greater is the loss in fidelity to the waveform.

Sampling frames may be of set length, 10 to 25 msec, or of varying lengths determined by the rapidity of change in the sound wave. Vowels, for example, because of their fairly long "steady state" do not need to be sampled as frequently as consonants. Whether of set or varying length, the frame becomes the basic unit of analysis of the wave whose characteristics are to be measured and stored.

The fundamental frequency and voicing characteristics are important pieces of information to be obtained from this frame. The fundamental frequency reflects the rate of vibration of the vocal folds and is an important piece of information to obtain because humans are sensitive to even minor fluctuations in it. The second important distinction—voiced or unvoiced—is also determined largely by vocal-fold vibration. A phoneme is voiced if the vocal folds vibrate during its production, as with most vowels. It is unvoiced if the vocal folds do not vibrate, as when some consonants are produced. It is an important distinction to the human perception of speech sounds and for the computer because the two types of sounds—voiced and unvoiced—are synthesized differently by computer.

Breaking the sound wave into frames and making these two distinctions about it lead us to two approaches for further analysis. These are commonly referred to as *modeled* and *unmodeled* approaches.

The modeled approach to storing and reproducing the sound extracts additional pieces of information about each frame. In addition to the fun-

Fig. 12-1. Digitizing an analog waveform.

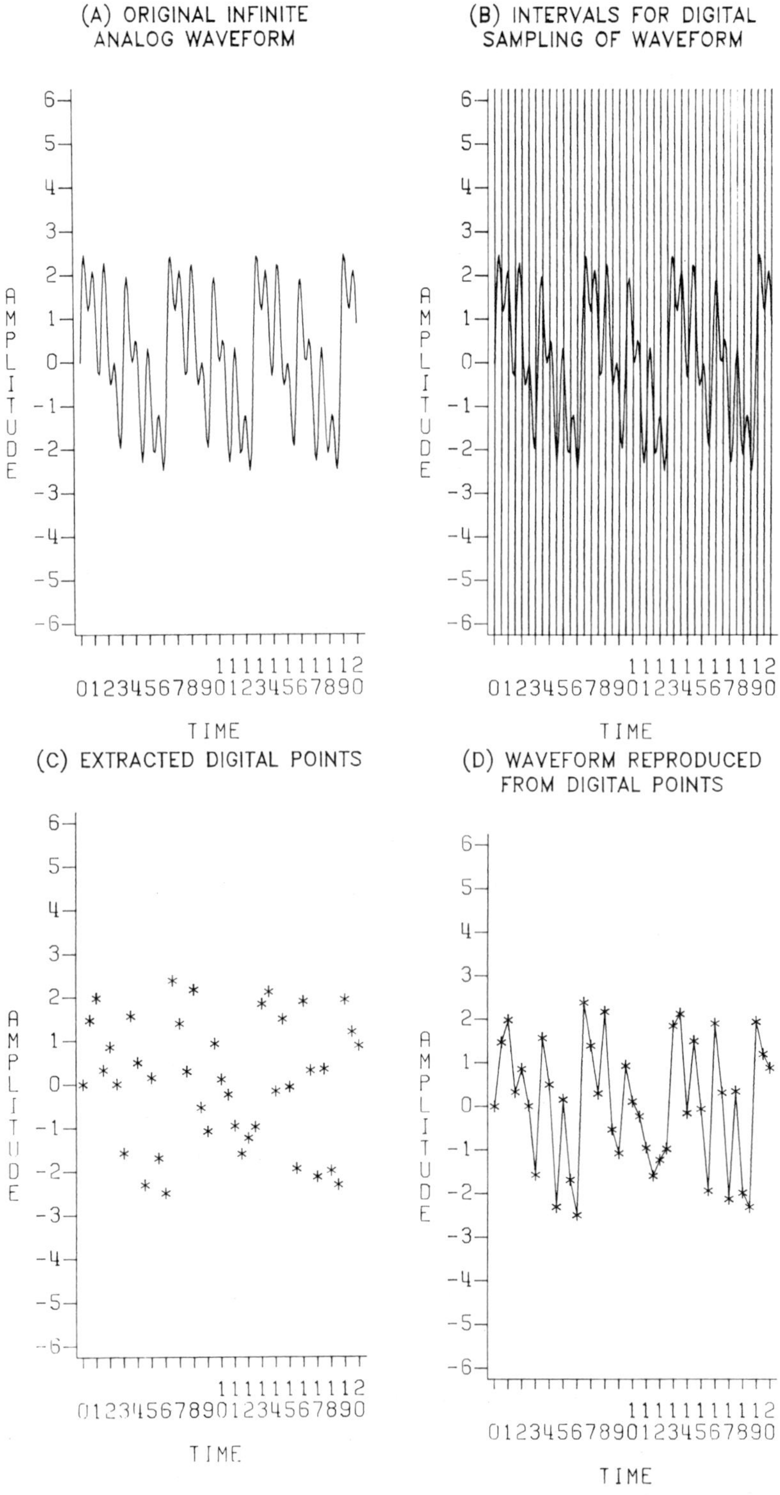
(A) ORIGINAL INFINITE ANALOG WAVEFORM
(B) INTERVALS FOR DIGITAL SAMPLING OF WAVEFORM
(C) EXTRACTED DIGITAL POINTS
(D) WAVEFORM REPRODUCED FROM DIGITAL POINTS
AMPLITUDE
TIME
6 5 4 3 2 1 0 -1 -2 -3 -4 -5 -6
0 1 2 3 4 5 6 7 8 9 10 11 12 13 14 15 16 17 18 19 20

damental frequency and voiced characteristics, the loudness of the signal and, typically, ten reflection coefficients are obtained. The reflection coefficients define the shape of the vocal tract needed to produce the sound. These coefficients can be used in a linear predictive coding equation, similar to a regression equation, to reproduce the original sound wave (Doddington and Schalk, 1981). This method of encoding the digital information about the wave allows an intelligible reproduction of the original sound from a greatly reduced number of bits of information. Often the number of bits per frame can be reduced from approximately 100,000 to 2000 and, because the vowel sounds can carry across several frames, further reduced to 1200 without substantial loss of reproducibility of the sound (McDermott, 1983).

The other approach to storage and retrieval is an unmodeled one. It uses the same basic information about the sound, but makes a different analysis of it. The unmodeled approach uses a mathematical technique called waveform encoding, which relies on Fourier transforms. Through fast Fourier transforms a waveform of any shape can be expressed as a series of sine waves occurring at the fundamental frequency and its overtones (McDermott, 1983). Figure 12-2 shows a waveform reduced to sine waves. These sine waves occur at its fundamental frequency and overtones. The original waveform can be reproduced by simply adding together points taken from each of the sine waves at each period in time. Therefore, the information stored about the wave can be stated as the fundamental frequency and the relative amount of energy occurring at each of the overtones. The wave can then be reshaped for further economy, and approximately one-twelfth of the original data obtained is sufficient to reproduce the sound.

Both of these approaches have as their goal the ability to store and faithfully reproduce speech sounds on a microcomputer. To achieve this goal

Fig. 12-2. An example of Fourier's theorem. Any complex waveform (left) can be expressed as a series of component sinusoids (right four waveforms).

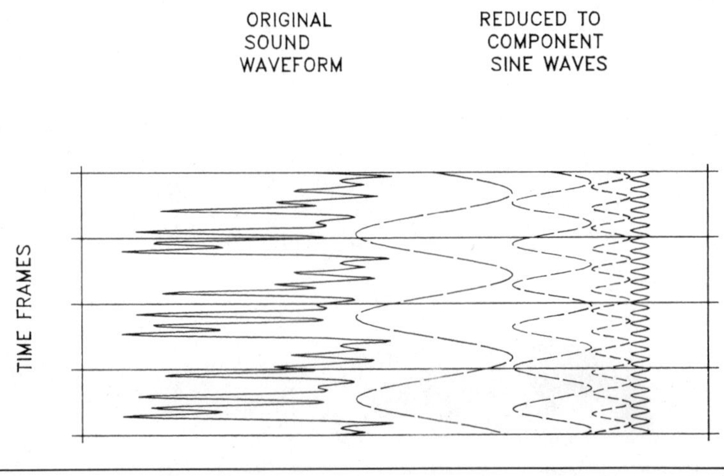

the original speech signal must be converted from an analog to a digital signal, and then reduced to the minimal number of bits that will allow the faithful reproduction of the sound. Even having done this, the amount of speech that can be stored on a microcomputer is limited. After reduction, only a couple of minutes of speech, or approximately 200 words, can be stored in 128 K of computer memory at any one time.

SPEECH SYNTHESIS

Two very different processes are commonly referred to as speech synthesis. The first process involves the recording, storage, and playing back of human speech. We call this a voice-record-playback system. It has advantages in intelligibility and "humanness" of the speech produced. Its major disadvantages are a need to "teach" new words to the computer, and a limited vocabulary size. The vocabulary size, normally restricted to between 50 and 500 words, is imposed by computer memory limitations and disk storage-access capabilities. This type of speech storage and synthesis is subject to the limitations imposed by the interval used for waveform sampling and the approach—either modeled or unmodeled—it uses to store and reproduce the speech sound.

A second process called *speech synthesis* takes some form of typed text and pronounces it according to a set of pronunciation rules. This form of synthesis we refer to as *text-to-speech synthesis*. Its major advantages include versatility of application and an essentially unlimited vocabulary. The disadvantages are the production of speech that is less immediately intelligible and the mispronunciation of words that do not follow the pronunciation rules. While this type of speech synthesis does not require the teaching of new words to the computer, it frequently does require training the computer user to understand what the computer has said.

Synthesis by rule turns text into speech. This approach uses some form of text as input and generates speech output based on a set of rules, or algorithms, controlling two types of sound generators. Voiced sounds for vowels and some of the consonants, such as /v/ and /z/, are produced by a voiced sound generator. A separate fricative generator produces the source for consonants like /s/, /k/, /f/, and /th/. The signals from these two generators are fed through a vocal-tract simulator and a set of filters. These perform the transfer function of the human vocal tract and filter out extraneous noise. The output from these filters passes to a digital-to-analog (DA) converter and then to a smoother. The DA converter changes the discrete sound signals into a wave that can then be smoothed. The smoother builds the transitions between the sounds. It slopes the beginning and ending of each of the sounds and blends them into each other. The smoother produces the rising and falling pitch of the words and adds any vocal inflections to their expression. Figure 12-3 illustrates a model of the general process of generating speech with a text-to-speech synthesizer.

The basic software, or program, for a text-to-speech synthesizer defines the set of rules that determine how text entered at a keyboard as a string of letters should be pronounced. Four hundred rules are adequate for the correct pronunciation of 96% of the 1000 most commonly used English words (Anderson, 1982). In addition to relying on these rules, frequently used

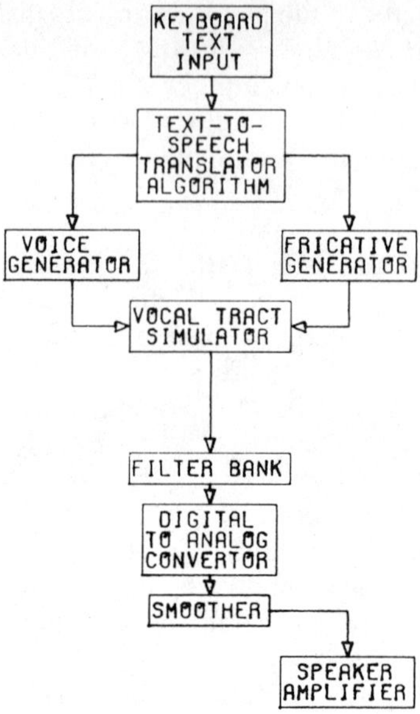

Fig. 12-3. An example of the components and sequence of operations in text-to-speech synthesis.

words and words that do not follow the rules can be placed in a dictionary from which they are looked up to determine the correct pronunciation.

Before it can use these pronunciation rules, the speech synthesizer must first chunk the incoming text into some standard-sized pieces. These pieces could either be letters treated as phonemes, or morphemes or words. Morphemes—word roots, prefixes, and suffixes—reproduce English more accurately and intelligibly than phonemes do. The phonemes are more susceptible to pronunciation changes owing to word context or syntax. Nevertheless, it takes 12,000 morphemes to reproduce the English language roughly, but only 48 to 64 phoneme-like sounds to do the same (Songco, Allen, Plexico, and Morford, 1980). Therefore, most microcomputer synthesizers use the phoneme rather than the morpheme. The synthesized speech may not be as clear and intelligible, but its defining characteristics can be stored in much less memory.

The other important programming consideration is the *smoothing algorithms* used to blend one phonemic sound into the next. Adjacent phonemes, when produced by humans, overlap and run together in ways that change their sound patterns. Smoothing algorithms have to provide for these changes in sound, not only to produce a more natural sound, but also to produce one quickly enough and with adequate intelligibility. In normal conversation humans produce about 1400 phonemes a minute. If produced one after the other, only about 600 to 900 of them could be generated in that minute. If the program's synthesis does not account for this fact, its speech will be unbearably slow, fragmented, and unintelligible. So smoothing is not a process for dressing up the sound sequence, but a necessary step for producing an acceptably intelligible one. In short, the smoothing algorithm is a model of coarticulation effects.

The final step in generating the speech sound is to add prosody. Prosody includes changes in pitch, intensity, and timing, as well as the hesitations and vocal jitters that occur in normal human speech. Listeners use prosody to aid their interpretation of the meaning and emphasis of an expression. It is the most difficult aspect of speech to define with a set of rules, however, and consequently the most difficult to program a computer to produce. Lack of adequate prosody is what makes computer-generated speech sound stilted, monotonous, sing-songy, and plodding—in short, machine-like. Most current text-to-speech synthesis systems give the user some means of adjusting the prosody of the speech produced. This frequently involves adding punctuation to the text to control the duration of phonemic sounds, length of pauses, pitch, and rhythm. The insertion of correct punctuation to make the speech sound natural, however, can be tedious, even with practice.

CURRENT SPEECH-SYNTHESIS SYSTEMS

The available speech synthesis systems for microcomputers can be divided into three types. Two of these use some form of prerecorded human speech. The third uses the text-to-speech synthesis approach. Some systems combine approaches, but are predominantly of one type or another. A combination system might generate most words by rule but also provide a pronunciation dictionary for the common rule-breaking words, or produce most of its words and expressions from an internal dictionary but include a set of rules to overcome limitations of that dictionary.

One approach to speech synthesis provides a prerecorded vocabulary that is played back from read-only memory (ROM). This type of system generally provides the most intelligible speech, but offers the most limited vocabulary. ROM is expensive, limited, and the user is not able to modify it.

A second type of voice-record-playback system works in conjunction with speech-recognition software to allow a user to create a vocabulary of words and expressions in random-access memory (RAM). The computer can later reproduce this stored speech. The speech generated by this system is usually a little noisy because user-recording conditions tend to be noisy. Most computer users do not have access to sound-proof recording studios and professional-quality microphones. This type of voice-record-playback system also requires a significant amount of "training" time to enter the words for the recognition vocabulary. The advantage is that the vocabulary of stored words can be larger and more specifically oriented to the applications of the user. The vocabulary is still limited, however, to several hundred words. So the words placed in the vocabulary list must be carefully chosen.

Text-to-speech synthesis offers an unlimited vocabulary and requires no training period for building the vocabulary into the computer. It does demand a little more user patience and attentiveness to become accustomed to the speech. Although its pronunciation accuracy rate is often cited as 95 or 96%, any errors it does make are generally quite noticeable. Accuracy rate can also be expected to drop some when it tries to pronounce words from a highly specialized or technical area. The user should be aware that text-to-speech synthesizers produce a dialect of English that is not familiar to English listeners. It is not instantaneously intelligible, and most listeners will require a substantial "normalization time" before they can achieve 95% recognition rates. Some manufacturers will forward demonstration tapes of the speech output by their synthesizers. While these are helpful for evaluating intelligibility, the potential user must keep in mind that the nature of the *message* synthesized can lead to an overestimate of intelligibility. The Gettysburg Address or a well-known passage from Shakespeare can make a synthesizer sound more intelligible than it would be for the less-predictable speech occurring in normal conversation.

One consideration that affects the quality of the output of any of these types of speech-synthesis systems is whether a system comes equipped with its own speaker and other essential hardware or must use the speaker supplied with the microcomputer. Those systems that supply their own speakers tend to produce better quality sound and to be more expensive. Whether the difference in sound quality is important depends on the particular project for which the speech synthesizer is to be used. The importance of the quality of sound produced, the type of microcomputer on which the system is to work, and the amount of training available to users are important issues to be considered before purchasing a system. See Appendix B for more detailed information about some of the speech-synthesis systems currently available for microcomputers.

SPEECH RECOGNITION BY MICROCOMPUTER

Limited speech-recognition capability is now available for many microcomputers, and the mainframe-to-mini-to-micro "trickle down" phenomenon is beginning to assert itself. By and large, however, most speech-recognition schemes currently available are capable only of recognizing isolated words from among a small, predetermined vocabulary. Typically, the vocabulary size for reasonably priced systems ranges from 20 to 80 words. For at least some speakers, some of these systems show good hit rates, ranging from 95 to 99% correct identification of carefully spoken individual words. Although these current capabilities are a long way from being able to recognize unconstrained, running speech, it has occurred to several manufacturers and vendors that even such limited abilities can be useful in many software packages.

The claim has been made, and sometimes verified, that data and text processing can be done more quickly, more accurately, and less stressfully when the operator can enter verbal rather than keyboard commands. Therefore, commercially available systems concentrate on building vocabularies of commands for word-processing, spread-sheet, and data-base software. However, no one to date has developed a system based exclusively on the use of verbal commands. Generally, the state of the art allows verbal commands to work in conjunction with a set of keyboard commands. There is considerable optimism that most microcomputer users will find this to be of more than gimmick value, and many predict that speech-recognition devices will flourish in number and application over the next decade as the necessary hardware and software are developed and become less expensive.

In any event, what is available today is impressive, and it is clear that some aspects of current limitations will yield to greater computational power—memory, disk access, and processing time—and the development of more sophisticated algorithms for reaching decisions about the identity of the incoming sound waveform.

TYPICAL SPEECH-RECOGNITION STRATEGY

Imagine that you are given a dictionary that translates Chinese characters into their English equivalents. You have in your possession a large group of known patterns. These are stored versions of the physical characteristics of all possible Chinese patterns and their meanings. Suppose now that you are given a piece of paper containing one Chinese character whose meaning is unknown to you, but that you have a fairly strong motive to recognize it. You must extract its meaning and make it "known" to you. How do you proceed? You are likely to try to match this unknown pattern against each of the known patterns until you arrive at a satisfactory match. When you do, you can assume that the meaning of the unknown character is the same as the meaning of the known character.

Speech-recognition devices work just this way, using some variant of this "compare the unknown to a series of knowns and look for a satisfactory match" strategy. Some systems use extra decision steps before a final

Fig. 12-4. An example of the components and sequence of operations in a typical speech recognizer.

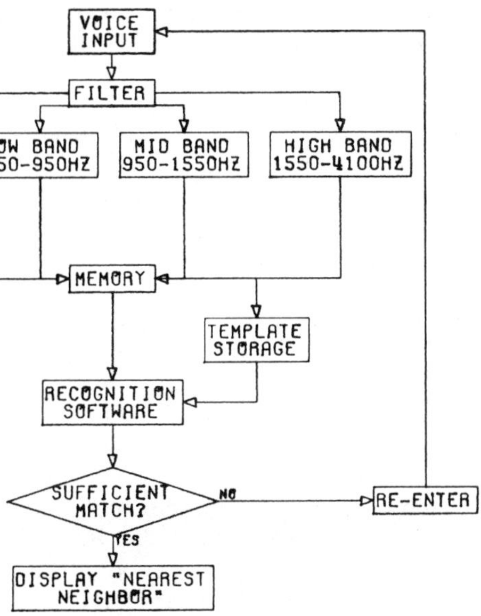

recognition is made, but all face the task of analyzing the incoming signal and comparing it to a stored set of reference or known patterns. Figure 12-4 is a representation of a typical approach taken by speech-recognition devices. The *voice input* represents a microphone, which converts the incoming acoustic waveform to a voltage. Some recognizers will work with virtually any microphone. Others are supplied with specially adapted microphones. For example, a low-sensitivity, highly directional microphone might be supplied if the system is intended to function well in a noisy environment.

The voltage waveform generated by the microphone is usually filtered, in part to remove spurious nonspeech noise, but in larger part to perform an acoustic analysis of the incoming waveform over time. Figure 12-4 shows four bandpasses. Many common recognition devices will split the incoming signal into as many as 16 frequency regions.

The signals present at the output of each bandpass are a reflection of the amount of energy present in the input signal within that bandpass at any given moment. The signals, however, are usually in analog form. They need to be digitized before they can be represented in the speech recognizer's memory. The AD conversion (not depicted in Figure 12-4) may use one of the techniques discussed in the preceding section. Linear predictive coding (LPC) techniques appear to be increasingly attractive to the developers of these systems. LPC allows time-frame samples to be digitally represented in relatively few data points. Hence, less computer memory is necessary to represent the parameters of the vocal-tract configuration necessary to produce a waveform the same as that present in a given frame. Alternatively, some recognizers use zero-crossings and the fast-Fourier transform to obtain a digital version of the amplitude spectrum in the time frame. In this way, formant values present in the output of each filter can be represented over time. Whichever technique is used, the outcome is a set of digitally extracted features of the input analog signal that can be stored in the speech recognizer's memory. The next step is to compare the representation of the unknown signal with a group of previously stored patterns, shown as *template storage* in Figure 12-4. It is, of course, critical that the features representing the stored templates be in the same form as those representing the unknown. The comparison is achieved by *recognition software* that computes the degree of match between the unknown pattern and each of the stored templates read into computer memory. Since both the unknown and known templates are represented by a large number of digital points, recognition software must make point-by-point comparisons and have a way of estimating the degree of similarity of each pattern match. This is usually accomplished through multidimensional analysis techniques that yield statistical *distance apart* estimates between the unknown and each of the knowns. The computer must then keep track of all the similarity estimates obtained for each comparison, choose the closest match—"nearest neighbor"—and decide whether the match is close enough to be considered an identification.

If the match is sufficient, and sufficiently distinctive from other comparisons, an identification is made. The word represented by the nearest-neighbor stored template may appear on the host computer's terminal, or be sent as a keyboard-emulated command to some application software currently running on the host computer. In this scheme, the best performance is obtained when the speaker is trained and the voice input is a carefully articulated, isolated word. The stored templates are digital representations of the time-distributed acoustic features of whole words. The recognizer has not attempted to break the incoming waveform into component phonetic features or done any other form of linguistic analysis. It has only received and compared digital patterns representing the acoustic waveforms of sound across time and chosen the best match.

To do this, speech-recognition devices have hardware components—microphones, filters, central processing units (CPUs) with given amounts of memory, and a means to store and retrieve template patterns—and software—programs to execute matches and reach decisions. Integration techniques have allowed many of these components to be placed on chips. The chips can be mounted on boards and inserted in an expansion slot on a microcomputer. Alternatively, the components can be housed in a standalone cabinet and interfaced to the computer, typically through a serial (RS232-type) interface. In either configuration, the speech-recognition device can be thought of as a dedicated microcomputer with ROM-based recognition software.

One of the major distinctions made about types of speech recognizers has to do with the stored templates. In speaker-dependent systems, each individual speaker who intends to use the system must enter his or her own template patterns. This process is known as *training* or *enrolling* the speech recognizer. If the targets to be recognized were the digits from zero through twenty, the speaker would be prompted to produce several repetitions each of these words. The speech recognizer would average the features extracted over each pronunciation of each target, and store those average representations as the *known* templates. Since enrollment can be a time-consuming process, and since it may be desirable to have several speakers enrolled on the system—a memory-consuming process—the known templates are usually written on floppy disks, from which they can be loaded to memory as needed by each system user.

The second approach is called *speaker-independent* recognition. In this scheme, the stored templates are obtained from a large group of speakers, averaged, and usually stored on a ROM chip. These systems are less time-consuming to set up, since no individual enrollment need occur. They are also potentially more flexible, as they purportedly recognize unknown words from a broad range of speakers. Speaker-independent systems, however, are usually less accurate than speaker-dependent systems (White, 1984), require more matches between known and unknown, require more memory-consuming recognition software (Levinson and Liberman, 1981), and are usually quite restrictive of vocabulary size.

Speaker-dependent systems have several advantages. The user can establish his or her own vocabulary file and often may have several sets of them. The language used need not be English. Even when it is, the dialect of the speaker need not be a mainstream version of English. The performance levels of some speaker-dependent recognition systems that work at the "whole-word" level have been very good. As noted by Doddington and Schalk (1981), however, there is no agreed-on protocol for establishing performance capabilities for comparative purposes. Their experience with evaluating specific systems showed that men are generally recognized better than are women. There is also considerable interspeaker variation. There are some speakers who cannot seem to enter "unknown" versions of a word that are sufficiently like the "known" version they produced themselves in the enrollment period. They just cannot seem to say the same word close enough to the same way consistently enough to be recognized.

LIMITATIONS OF CURRENT RECOGNITION SCHEMES

Two of the principal constraints on the performance of current systems are vocabulary limitations and poor (or no) ability to recognize words in continuous speech. Although a 40-word vocabulary might be sufficient to allow verbal control of a software program, it is clearly constraining considering the vocabulary range most adults can recognize in continuous speech. Levinson and Liberman (1981) estimate that most adults have a working receptive vocabulary of over 100,000 words.

Most of us could learn to input continuous text as a series of well-isolated—separated by 200 msec or so—carefully articulated words. Nevertheless, it would be a laborious task, and most nonhandicapped users would find it quicker to enter the text at the keyboard. Private and corporate research and development teams are well aware of these limitations and are beginning to implement hardware and software solutions—largely on mainframe and minicomputers—to overcome them. Vocabulary size is constrained at present by several inter-relating factors.

1. As vocabulary size grows, so does the probability that some pairs of words in the vocabulary are acoustically similar and therefore likely to be confused by the recognition software. One way a manufacturer can attain larger vocabulary files is by selecting words that are highly dissimilar to one another. Given the limits on word length that currently exist, however, it is inevitable that the potential for confusibility will increase as a vocabulary gets to some given, but still fairly limited, size.
2. As the vocabulary grows, so do the memory requirements for the microcomputer. Although available RAM for microcomputers has grown rapidly in a short time, it still imposes serious constraints on vocabulary size.
3. As vocabulary grows, so do the number of stored templates and the number of comparisons that must be made against each unknown template. This can lead to increased processing time for each comparison. If the computer's response lag for a verbal command is considerably longer than that for an equivalent keyboard command, the verbal command loses its advantage, and most users will choose the keyboard.

Unlike humans, speech recognizers have a more difficult time identifying a word in continuous speech than in isolation. The limitations of speech recognizers for identifying words in continuous speech derive from two main sources. Words in continuous speech do not have well-defined onset and offset boundaries. The software cannot rely on periods of relative silence to detect them, as it can when isolated words are input. These onsets and offsets are also subject to the great variability caused by the prosodic and coarticulation effects described earlier. Although enrolling words in the contexts in which they will occur helps overcome this problem, such a procedure is memory-consuming. Moreover, if the unknown sequences are entered with much variation in rate or tempo as compared with the known versions, temporal misalignments can "fool" the recognizer.

There are a number of hardware refinements on hand and on the horizon to address some of these limitations. One is to extract more acoustic features. Potentially, the confusibility inherent in large lists of words could be reduced if a more fine-grained digital representation of words could be accomplished through more detailed spectral analysis of the signal. More filter pass-bands could be used, and digital sampling rates could be increased. A second solution would be to increase RAM so that more stored templates can reside in memory at any given time.

Several vocabulary sets can be represented in RAM at once through disk emulators—RAM spoolers. Switching from one set to another does not involve the access and loading time problems inherent in conventional disk storage. The continued evolution of very large scale integration (VLSI) technology should also contribute to substantial reductions in accessing and processing time. Although such developments should allow considerably increased vocabulary size, most observers agree that there will be an upper boundary to vocabulary size given hardware developments alone. Even if hardware developments allowed very large (say 10,000-word) vocabularies, think of the time it would take each individual to enroll the speech recognizer!

SOFTWARE DEVELOPMENTS

Equally important in the solution to the current limitations of speech recognizers are developments in recognition software.

Temporal Normalization

Isolated word recognizers using whole-word templates can achieve better hit rates when the stored templates are adjusted to the duration of the unknown utterance. It is relatively easy to adjust known templates in a uniform way—through recognition software—for words that are bounded by relative silence.

Dynamic Programming

Dynamic programming (Kato, 1980; White, 1984) is a technique for nonuniform time normalization that has proved to be useful in the recognition of words in continuous utterances. Dynamic programming allows the segment durations of stored templates to be adjusted in a nonuniform way to obtain a "best temporal fit" to the unknown template. Hence, it represents a form of tempo normalization for the speech recognizer.

Different Units of Analysis

It has already been noted that a large number of known templates would be required to represent unconstrained speech. More finite representations of speech could be obtained through segmenting the speech input into other units. For example, there are 20,000 or so syllables in our receptive vocabularies. This is still a large number, so a more attractive candidate is the phoneme. If software could impose boundaries on the acoustic features extracted from hardware and use those boundaries to recognize individual phonemes, one could represent incoming speech as a se-

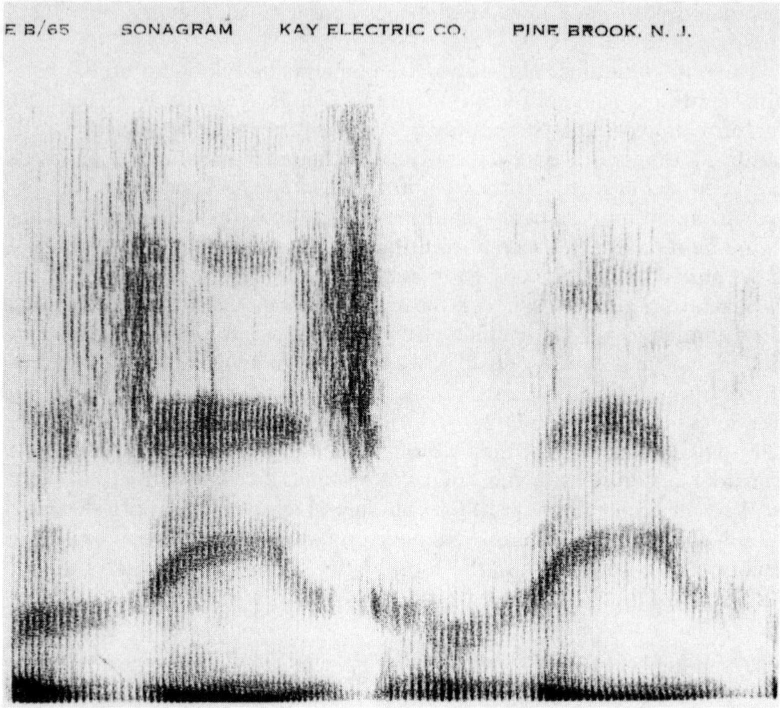

Fig. 12-5. Wide-band spectrogram of the nonsense utterance "Washahwaf."

quence of the limited number of phonemes in the language. However, there are many residual problems in this approach. Because of the great variability in speech production, phonemes are actually realized as a great number of allophones. No one knows exactly how many allophones there are in English, or how they are represented acoustically. Moreover, the boundaries between one sound and another are not distinct in human speech (see Fig. 12-5 for confirmation). Finally, it appears that human listeners can override the preliminary decisions they make at the phonetic level by searching for meaning. They can invoke semantic, syntactic, and pragmatic knowledge.

Recognition Software

Recognition software can use additional "linguistic" information in reaching a final decision on the identity of the continuous-speech input. An example of this approach is HARPY (Reddy, 1980), a minicomputer-based continuous-speech recognizer. HARPY is similar to conventional microcomputer systems in that it is speaker dependent and has hardware to convert continuous input into digitally represented acoustic segments. In addition, however, it has a phonetic segment algorithm that segments the acoustic representation into phone-sized templates. The initial comparisons are then made for individual sounds rather than for whole words. Like other recognizers, the comparisons yield a goodness-of-match estimate, or a probability that a given stored template represents the correct identity of the current unknown. HARPY's speech-recognition algorithm also uses rules of syntax and vocabulary to modify the probability estimates obtained by the phone-matching section. This information is in the form of probabilities of occurrence of the sentences that could be constructed from its 1000-word vocabulary. In this way, a phone or phone sequence with a low probability at the initial pattern-matching level could be selected by the recognizer if that sequence yielded a higher probability for the occurrence of the entire sentence. Other approaches to the recognition of continuous speech, such as that described by Kaplan (1980), are not so heavily linguistic as HARPY, but do use probabilistic data to select among possible alternatives represented by the unknown continuous-speech input.

These approaches are all guided, to some extent, by the human perceptual strategy of making a series of tentative decisions about the nature of the syllabic structure and phone identity of an utterance as it unfolds. This necessarily includes the ability to change those decisions on the basis of subsequent categorizations at the semantic and syntactic levels.

These hardware and software strategies will continue to evolve and should make it possible for microcomputers to recognize words in continuous speech in the near future. That is not to say that the speech input will be unconstrained, however. The sort of speech that microcomputers will recognize in anything like the near future may be restricted to a vocabulary in the low thousands of words, presented in constrained syntactic patterns, and require careful articulation by the speaker. Capabilities beyond that will come slowly.

Speech scientists still do not have a very explicit or detailed model of all the information humans bring to bear on extracting the meaning of speech utterances. Software developers cannot program what is unknown to them. Research on speech perception in humans has demonstrated that it is more than a signal-processing, template-matching operation. The boundaries in speech are fuzzy, and humans seem to resolve fuzziness on the basis of cognitive information that is not yet well understood. Increasingly, speech recognition by machine is being viewed as in large part a problem in artificial intelligence. White (1984) recently noted that,

> Speech recognition is not a typical engineering problem. It is a scientific Gordian knot. It draws on LSI (large-scale integration) and VLSI (very large-scale integration) chip design, signal processing, acoustic phonetics, natural-language theory, linguistics, mathematics of stochastic (probability) processes, and computer science techniques. Because of its multidisciplinary nature and because many competent minds have pondered the problem for years, we should not expect a breakthrough in speech-recognition capability. Progress will be made, but it will be evolutionary, not revolutionary. Naive enthusiasm from novices in the field sometimes leads to proclamations that dramatic progress is imminent. Such views fail to consider the interdependence of disciplines required to produce a commercially viable product.

SELECTION OF SPEECH RECOGNIZERS

Some of the currently available components that allow some microcomputers to act as word recognizers are presented in Appendix C.

Applications

Individuals spending a great deal of time using application software may indeed profit from using verbal commands as adjuncts to keyboard commands. Many manufacturers provide predefined vocabulary files that can be custom-tailored to some of the more popular word-processing, spreadsheet, and data-base management software currently available for microcomputers. The user would be well advised to obtain vocabulary files that are compatible with his or her application software.

Installation

One can safely assume that installation will require more than obtaining the right cable and loading a disk. One may have to obtain an interface to the microcomputer, such as an RS232, or mount a board on an internal expansion slot and interface the microphone to the board. Some disk-based software is usually included with recognition systems. Nevertheless, as with other hardware and software for microcomputers, the systems may not be free of bugs when they first appear in the marketplace. It will be necessary to spend some time with manuals, the quality and detail of which may vary considerably from system to system.

Enrollment and Testing Time

Available systems vary in the length of time required to train them. The amount of training time necessary depends largely on the size and number of vocabulary files, the number of repetitions of each target the system requires, and the manner and speed with which it prompts the user to repeat targets. Some speakers on some systems may require rather frequent re-enrollments as well. Enrollment should be made in the same environment as the entry of unknowns. It would be a mistake, for example, to enroll the system in a sound-treated room if it will be used on a production line.

Flexibility

It may be advantageous to be able to alter vocabulary files in a fairly simple way. If a predetermined vocabulary file supplied by the manufacturer has especially confusible words—such as *go* and *no*—and you intend to use those commands to control application software, disastrous consequences could follow from errors made by the recognizer interchanging these words and performing the wrong action. If *go* could be changed to *leave* by the user, the problem might be avoided. Not all acoustically confusible words are as immediately obvious to a human, for whom the distinctions are implicitly based in linguistic knowledge, as they will be to a computer working without this knowledge. Users are well advised to test their speech-recognition systems with less-than-precious data to discover and alter confusible commands.

Rates and Types of Errors

One of three things can happen when an utterance is entered into most speech recognizers. It can be correctly identified (a hit). It can be recognized as a different word in the vocabulary file (a false-positive or substitution). It can be rejected on some programmed criterion. In some recognizers, the rejection threshold can be adjusted by the user. This can be a convenient feature, especially if the system is to be used by several individuals, or in a difficult or highly variable acoustic environment. Setting recognition thresholds so that fewer rejections are made should improve the system's hit rate but at the expense of a rise in substitution errors (Doddington and Schalk, 1981). For some applications, this may prove to be an unsatisfactory trade. If the recognizer is acting in some way as a keyboard emulator, a high reject rate may slow the user's application, but at least not at the expense of entering undesired text, data, or commands.

The selection of speech-recognition devices should be done with the same caution a person would exercise in the selection of any microcomputer hardware or software. A clear notion of the applications desired, a good working knowledge of one's current hardware and software (and the extent to which available speech recognizers are compatible with them), and a strong commitment to spend the time necessary to investigate, choose, install, and become familiar with the system are necessary. Preliminary hands-on experience and inspection of the documentation also help considerably in making an informed decision.

APPLICATIONS FOR THE HANDICAPPED

It has been estimated (Dahmke, 1982) that some 500,000 Americans could use some form of synthetic speech as a prosthesis for nonfunctional motor speech. When one adds other handicapped populations that could potentially profit from speech-synthesis and speech-recognition devices—the visually impaired, the hearing impaired, and the mentally retarded—it is clear that the handicapped population that could derive benefit from these technologies is large and underserved.

Many of the devices listed in Appendices B and C, although not specifically intended for the handicapped, can nevertheless be used as is for some handicapped individuals. Visually impaired individuals could profit from the use of a speech synthesizer that provides text-to-speech synthesis. They could hear the commands and text entered at the keyboard, or have telecommunication text read as it is received by the terminal. Individuals with motor impairments who retain enough manual ability to work a keyboard could use either type of conventional speech-synthesizer system. Conventional speech recognizers may be useful to those with severe motor handicaps not affecting the oral mechanism. As previously mentioned, virtually any microcomputer can be made to talk, and most can be made to recognize speech to some limited capacity. There are frequent articles (e.g., Demasco and Foulds, 1982) detailing the particulars of interfacing a given microcomputer with a speech synthesizer or recognition system.

For individuals whose handicaps are so severe that they cannot access a conventional keyboard quickly or reliably enough, an increasing array of specially modified synthetic-speech devices is available. Appendix A contains a representative sampling of some of these devices. These devices can be divided into three general groups: portable dedicated speech synthesizers, nonportable communication boards, and talking terminals.

Portable Dedicated Speech Synthesizers

Dedicated, portable, prosthetic speech synthesizers are battery operated and usually use a flat membrane keyboard divided into a matrix of rows and columns of square cells. Each of these cells is a key corresponding to some stored segment of speech—words, phrases, sentences, phonemes, etc. Each cell in the matrix is labeled in some way on the keyboard. This is usually done with an orthographic or pictographic representation. The more elaborate—and expensive—of these devices use several registers for the keyboard. These registers can be thought of as separate vocabulary files. Keyboard overlays represent the currently selected file. A membrane keyboard with 128 cells and 5 registers can store 5 vocabulary files of 128 utterances each. Often, one or two of these registers can be programmed by the user. Some of these systems will store sequences of keys in buffer memory and allow their playback as a concatenated string, often with overlaid prosodic information. A few allow speech to be represented as a phoneme code and contain synthesis algorithms capable of doing text-to-speech synthesis so that the user can program any message within his or her linguistic capability. Most of these systems must be accessed directly by the user, through a finger-touch or mounted pointer stick, and many are supplied with keyboard guards to help prevent spurious cell selection.

Nonportable Communication Boards

Nonportable communication boards are in many ways similar to the portable devices just discussed. What is lost in portability is gained in terms of flexibility. Individuals whose motor impairments are such that they cannot use a direct-access mode of selection on any keyboard often retain the ability to control some switching mechanisms in a reliable way. Many of these electronic boards allow cell selection through a switch-controlled optical-scanning scheme. The user can use the switch to operate the keyboard indirectly. Some of these boards are supplied with speech synthesizers, and some allow the addition of an outboard synthesizer as an option. Some of the more sophisticated systems can be interfaced with other devices, such as microcomputers or environmental-control systems. Thus an individual with sufficient cognitive ability can gain access to the operations of microcomputers for programming, writing text, accessing information networks, running application software, and controlling aspects of the environment such as light, heating, and the like. Not surprisingly, some of these boards are rather expensive. For some individuals, however, they can lead to dramatic improvements in terms of independence and social and vocational horizons.

Talking Terminals

These are essentially conventional microcomputers that have been outfitted with speech-synthesis devices that allow spoken output of what appears on the microcomputer's monitor. Unmodified, they are especially useful for the visually impaired. We have referred to these as MICRO devices in Appendix A.

Selection Considerations for the Handicapped

Many considerations, as outlined by Silverman (1980), should go into the selection and implementation of a speech prosthesis. Ideally, thorough evaluations should be performed in order to obtain valid estimates of each individual's cognitive, linguistic, motor, vocational, and social abilities. Such estimates are useful in determining the complexity, flexibility, and portability characteristics of a system suitable for that individual. Particular care needs to be exercised in "interfacing" the individual to the system—many switch types and mounting arrangements are possible, and particular choices may have to be arrived at empirically. For these reasons, individual clinicians should seek multidisciplinary assessments for candidates for these systems, including trial fittings, from individuals who are well-informed and well-experienced in selection and "installation." Several regional centers offering these services have evolved over the last few years, and clinicians should be informed about what is available in their geographic areas.

Finally, it is important that clinicians, clients, and their families have realistic expectations about speech prostheses. The synthetic speech they generate is usually based on some of the popular chips employed in the devices listed in Appendix B and is subject to the same limits of quality. They also require a normalization period on the part of the listener, as discussed in the section on speech synthesis. An additional limitation of devices for the handicapped has to do with access and assembly time for constructing messages. We are accustomed to very short response times in the give and take of conversation, and as Vanderheiden (1983) cautions, the quality and timeliness of the synthetic speech available in most prostheses severely constrain their easy use in conversation.

For the present, meeting a handicapped individual's communication needs in an adequate way may entail several systems: a prosthetic voice, a nonportable system for school or vocational work, a telephone transmitting device (TTD) for telephone use, and a portable note writer for quick business or consumer situations. As with speech synthesizers and speech recognizers for microcomputers, the immediate future will show some evolutionary improvement in quality and access time.

CONVERSING WITH COMPUTERS

Computer synthesis and recognition of speech have advanced remarkably during the past 5 years, both in sophistication of technique and in commercial availability of inexpensive products. These factors have led to a growing interest in computerized communication devices. Speech facilities are being added to many popular software packages, and a multitude of computerized devices are being designed for the speech impaired and handicapped. Computer recognition of continuous speech, however, is still a problem that will require major advances in the fields of artificial intelligence and speech science.

Speech synthesis and limited recognition capabilities are available for several software packages. The Echo II speech synthesizer, for example (see Appendix B), has been incorporated into a talking word processor, a data-base manager, a check register, a calendar, a filing system, and an intelligent terminal program. Many more talking products are likely to appear on the market within the next few years. Speech synthesis may even be a standard option on future computers and terminals.

As microcomputers expand in memory and processing ability, speech synthesizers can represent more detail in source and filter representations of speech sounds, more detailed models of coarticulation effects in smoothing algorithms, greater flexibility and realism in prosodic patterns, and a larger and more detailed inventory of exceptions in the pronunciation dictionary. The human data base to guide such improvements is substantially in place. Improvements in text-to-speech synthesis largely rest with hardware improvements.

Speech recognition presents a more difficult and complex problem, and the advent of the truly conversational computer awaits a major breakthrough in that area. Even so, the limited speech recognition capabilities currently available are finding useful applications in the fields of business, industry, banking, and rehabilitation. Speech-recognition systems typically require less user training, are more convenient, and can receive data faster and more accurately than the traditional method of typing on a keyboard. Such systems might also be useful for voice verification and user recognition as part of a computerized security system (McMahon, 1984). All of these applications can be implemented using the current technology. Computer recognition of continuous human speech cannot, however, be so implemented.

In the realm of speech recognition we can expect to see larger vocabulary files and faster access of those files. These combined advances in storage and access capabilities should lead to higher recognition rates and perhaps even some limited ability to recognize words in context.

The achievement of computer recognition of continuous speech will require a major advance in the field of artificial intelligence. The current recognition strategies cannot be merely modified and improved in an evolutionary fashion until they come closer to the human ability to understand speech (Zadeh, 1984). Today's methods have still not dealt with the difficulties pointed up by Pierce in 1969 and Lea in 1970. The basic problem is not one of limitations in computer hardware or in programming technique; it is a speech-science problem rather than a computer-science problem.

A human being has "a general sense of what a conversation is about," is able to abstract a pattern of relevant information from a large mass of acoustic data, and can decipher a meaningful utterance (Pierce, 1969, p. 1049). This human process includes summarizing incoming data, associating it appropriately with already accumulated data, making a series of assumptions about the speaker, resolving ambiguities, and arriving at some meaning. Traditional computer techniques for processing information are not good at summarizing, working associatively, resolving ambiguities, or arriving at meaning. There needs to be a radical shift in the way computers are designed and programmed to achieve these capabilities but, because the process by which the human brain accomplishes these tasks is so little understood, that shift is not likely to occur in the foreseeable future.

REFERENCES

Anderson, J. Talk is getting cheaper. *Creative Computing*, pp. 137–147, Dec. 1982.

Dahmke, M. Let there be talking people too. *Byte*, pp. 7–8, Sept. 1982.

Demasco, P., and Foulds, R. A new horizon for nonvocal communication devices. *Byte*, pp. 166–182, Sept. 1982.

Doddington, G. R., and Schalk, T. B. Speech recognition: Turning theory into practice. *IEEE Spectrum*, pp. 26–32, Sept. 1981.

Kaplan, G. Words into action: I. *IEEE Spectrum*, pp. 22–26, June 1980.
Kato, Y. Words into action: III. A commercial system. *IEEE Spectrum*, p. 29, June 1980.
Lea, W. A. Evaluating speech-recognition work. *J. Acoust. Soc. Am.* 47:1612–1614, 1970.
Levinson, S. E., and Liberman, Y. Speech recognition by computer. *Sci. Am.* 244:64–76, 1981.
McDermott, J. The solid-state parrot. *Science 83*, pp. 59–65, June 1983.
McMahon, M. TI's Mike McMahon discusses speech technology. *Personal Computing*, pp. 237–241, Jan. 1984.
Pierce, J. R. Whither speech recognition? *J. Acoust. Soc. Am.* 46:1049–1051, 1969.
Reddy, R. Words into action: II. A task-oriented system. *IEEE Spectrum*, pp. 26–28, June 1980.
Shane, H. C., and Bashir, A. S. Election criteria for the adoption of an augmentative communication system: Preliminary considerations. *J. Speech Hear. Disord.* 45:408–414, 1980.
Silverman, F. S. *Communication for the Speechless*. Englewood Cliffs, N.J.: Prentice-Hall, 1980.
Songco, D. C., Allen, S. I., Plexico, P. S., and Morford, R. A. How computers talk to the blind. *IEEE Spectrum*, pp. 34–38, May 1980.
Vanderheiden, G. C. Non-conversational communication technology needs of individuals with handicaps. *Rehabil. World* 7:8–12, 1983.
White, G. M. Speech recognition: An idea whose time is coming. *Byte*, pp. 213–222, Jan. 1984.
Zadeh, L. A. Coping with the imprecision of the real world. *Commun. ACM* 27:304–311, 1984.

APPENDIXES TO CHAPTER 12

These appendixes provide sources of information about some of the speech synthesis and recognition systems and devices for the handicapped currently available for microcomputers. We do not intend to review or endorse any of the products listed or to purposely exclude any product which might not be listed. We intend only to provide information so that your search for an appropriate device is informed, quick, and easy.

Most of the information in these appendixes was obtained from independent product reviews and manufacturers' specification sheets or promotional literature. While we have tried to ensure the accuracy of the information at the time we obtained it, the computer hardware and software marketplace is unstable. Rapid change in product enhancements and capabilities almost ensure that some inaccuracies will exist. We recommend that you call or write a manufacturer or vendor, carefully read their promotional literature, and perhaps discuss your particular application with them before you purchase any device.

Such publications as *Communication Outlook* and *PRC Current Expressions* (see the Selected Reading list at the back of this book) are good additional sources for product information.

Appendix A lists synthetic speech devices developed as aids for the handicapped. Many of the devices listed in Appendix B and Appendix C could also be used by the handicapped, though some modification may be necessary.

Appendix A. Speech Synthesis Devices for the Handicapped

Product	*Company*	*Type*	*Comments*
AVOS System	Avos Inc. 1485 Energy Park Dr. St. Paul, MN 55108 (612) 646-1515	MICRO	Avos Z-80 based micro, 64K, 2 disk, CP/M voice driver speaks words as they appear on screen. Intended for visually impaired. Price: $3000 (Review: *Creative Computing*, Dec. '83, 332–333)
ALLTALK	Adaptive Communication Systems Box 12440 Pittsburgh, PA 15231 (412) 264-2288	DPSP	Memory sufficient for 800 words. 128 squares accessed on membrane keyboard using magnetic sensor. Overlay available.
COMPUDAPTER	R/M Systems 22903 Fern Ave. Torrence, CA	BOARD	External keyboard emulator for Apple II. Allows keyboard to be controlled by 3 touch controls. Intended for motorically impaired.
EXPRESS 3	Prentke-Romich Co. 8769 Twp. Road Shreve, OH 44676 (216) 567-2001	BOARD	Communication board 8 × 16 matrix, can be direct selected or switch controlled. 18K user programmable characters. Optional Apple interface and speech output. Price: $3780; speech output, additional $825
FORM-A-PHRASE	Sci-Tronics, Inc. 114 Stillwood Dr. Coraopolis, PA 15108 (412) 264-2288	DPSP	Main unit with speech synthesizer. Control units available (keys, number board, word board). Vocabulary supplied in ROM. 128 utterances. Price: main unit $1450; each control unit $130–$800
MINSPEAK	Prentke-Romich Co. 8769 Twp. Road Shreve, OH 44676 (216) 567-2001	BOARD	Language prosthesis board with software. Requires keyboard emulator & speech synthesizer. Uses Ideographic symbols. Flexible & expandable. (Review: *Communication Outlook*, Fall '83, 8–11)

SAY IT	Schneier Communication 1603 Court St. Syracuse, NY 13208	BOARD	Software allows single switch control of Apple II. Output printed or spoken. Price: $40 Also markets QUICK TALK word & sentence generator.
SPECIAL FRIEND	Shea Products Inc. P.O. Box 184 Clawson, MI 48017	DPSP	Membrane keyboard allows text-to-speech synthesis. Can program keys to store messages. Overlap available.
TALKING TRANSEND	Transend Corp. 2190 Paragon Dr. San Jose, CA 95131 (415) 424-0900	MICRO	Modified electronic communication package for Apple II & IIe. Includes modem, Echo II synthesizer (see Appendix B).
VOXTRAN TRANSEND	Texas Instruments P.O. Box 402430 Dallas, TX 75240 (800) 527-3500	DPSP	Membrane keyboard with several overlays (36 locations each). Stored speech not user programmed. Can spell out any message.
VOIS-130	Phonic Ear, Inc. 250 Camino Alto Mill Valley, CA 94941 (415) 383-4000	DPSP	Membrane keyboard, synthesizer. Has over 350 words, phrases, and morphemes stored. Can also work with text to speech. Bliss symbol/word overlap available. Price: $3000
WORDS + PORTABLE VOICE	Words + Inc. 6225 Fair Oaks Ave. Sunnyvale, CA 94086 (408) 730-9588	MICRO	Epson MX20 portable computer & text-to-speech synthesizer. Flexible version has external switch panel to control keyboard. Price: $1450

Terms: DPSP (dedicated, portable, speech prostheses); MICRO (allows synthetic speech to be output from computer or terminal); BOARD (allows synthetic speech and/or ability to control microcomputer through modified control unit).

Appendix B. Some Currently Available Speech Synthesis Hardware and Software for the Microcomputer

Product	*Company*	*Type*	*Microcomputer/Comments*
Cognivox VIO-1003	Voicetek POB 388 Goleta, CA 93116 (805) 685-1854	Voice record playback	Apple II 32K, disk, DOS 3.3 externally housed unit with microphone & power supply; voice recognition & synthesis. Price: $300 (Review: *Byte*, Sept. '82, 231–235)
COMVOICE	Genesis POB 1143 Bethlehem, PA 18018 (215) 861-0850	Text to speech	Commodore 64, VIC 20. Speaker/amplifier included.
DECtalk	Digital Equip. Corp. 1 Burlington Woods Burlington, MA (617) 273-6500	Text to speech	RS232 serial, self-contained. Telephone interface/touch-tone business applications. Price: $4000 (Review: *InfoWorld*, Jan. '84, 21–23; *Mini-Micro Systems*, Mar. '84, 52–54)
DX-1 Sound Process System	Decillionix POB 70985 Sunnyvale, CA 94086 (408) 732-7758 [call (408) 735-0410 for phone demo]	Voice record playback	Apple II uses 24K, music, etc. Price: $150
ECHO	Street Electronics 1140 Mark Ave. Carpinteria, CA 93013 (805) 684-4593	Text to speech	ECHO II—Apple board, disk, 48K, 700 words, woman's voice. Uses Applesoft, PASCAL, or graFORTH; data-base manager & word processor available. Prices: $150; ECHO PC–IBM, RS232 serial port $200; ECHO GP–general-purpose, speaker, RS232 & cable interface $200 (Review: *Creative Computing*, Dec. '82, 120–130, 137–147; *Computing Teacher*, Apr. '84)

INTEX-TALKER	Intex Micro Systems 725 S. Adams Rd. L8 Birmingham, MI 48011 (313) 540-7601	Text to speech	Self-contained with speaker jack, RS232 serial & 34-pin parallel-edge connector. Price: $300
MICROVOX	Micro Mint 561 Willow Ave. Cedarhurst, NY 11516 (516) 374-6793	Text to speech	Build-your-own (Ciarcia's Circuit Cellar, *Byte*, Sept.–Oct. '82). Price: assembled $300; kit $219; 3K-buffer $15
PC Parrot	Dragon Data Systems 1068 Homer St., Suite 110 Vancouver, BC, Canada V6B 4W9 (604) 255-0584	Voice record playback	IBM PC needs: disk drive 64K. Price: $40
PROSE 2000/2020 CALLTEXT 5000	Speech Plus 461 N. Bernardo Ave. Mountain View, CA 94043 (415) 964-7023 [call (415) 969-6257 for phone demo]	Text to speech	Small business computers using multibus standard IBM PC or compatible RS232 serial port. Telephone interface for touch-tone access. Price: $2700 (Review: *PC Magazine*, Jan. '83, 68–69)
S.A.M. Software Automatic Mouth	Don't Ask Software 2265 Westwood Blvd. Suite 150 Los Angeles, CA 90064 (213) 397-8811	Text to speech	Atari 400, 800 32K, 1 disk. Apple II, II+, 48K, 1 disk Blanks out screen during vocal output. Price: $60; circuit board & speaker incl. $125 (Review: *InfoWorld*, 5:41–42; *Creative Computing*, Dec. '82, 137–147)

Appendix B. (continued)

Product	*Company*	*Type*	*Microcomputer/Comments*
Speech Master	Tecmar Inc. 23600 Mercantile Rd. Cleveland, OH 44122 (216) 464-7410	Text to speech	IBM PC Prices: Speech Master Board $400; Speech Master Software $100 (Review: *InfoWorld*, Feb. 13, '84, 68–69)
Type-N-Talk	Votrax Inc. 1394 Rankin Troy, MI 48083 (313) 588-2050	Text to speech	TRS-80 Models I, II, III, Color; Apple II needs serial card; Atari 400, 800; 850 interface module required; IBM PC needs RS232 serial port; IMSAI 2SIO (Review: *PC Magazine*, Jan. '83, 308–312; *Creative Computing*, Dec. '82, 120–130)
VOICEBOX	The Alien Group 27 W. 23rd St. New York, NY 10010 (212) 741-1770	Text to speech	Commodore 64 disk or cassette; VIC 20 cassette, 2K RAM used. Price: $130 (Review: *Creative Computing*, Dec. '82, 137–147)
Voice Master	COVOX Inc. 6/5-D Conger St. Eugene, OR 97402 (503) 342-1271 [call for phone demo]	Voice record playback	Commodore 64; microphone supplied; 64 words-in-memory limit. Price: $90

Terminal Emulator II	Texas Instruments Speech Department M/S 6426 9901 S. Wilcrest Houston, TX 77099	Text to speech	Can be interfaced with many micros; voice synthesis processor and memory computer chips available.

Voice Synthesis Processor and Speech Development System Regional Technology Centers:
Information, Customer Support, One-Day Instructional Seminar:
Speech Synthesis Technology Course No. ATS-400. Price: $150

BOSTON 400-2 Totten Pond Rd. Waltham, MA 02154 (617) 890-6671	CHICAGO 515 W. Algonquin Rd. Arlington Heights, IL 60005 (312) 640-2909	DALLAS 1001 E. Campbell Rd. Richardson, TX 75081 (214) 680-5066
ATLANTA 3300 N.E. Expressway Atlanta, GA 30341 (404) 452-4682	NORTHERN CALIFORNIA 5353 Betsy Ross Dr. Santa Clara, CA 95054 (408) 748-2220	SOUTHERN CALIFORNIA 17620 Fitch Avenue Irvine, CA 92714 (714) 545-5210

Appendix C. Some Currently Available Speech-Recognition Hardware and Software for the Microcomputer

Product	*Company*	*Type*	*Microcomputer/Comments*
APPLE VOICE INPUT MODULE	Future Solutions 3198-7 Airport Loop Costa Mesa, CA 92626	Speaker dependent/ isolated words	Apple II, Plus, IIe; DOS 3.3, 48K, 1 disk; add-on board supplied; 80-word max. Price: $920 (Review: *Electronic Education*, Jan. '84, 40–43)
AURICLE	Threshold Technology 1829 Underwood Blvd. Delran, NJ 08075 (609) 461-9200	Speaker dependent/ isolated words	Hewlett Packard PC through IEE-488; 120-word max vocabulary. Other micros: 80-word max. Price: $1500
COGNIVOX V10-1003	Voicetek Box 388 Goleta, CA 93116 (805) 685-1854	Speaker dependent/ isolated words	Apple II, 48K, 1 disk; built-in speaker; 32-word max. Price: $300 (Review: *Byte*, Sept. '82, 231–235)
SCRATCH PAD with VOICE DRIVE	Supersoft Box 1628 Champaign, IL 61820 (217) 359-2112	Speaker dependent/ isolated words	Recognition board supplied. Spread-sheet applications; 100-word max. Prices: IBM PC $1500; TI Professional $2600 (Review: *PC World*, Dec. '83, 38–43; *Personal Computing*, Apr. '84, 24–26)

SPEECH COMMAND SYSTEM	Texas Instruments POB 402430 Dallas, TX 75240 (800) 527-3500	Speaker dependent/ isolated words	TI Professional, MS-DOS 256K. Recognition board supplied. Spread-sheet applications; 9–50-word max vocabularies. Transparent keyboard util. Price: $2600 (Review: *Computers & Electronics*, Dec. '83, 40–43; *Popular Computing*, Feb. '84, 142–150)
VOICE BASED LEARNING SYSTEM	Scott Instruments 1111 Willow Springs Denton, TX 76201 (817) 387-9514	Speaker dependent/ isolated words	Apple II, IIe; 48K, DOS 3.3, 2 disk; authoring software for training material develop; 40-word max vocabulary.
VOICE INPUT MODULE INTROVOICE	Voice Machine Comm. 1000 S. Grand Ave. Santa Ana, CA 92705 (714) 541-0454	Speaker dependent/ isolated words	Includes 8K RAM memory; 80-word max; mod II: 160 max. Prices: Apple & Franklin $850; 1 disk, has board $1000
V8500	Votan 4487 Technology Dr. Fremont, CA 94538 (415) 490-7600	Speaker dependent/ isolated words	IBM PC can be used with IBM applications programs; 256-word max. Price: $10,000 (Review: *Computer Decisions*, Feb. '83, 49–51; *Popular Computing*, Feb. '84, 142–150)

13

Microcomputers and Hearing Aids

James Curran and
David Preves

An emerging recognition of the need for better systems of hearing aid amplification, better methods of application, and better procedures for assessing the satisfaction, benefit, and use of amplification has arisen at a time when microcomputers and microprocessor technology are beginning to flourish. The everyday use of the microcomputer and familiarity with digital techniques will soon be a fact of life for both clinical and research activities. The obvious advantages that accompany the use of a microcomputer and associated technology in the clinic or laboratory setting have been summarized in other chapters in this text. The barriers of initial high cost, unfamiliar technology, inordinate expenditure of time to learn, and inadequate processing power are all rapidly falling away. Clinicians faced with real-world needs to incorporate a more powerful, precise, and efficient procedure into their clinical and research activities will find it increasingly easier to do so with personal computers.

The application of microprocessor technology to the measurement, design, selection, and fitting of hearing aids is a fairly complex area. The utilization of digital circuitry and microcomputers is not only obviously applicable to the development of computer-assisted hearing-aid fitting programs, but also is integral to the design and development of hearing aids and the acoustic measurement instruments used for analyzing their performance. Digital technology may be used to form portions of the circuitry of hearing aids, especially microcomputer-controlled programmable hearing aids.

COMPUTER-ASSISTED HEARING AID SELECTION AND FITTING PROGRAMS

One of the most evident applications of the personal computer is in the development of programs for the selection, evaluation, and fitting of hearing aids (Agnew, 1983). The audiologist has many different methods or strategies from which to choose. For instance, a program can be used that calculates the estimated required gain at a given use setting based on a given formula, after which the computer proceeds to search its memory to select hearing aids that fulfill the criteria (Berger and Gans, 1984; Glascoe, 1984). Or, a program may be developed not only to list all appropriate aids, but also to rank them from most to least appropriate. Computer software programs are available that predict aided thresholds using a trial

The authors wish to express their appreciation to Barry Voroba, Ph.D. and Gerald Popelka, Ph.D. for their contributions in the preparation of the manuscript. We are grateful to William Austin, President, Starkey Laboratories, for his personal support of this project.

hearing aid and attached custom ear mold, which may then be compared to functional gain measurements to show both the desired and actual aided hearing-threshold change. Another hearing aid evaluation method incorporates probe microphone measurements into the fitting protocol. The desired aided response is compared to actual performance with the computer as adjustments and modifications are performed on the hearing aids and ear molds (Preves, 1982; Rasmussen, 1984). Any number of additional approaches or methods are available to the audiologist for implementation. With imagination and planning, any of the common hearing-aid evaluation and fitting strategies in use today can be adapted in such a way that a personal computer can be utilized in the administration of the protocol.

The *Preliminary Hearing-Aid Selection System* (PHASS) (Craig and Siegenthaler, 1981) is an example of a type of preparatory program that might be considered useful for selecting an aid or group of aids for further evaluation in the clinic. The program was developed to minimize problems related to inventory control, human error, bias, and inconsistency in the initial selection process. Recognizing that the busy clinician ordinarily does not have time to perform an exhaustive search for appropriate models, the PHASS selects aids according to ten descriptors including gain, output, and reference-test gain. The features and performance of the desired aids are determined by the clinician. This type of program depends entirely on the skill of the audiologist in correctly selecting the appropriate hearing aid characteristics; the computer program merely identifies those aids in stock that possess all or most of the features and performance characteristics desired. Preselection of hearing aids from stock, using this approach, is primarily a housekeeping program with the added benefit of quickly reducing to a small pool those aids under consideration for the client during the evaluation process.

Another program, *Hearing Aid Manager* (Glascoe, 1984), is similar to PHASS. It also is designed for any facility that has to handle a large number of aids. It differs from PHASS in that aids are entered into memory according to 27 or 28 individual features, or descriptors, rather than 10. The descriptors are taken directly from the specification sheets, or from hearing aid test-box results.

One of the earliest reports of a specifically dedicated computer-assisted hearing aid fitting program was by Glascoe and Johnson (1975). With the use of a minicomputer, a program was developed that utilized two thirds of the speech reception threshold (SRT) to find the lower limits of desired gain and used average maximum power output (MPO) – 10 dB to define the upper limit of the gain range. Instruments whose full on-gain values fell within this range were selected as appropriate for the subject.

Recently, a rash of microprocessor-based computer-assisted fitting programs has become available. A typical example was reported by Gans, Ver Hoef, and Berger (1983). Based on the Berger formula (Berger et al., 1980), the program requires the entry of pure-tone thresholds, the air-bone gap, and uncomfortable loudness level (UCL) measurements to yield a generic prescription (i.e., desired gain values that constitute an initial "ball park" estimate).

Essentially, the program relieves the operator from the hand computation the Berger formula requires. In its original form the program had no provision for search and selection of appropriate instruments, nor did it provide a recommendation as to which would be most suitable. Recently, however, Berger and Gans (1984) reported an updated version that includes capability for searching the memory for instruments that have the performance characteristics that satisfy the criteria as developed by the formula. A feature of the program is the incorporation of an adaptive "goodness-of-fit" algorithm—that is, the computer continually searches memory for instruments that fit the desired gain values. If the user wishes to find the three instruments that are most compatible, the program initiates a continuous search until the three best-matched instruments are found. If no instrument is found that matches very precisely the desired target gains, the computer adjusts automatically to a wider acceptance criterion and continues the search using the expanded window of acceptability until three matches are located. There is a provision for in-the-ear, behind-the-ear, monaural, and binaural selections, as well as of signal hearing aid CROS selections, and any number of instruments can be added to or deleted from memory according to the wishes of the operator.

Glascoe (1984) has developed *Hearing Aid Selector* (HAS) that also utilizes the Berger formula to obtain desired gain values. It can be used in conjunction with his *Hearing Aid Manager* to select desired instruments from a large pool of aids stored in memory. A program has been developed by Stacey (1984) in Great Britain that incorporates a data base of response curves of hearing aids, based on 2-cm^3 coupler measurements. An automatic comparison between the optimal desired gain values (again based on the Berger formula) and the individual aid responses is initiated after target gain values are derived, in order to ascertain the best matches.

Recently, Moomaw (1984) introduced the *Systematic Hearing Aid Prescription* (SHAP) program. After entering pure-tone thresholds and UCL for selected frequencies, the operator then selects from a menu of options, including compression versus linear instruments, type of instruments required, type of ear mold required, and criteria in decibels for an acceptable match. The gain is calculated from the patient's audiometric data, and an algorithm based on the POGO method is used (McCandless and Lyregaard, 1983). POGO is a modification of the half-gain rule that utilizes insertion gain values rather than 2-cm^3 coupler gain values. Frequency response changes (based on averaged corrections), which result as different ear molds are specified, are automatically added to the target gain values. Provision for adding or deleting a hearing aid from the file is included. A built-in set of correction factors converts 2-cm^3 coupler data to insertion gain values. A display and printout shows the operator which aid(s) most closely match the desired gain and SSPL90 as determined by the algorithm, and the distinctive features for each acceptable instrument are listed.

Another commercially available computer-assisted fitting program, *Computer-Assisted Hearing Aid Fitting and Sales Program* (Katz, 1983, 1984), takes a slightly different approach to the fitting process. The program stores 2-cm^3 coupler responses of instruments and then calculates the amount of insertion loss, average corrections because of ear mold type, and pinna and concha effects. After entry of pure-tone thresholds, most comfortable loudness (MCL), and UCL, the clinician decides the amount of threshold shift desired at each frequency. The computer searches its list of aids (up to 600 can be stored), displays full on-gain values by frequency for each aid considered acceptable, and reports the amount of volume control rotation in percent required to provide the gain desired by the clinician. It also rates the closeness of match between desired gain and available gain in the aids. In addition, the individual audiogram can be displayed, and the combined frequency response of the selected hearing aid and ear mold can be superimposed on the hearing loss to provide a visual display of the presumed correction that will be provided. All data can be printed out, if desired.

An interesting feature of the *Computerized Fitting Analyzer* program (Preves, 1984) is the incorporation of a proprietary response selection procedure for in-the-ear aids. Values for selection of the appropriate frequency response for in-the-ear aids are provided by an algorithm Starkey Laboratories utilizes in its daily design of custom circuits. Provisions for selecting optional features such as Select-A-Vent, automatic gain control (AGC), and tone controls are also available. The printout is provided in a generic format and displays SSPL90, peak gain, and response-curve slope values. Behind-the-ear aids are selected by the use of a formula based on the combined averaged values of three traditional hearing aid selection procedures.

Another proprietary computerized fitting system has been reported by Feldman (1982). The Beltone *Certifit* method involves the use of time sharing and teleprinter terminals placed in dispensing offices for transmission and reception from a central computer. The central computer is programmed to recommend an instrument based on a goodness-of-fit approach, and the criteria for the match are selected by the dispenser. Either a computer-generated algorithm for gain and response selection based on the modified Berger approach is available to the dispenser, or the operator can select a 5-dB per octave or other slope response. Pure-tone thresholds, UCL, MCL, and discrimination scores are used to generate the final recommendation. Data from all fittings are stored in the central computer and are readily available for retrieval and analysis of long-term trends.

Lauridsen and Nielsen (1981) constructed a real-ear hearing-aid fitting system around a Hewlett Packard 9815 desk-top computer. An analog-to-digital converter converts the output of a probe-tube microphone to digital form, and subtractions are performed to determine the etymotic or insertion gain response. The computer is also used to set up control sequences for each type of measurement. The project has been extended by the authors to make available a commercial system (Rastronics Computer System CCI-10) that performs the same functions (Nielsen, 1984; Rasmussen, 1984).

Popelka and Engebretsen (1983) developed a comprehensive computer-based program that attempts to account for as many of the factors influencing individual performance and corrections as possible. Earphone measurements of the auditory system, sound-field measurements involving hearing aids, and coupler measurements of hearing aids can all be expressed on a single graph providing a reasonable representation of what is happening at the eardrum of an individual wearing a particular hearing aid. Many of the factors associated with the *individual* coupling (canal geometry, ear-mold effects, venting, etc.) can be accounted for on an individual basis. Currently, the program uses functional gain, but probe microphone or probe tube approaches can also be employed.

The Central Institute for the Deaf CID Computer Software–Phase IV (1985) program displays results by showing what the hearing aid is doing to the incoming sound, rather than showing what the hearing aid is doing to the auditory system. In an audiogram format, thresholds are shown in the same place on the graph for both the unaided and the aided conditions (aided thresholds are not shown). A typical speech spectrum at normal conversational levels is used for the unaided condition. The results of a hearing aid are depicted by placing the speech spectrum farther down the audiogram, depending on the actual gain (at the eardrum) at each frequency region. The program can be used for any hearing aid and any magnitude or type of hearing loss. In addition, it can show the SSPL90 of an aid at the eardrum (rather than in the coupler). The program does not rely on any specific fitting strategy. One could choose any available method and use the CID program to verify (at the eardrum) that the fitting procedure was being implemented accurately.

Popelka advocates a fitting procedure (Pascoe, 1980) that brings the speech spectrum to the MCL range and limits the amplified spectrum from entering the UCL range over a wide bandwidth (Skinner and Miller, 1983; Skinner et al., 1982). Thus, if MCL and UCL are entered, the computer program can determine if the Pascoe method is being properly implemented. The computer program, however, does not require that one use this fitting philosophy exclusively. For example, a fitting strategy stating that the speech spectrum should just be audible could be used. In this case only thresholds need be entered into the computer; MCL and UCL could be omitted. The computer facilitates the many transformations required, for it easily handles all correction factors, data analyses, and reference values.

Voroba (1982) has recommended an approach to computer-assisted hearing aid fitting that represents a marked departure from prescriptive methods. In his system, the hearing-aid response is not determined through algorithms based on audiometric parameters. Amplification is, instead, selected by the hearing-impaired listener within the framework of the method of paired comparisons, a classic psychophysical task. His rationale arises from the recognition that there exist significant limitations in the understanding of relationships between audiometric data and effective amplification. Moreover, in the case of in-the-ear aids, even the best prescriptive algorithms are vulnerable to many intervening decisions and variables in the manufacturing process that typically alter the hearing aid's output.

With the development of a computer-based programmable auditory comparator, Voroba (1984) addresses these concerns with reference to in-the-ear aids by providing exact correspondence between the amplification preferred during the hearing aid evaluation and that provided by the delivered instrument. An essential factor in achieving this correspondence is the use of the identical canal aid shell and transducers for both the test module worn during amplification selection and the final hearing aid. The test module becomes the finished hearing aid once the amplifier circuit is added. Thus, any variation in earshell acoustics that might have occurred during manufacturing are avoided.

Another aspect of the "principle of correspondence" involves the use of real-world sound-field stimuli during the amplification-selection process. Pretaped specimens of the listener's actual work, home, or play environments serve as the background within which the preferred amplification is chosen. A second channel provides the listener with a target speech signal of connected discourse. Both stimuli are presented to the subject while the test module is worn. The listener monitors a console as each of two hearing-aid amplifier circuits is switched into the test module via an umbilical cord. The subject must adjust the level of amplification for maximal comfort and choose a preferred circuit by pressing a button below the display window.

The microcomputer in this system enters the preferred circuit coordinates in its memory and, based on preprogrammed rules and instructions, presents the subject with a different pair of amplifiers for the next tournament evaluation. When a final amplifier preference has been determined, a duplicate circuit is installed in the test module, thereby transforming it into the finished hearing aid. Internal programmable digital circuits are visualized as being more appropriate than duplicate circuits; the eventual use of these circuits is expected to increase the correspondence between the test instrument and the one actually worn.

Practical Decisions

A key aspect of any hearing aid evaluation procedure includes decisions and information pertaining to monaural versus binaural fittings, directional versus nondirectional instruments, AGC versus linear circuitry, new versus old user, need for telephone coil, and choice of type of aid (in-the-ear, behind-the-ear, eyeglass, or body). These choices are often difficult to make, for clear-cut criteria are not always apparent from an examination of the patient's history or circumstances.

In exactly what manner can the microcomputer be used to resolve these issues? The trite saying, "garbage in, garbage out" is never more true than in this instance. The program author must have a definite idea as to what outcomes are expected *before* program development. To expect a computer magically to produce answers to problems of hearing aid evaluation that have escaped easy resolution by audiologists since the beginning of the profession is extraordinarily naive. The computer is capable only of rapid numeric computations and will not provide an answer to a fitting problem that has not been addressed by the creator of the program.

A brief examination of the actual chain of events involved in the design of a typical computer program may assist the clinician interested in developing his or her own program, and may help in the analysis of commercial programs.

The steps involved in developing a computer program include, but are not confined to, the following:

1. *Defining the problem.* This includes identifying the variables and formulating an exact statement of the problem.

2. *Developing the algorithm.* This is simply a step-by-step specification of the solution to the problem.
3. *Making a flow chart of the algorithm.* A flow chart diagram is an illustration of the sequential actions and decisions performed by the computer program.
4. *Programming the algorithm in the language of choice.* The actual generation of the program code may be executed by the clinician after some familiarization, or it may be done by a computer professional.

Thinking clearly about each step of the task at hand is an absolute prerequisite to program writing. Once the program is formulated, a specific algorithm must be developed to provide a solution. The solution to the problem, however, is only as good as the original thought processes of the author.

The following discussion provides an illustration of the types of problems that are typically encountered and must be resolved in the design of any computer-assisted fitting program. The prescriptive strategy where the hearing aid's electroacoustic performance is selected on the basis of threshold and similar measures is analyzed because it appears to lend itself to easy computerization. Whatever strategy is eventually chosen for computer implementation will present its own unique set of issues that will mandate carefully arrived at decisions by the author. The eventual compromises employed in the program will determine the level of predictive utility that can be expected when it is put into effect in the clinical or research setting.

Predicting Electroacoustic Parameters from Pure-Tone Thresholds

A common strategy for incorporating the microcomputer into the fitting process uses pure-tone thresholds, as well as MCL, UCL, and other values as predictors of appropriate gain and saturation sound pressure level (SSPL 90). The programs are designed to provide an approximate estimate of desired, or target, gain levels that can be used to order custom in-the-ear or canal aids. Alternatively, the computer may be asked to find a number of aids in memory that satisfy the criteria. The clinician is then relied on to adjust the instrument(s) and ear mold(s) to the perceived needs of the subject. Aided thresholds (functional gain measurements), speech audiometry, or other measures may be used as criteria of sufficient fit.

This appears to be a common-sense approach to computer-aided fitting and is a perfectly adequate strategy for the initial selection of an instrument. Any attempt to force or impute a higher level of predictive rigor or precision, however, simply fails in light of what is known about aided performance on the individual.

Many factors have been identified as tending to influence the performance of the individual with the hearing aid (Pascoe, 1980). They are not all accounted for in the simple predictive relationship mentioned above. Several modify the distribution of energy at the eardrum in the aided condition, and each plays a part to a greater or lesser extent in the essential arrangement of spectral energy. The contributions of each factor in many respects is unknown in terms of amount of influence exercised. Moreover, each is subject to systematic, predictable, control by the clinician to only a limited degree. These reflections should not be overlooked in considering the development or purchase of a computer-based hearing aid fitting program that uses pure-tone thresholds as the independent variable.

Factors that tend to produce output differences when the aid is worn and that cannot be predicted or controlled with any measure of accuracy include (1) position of the microphone, (2) intramodel electroacoustic performance variations, (3) ear hook and tubing properties, (4) ear-mold configuration, (5) ear-mold circumference leak, (6) space between the tip of the ear mold and the tympanic membrane, and (7) impedance of the middle-ear system.

An associated area of concern regards the manner of storing the electroacoustic performance of each instrument in memory. When entering the gain, SSPL90, and other parameter values of a specific model into the computer, the author can either record the published full on-gain (or insertion gain) and SSPL90 values in the normal condition as obtained from specification sheets, or, alternatively, measure each given aid individually. In addition, the effect of the volume-control position and taper on the gain (full on, or insertion, or reference test?) could be entered, all or in part, depending on the perception of the author. Similarly, the change in output spectrum that occurs as the individual controls are varied (such as reduction of the SSPL90 or low-cut trimmers), and the effect of automatic gain control circuitry on the performance of the instrument could also be considered for storage. The choice of parameters, the method of entry, and the rules followed will materially affect which instrument(s) are selected for trial by the computer program.

When one considers the foregoing, one must conclude that any computer-based program developed to assist hearing aid selection and fitting that uses pure-tone thresholds as a predictor of gain and response must somehow deal with the questions and considerations cited in order to provide an acceptable level of fitting success (Donnelly, 1982). Similarly, *every* method of hearing aid evaluation, on close analysis, will reveal its own sources of error, which have the potential to affect validity to a greater or lesser degree. The likelihood of coherent outcomes will increase in direct proportion to the quality of the decisions the author makes as each source of error or difference is scrutinized and evaluated. Failure to acknowledge this core understanding may lead to the development of computer-based fitting programs that appear elegant and specific on the surface, but which in reality lack essential validity and, ultimately, clinical utility.

Clinician or Computer?

As previously stated, some determination is required, as part of the problem-analysis step, as to whether a computer is really necessary. Perhaps certain fitting decisions can be made simply and quickly by the audiologist without the involvement of the computer.

For example, regarding the issue of binaural versus monaural fittings, a clinician might write a set of arbitrary rules suggesting that binaural fittings are indicated only when (1) thresholds are symmetric and no greater than 15 dB apart in each ear, (2) both thresholds are greater than 45 dB hearing level (three-frequency average), (3) the user is under 18 years of age, (4) the discrimination scores for the two ears are better than 50% bilaterally, and (5) differences between discrimination scores for the two ears are no greater than 30%. A program could be easily constructed so that the entry of basic historic and audiometric data would automatically result in a computer-provided decision to fit or not to fit binaural instruments. Nevertheless, one must ask whether the decision to fit binaural aids could not have been made just as quickly and easily by the clinician after a simple, rapid examination of the data.

Suppose, instead of the explicit criteria outlined above, other, more complex and subtle considerations are believed to be critically important in arriving at a decision. These considerations might include (1) the candidate's need to function in an environment where binaural advantages are required (binaural summation effects, loudness squelch in noise, elimination of head shadow, localization), (2) the degree of motivation, (3) the presence of unhappiness with previously fitted monaural instruments, (4) the cosmetic appearance of the individual instruments, (5) the size of the ear, (6) the telephone-ear preference, (7) the person's desire to drive, or perhaps (8) the clinician-held belief that even when discrimination scores are poor, and the thresholds and scores are grossly asymmetric, more often than not trial with binaural amplification may still be desirable. Even in the situation described, it may very well be that the wisdom and experience of the clinician would *still* provide a quicker, more valid real-time decision than could the computer. In order to provide computer-assisted answers that would consistently concur with the experienced clinician's judgment of the situation, a very intricately designed algorithm would be required with quite specific ratings and values assigned to various degrees of behavioral and situational factors.

ASSESSMENT OF HEARING AID CANDIDACY

Current approaches to hearing aid selection assume that most individuals are candidates for amplification if they voluntarily initiate the evaluation process and hearing loss is, in fact, present. However, certain conditions or factors in the individual's hearing history may indicate that special procedures or precautions are required. Such conditions might be, for example, an external-ear anomaly that makes it difficult to attach a conventional behind-the-ear or in-the-ear instrument. An alternative fitting, perhaps a bone-conduction instrument, might be required. Or, as the history is obtained, it might become apparent that sufficient motivation is lacking. Some subjects seek confirmation of their own belief that an instrument is unnecessary, and when this attitude is coupled with borderline impairment, it may be justifiable to postpone a trial with amplification.

A subject may appear to be a good candidate audiometrically, but factors such as lifestyle or communication needs may make him or her a poor candidate. The reverse may also be true. In cases where little loss is apparent, the history may show an obvious need for amplification. The experienced audiologist knows that in evaluating hearing-aid candidacy the chances for eventual success are a combination of many factors, each of which must be weighed separately in the individual case in order to arrive at a beneficial judgment.

Given the subtle complexities that may enter into the decision, can a computer help a clinician make a better judgment? One attempt, reported by Fitch (1984), involves a computer-assisted program that requires the subject to answer a series of questions before being tested by the audiologist. The questions are an assessment of communication needs plus some of the "soft" factors involved, such as judgments of finger dexterity or sensitivity. After testing, the answers to the questions are combined with the audiometric results. The computer uses the results of the questionnaire and the test data to rate the individual from poor to excellent in terms of candidacy. One of the side benefits of the program is that summaries of patient histories, reports to referring sources, etc., also can be automatically generated based on the information obtained from the questionnaire and the audiometric tests.

The success or failure of such programs, however, depends not only on the thoroughness and appropriateness of the questions themselves, but also on the time spent entering the data (is it excessive?) in relation to the benefits obtained, and on the algorithm developed. Each question, clinical judgment, and test result must be assigned a value in order to provide an overall rating. The individual items can be arbitrarily selected, or perhaps derived from one of the well-known questionnaires used to assess communication needs.

CONSIDERATIONS FOR A COMPUTER-AIDED FITTING PROGRAM

One returns again to the vital question that should be answered before such a program is purchased or implemented. Is a computer really required to solve or help to resolve a specific hearing-aid selection and fitting problem? A brief set of considerations might point to an appropriate decision.

Expenditure of Time

Is speed of the essence? One can contrast a research-clinical or teaching environment, where the time required to derive and to input large amounts of data is available and is not an overriding issue, to the purely clinical environment where any time-saving assistance is enthusiastically welcomed, or where the expenditure of excess time is counterproductive. If efficient expenditure of time is extremely important, and repeated analysis of complex events by hand is impossible to perform routinely, obviously a well-designed computer program is invaluable.

The time required to input air and bone conduction pure-tone thresholds, MCL, UCL, probe-microphone measurements, and other results for storage in the computer's memory is a problem that must be considered. By the use of certain peripherals, notably digitizing boards or graphics tablets, time expenditure can be markedly reduced. These types of data-entry devices eliminate the need for keyboarding or following a relatively slow, menu-driven program. Those clinicians who have experienced the intense level of activity found in a busy, successful audiologic practice can appreciate how critical it is that any computer program be swift of execution, easy to operate, and not interrupt the normal flow of activities.

Trend Analysis

Will the data be used to identify trends over a period of time? A very powerful portion of any computer-assisted fitting program can be the ability to store recommendations of fittings and compare the fitting decisions and the electroacoustic parameters of the aid to both the audiologic measures entered at the time of initial fitting and to a measure of satisfaction or benefit that can be obtained at a subsequent time. In this way, one can begin to discern trends relating to successful or unsuccessful recommendations or fittings (Walden et al., 1982). Provision must be made for entering subsequent changes to a fitting, such as adjustment of trimmers and ear molds and similar acoustic modifications, in order to assure the accuracy of the findings.

Computer-assisted trend analysis may possibly be the most compelling argument for the development and installation of a computer-assisted fitting program. Such a program provides the capability to monitor quality and accuracy constantly by performing an ongoing analysis of events. It provides a major opportunity to increase precision in clinical skills, it is amenable to ongoing changes in delivery of services, and it is the perfect vehicle for upgrading and tracking efficiency.

Repeatability

Is there need for ensuring repeatability of decisions? Occasionally, on retrospective analysis, clinicians find that they specified dramatically different fittings for clients who presented nearly identical audiometric measures and needs at two different periods of time. Or, two audiologists engaged in dispensing in one facility may be making totally dissimilar recommendations for clients who have relatively similar findings. This lack of agreement suggests that no unified, reliable protocol or procedure exists that guarantees approximate correspondence in cases involving like characteristics. In this instance, the question of correctness or accuracy of the recommendation or fitting is not being examined (validity); rather the question of repeatability of decisions is under discussion (reliability). A necessary step to reduce random outcomes in hearing-aid selection, if this appears to be a desirable goal, requires the application of a protocol that assures repeatable results regardless of individual clinical bias. Providing for subsequent changes and modifications due to clinical judgment is also absolutely necessary, but the use of a computer-based fitting strategy has the potential to assure an initial set of recommendations or target values that serve as a common basis for the subsequent fitting (Correll, Ludvigsen, and Nielsen, 1983).

Patient Education and Counseling

Will a properly devised software program facilitate hearing-aid acceptance, orientation, and follow-up? The task of hearing-aid fitting does not cease with the evaluation; an especially critical period ensues when the patient decides whether to agree with the recommendations of the clinician. A computer-derived display or printout can both inform and persuade the client of the appropriateness of the fitting and help motivate him or her to accept and use the recommended aid(s). Moreover, a series of individually tailored lessons can be generated based on the specific patient's history, communication needs, and audiologic test results to provide systematic, controlled aural rehabilitation activities combined with constant reinforcement.

Report Generation

Can time and effort be saved and the quality of reports improved by use of a computer? The possibility of freeing the audiologist from routine, repetitious report writing to attend to other, more clinically important tasks is appealing. Form letters with the option for inserting individual data, findings, or recommendations are certainly possible to devise, but the risk of producing letters that are nearly identical save for pertinent data may not be considered an attractive alternative. An intelligent judgment concerning which reports could be best provided in computer format, as opposed to those requiring greater individual attention, is necessary. Report generation can be implemented with a word processor separate from the microcomputer. Or, by using a printout spooler, the personal computer can be used for data entry, while a separate document is being printed simultaneously.

Data-Management Requirements

Is there a need for fast, efficient handling of a myriad of complex, detailed data? In point of fact, computer-assisted hearing aid fitting programs offer as one of their main features—in one form or another—the capability of handling large amounts of data in a rapid, efficient manner.

The computer-based fitting program developed by Popelka (Pascoe, 1978; Popelka and Engebretson, 1983) involves the entering of a great deal of data. Although the time to fit one ear with this program is estimated to be approximately one hour, considerably more time would be required if all necessary computations were to be performed by hand. In this instance, it is very obvious that the need for data-handling capability is of such high priority that it would have been clearly unfeasible to contemplate such a fitting protocol without the use of the computer.

One of the valuable advantages provided by computer-aided evaluation programs is rapid manipulation of correction factors. Correction factors have been formulated for types of ear molds, amount of venting required, transfer of data from 2-cm^3 coupler response to insertion response, head and body baffle effects, etc. Other transformations related to the condition of audiometric and aided measurements must be generated depending on the formulation of the algorithm. For example, hearing thresholds obtained under earphones may have to be adjusted to reflect corresponding levels in a sound field, or coupler-derived gains may be displayed in terms of hearing level and then superimposed on the patient's audiogram. The popular formulas suggested for hearing-aid selection have some (but not all) of the necessary corrections and transformations already integrated into them. Parenthetically, many of the corrections utilized incorporate average values and do not account for specific individual differences. To be sure, a certain degree of approximation may be all that is desired; nevertheless, it is essential that all potential sources of variability be properly appreciated. Whether or not averaged correction factors are used, however, many numerically based transformations and other corrections are useful and necessary and lend themselves to easy and rapid handling by computer.

DIGITAL COMPUTERS IN HEARING AIDS

The incorporation of digital technology into such consumer devices as wristwatches and hand-held computers has not yet been paralleled in hearing aids (Cole, 1983). Hearing aid designers have been accused of not taking advantage of the latest technology available—namely digital signal processing—to solve some of the outstanding problems with current hearing aid fittings. However, incorporating a digital computer with adequate computing power for this application in a head-worn hearing aid that operates with a low-voltage battery is not a nontrivial packaging task. Available off-the-shelf microprocessor-integrated circuits powerful enough to be applied to this task are generally too large physically and require too much battery current to be housed in hearing aid cases of the size currently being marketed.

If digital computers could be packaged in hearing aids, it would be possible to perform digital signal-processing functions to eliminate the problems of environmental noise and acoustic feedback that plague current hearing aid fittings (Preves, 1982). A hearing aid with a digital computer would process input data under program control with software instructions written by programmers. Basic to such a mechanism are three steps: analog-to-digital conversion, adaptive filtering of the converted input signal by the central processor, and digital-to-analog conversion.

Nunley et al. (1983) have reported the development of a prototype digital hearing aid. The microphone, receiver, and power supply are contained in a behind-the-ear case and connected by a cord to the digital circuitry, which is packaged in a case worn on the body. The complete unit has been designed to provide adaptive filtering plus some type of noise suppression in real time.

Engebretson et al. (1984) have been awarded a 3-year contract from the Veterans Administration to design, implement, and evaluate a wearable, digitally based hearing aid at the CID. The goals are to formulate a digital hearing aid that can be programmed during the clinical evaluation process. The system will automatically determine the hearing threshold levels, most comfortable listening levels, uncomfortable levels, and calculate the required gain and SSPL values so that the mean sound-pressure levels of conversational speech fall within the MCL range and never exceed the UCL. The computer will be hooked to the digital hearing aid to shape the spectrum selectively and to provide frequency-selective output limiting. The algorithm is based on existing techniques that are currently implemented at CID by a four-channel analog-domain master hearing aid (Engebretsen and Miller, 1982; Skinner and Miller, 1983). Each channel consisting of a bandpass filter driving a hard limiter is followed by another bandpass filter to attenuate the harmonics generated by the peak-clipping process. For the evaluation process, the digital fitting system will generate speech and vary the amount of background noise. The digital hearing aid will be automatically programmed by the fitting selector. The hearing aids will have head-worn transducers housed in a conventional hearing aid case connected by wires to a belt-worn circuit module and battery pack. After preliminary field evaluations are completed, the goal is to package the unit entirely in a head-worn configuration.

Levitt et al. (1985) advocate using a powerful array processor controlled by a minicomputer to enable the hearing aid to perform extensive signal processing that could not be performed easily by analog electronics. Trade offs have been investigated in sampling rate and hearing-aid bandwidth versus amount of real-time signal-processing capability. It is surprising how little signal-processing capability remains with two such powerful computers when the sampling rate is only 25 kHz.

One of the reasons for the relatively low sampling rate utilized by Levitt (1985) is that not only is analog-to-digital and digital-to-analog conversion being performed, but also the array processor is being used to transform the sampled time signal waveforms into the frequency domain with a technique known as the Fourier transform. Although signal processing in the frequency domain presents advantages over that in the time domain, the fast Fourier transform (FFT) and its inverse take many cycles of computer time to accomplish, even for only 256 frequency points, which limits the amount of time available for signal processing before the next sample from the analog-to-digital converter arrives. Since this sophisticated and very large combination of two computers is many times more powerful than computers available in integrated-circuit size for packaging in small head-worn hearing aids, the immediate future does not look particularly bright for incorporating a similar digital computer assembly into a miniature hearing aid case and having it perform many significant functions.

The foregoing should not obscure the fact that custom microprocessor-integrated circuits (as opposed to standard, off-the-shelf circuits) can be designed specifically for hearing aid applications. By careful attention to design objectives, it is theoretically possible to fashion custom digital circuits today that can be used in hearing aids, although there still exist limitations of scope and practical difficulties related to power supply, size, etc. One example of a special-purpose digital computer totally packaged as a CMOS (complementary metal-oxide semiconductor) integrated circuit designed specifically for hearing aid use is the Graupe-Causey adaptive digital noise-rejection filter (Graupe, Beex, and Causey, 1982). The CMOS uses integrated circuit technology that results in very low current consumption by the battery. With this device, the signal itself is not converted to digital form in order to save space and achieve realistic size for hearing-aid use. However, sophisticated noise-rejection performance is still accomplished by the use of digital circuitry to control analog filters.

A prototype of the Graupe-Causey adaptive filter connected to a body-worn hearing aid has been evaluated for noise-rejection capabilities by a normal-hearing group and by groups with mild and moderate-to-severe hearing impairments (Stein and Dempesey-Hart, 1984). Speech discrimination scores were obtained with and without the filter in a quiet environment and with competing backgrounds of cafeteria noise, babble, and white noise. In general, all three groups of listeners demonstrated significantly higher speech-discrimination scores in noise with the Graupe-Causey adaptive filter than without it.

The Graupe-Causey circuit (to be introduced commercially as the Zeta Noise Blocker) is currently being tooled as a single CMOS integrated-circuit chip having dimensions approximately 4 by 5 mm. It has an *on-board voltage multiplier* and thus is capable of operating with conventional 1.3-volt hearing-aid batteries. The chip will have a drain current no greater than 300 μA. Because amplification is not included on the integrated circuit, an external preamplifier and power amplifier are still required in the hearing aid, which will make the package rather large. However, introduction of this device will mark the first use of a truly digital computer in a contemporary head-worn hearing aid case.

As mentioned earlier, the ultra-low current drain CMOS-type circuitry is not usable for the hearing aid application *unless* a higher battery voltage than that provided by existing head-worn hearing-aid (1.3-volt) batteries is available (Cole, 1983). Many CMOS circuit technologies operate at a minimum of 3 volts, which requires use of a voltage-tripler circuit (as used in the Graupe-Causey adaptive filter) or use of alternative battery technologies such as lithium-based batteries. However, most lithium batteries in use today for watches are designed for pulsed duty-cycle operation (current is drawn only briefly and periodically). Thus, these high-output impedance batteries can provide only relatively low amounts of the constant current required by hearing aid receivers in their continuous audio- and speech-processing applications. Some available 3-volt lithium batteries are now coming close to providing more than 100 hours of battery life, while supplying a constant current drain of over 1 mA.

Programmable Digital Hearing Aids

Although currently marketed hearing aids have considerable adjustment capabilities provided by SSPL, AGC, and tone-control potentiometers and switches, they are relatively limited because of physical space constraints as to the overall variation in performance that may be obtained. By replacing the adjustment potentiometers with a multiplying digital-to-analog converter, digital switches, and digital memory storage, a hearing aid conceivably could produce almost any realizable combination of gain, SSPL, and frequency response. Parameters for each hearing aid wearer's most desirable frequency responses and combinations of SSPL and gain could be stored within the digital ROM (read-only memory). In a further extension of this concept, EPROM (erasable programmable read-only memory) or EEPROM (electrically erasable programmable read-only memory) could be used to permit changes to be made in the stored parameters after the initial fitting, according to the changing requirements of the user.

Mangold and Leijon (1979, 1981) have designed and evaluated a hearing aid circuit that digitally stores several frequency-response contours that are considered desirable for the hearing aid wearer. The different frequency responses would be accessed by means of the wearer activating a push-button switch. The device is currently being tooled as two integrated circuits, one analog and one digital, for use in head-worn hearing aids.

Computer Simulation of Hearing Aid Performance

Modeling techniques used in computer-aided engineering (CAE) for representing transistors, resistors, inductors, and capacitors in electronic circuitry have been applied to represent the circuitry, transducers, and tubing in hearing aid fittings in terms of electrical components. In order to accomplish this task, basic electroacoustic analogs are utilized to convert acoustic components to electronic components. A frequently encountered situation requires converting the length and diameter of a tube protruding from a cavity of known volume to a series of capacitors, resistors, and inductors representing acoustic compliance, acoustic resistance, and acoustic mass, respectively.

De Jonge (1983) created such an electrical analog with 38 parameters for a hearing aid receiver connected to an ear hook 23 mm long, terminated by No. 13 tubing 46 mm long to the tip of the ear mold and driven by a constant voltage source. With a microcomputer, he simulated parallel vents of varying lengths and diameters in the ear mold, which terminated in the electrical equivalent of a modified Zwislocki ear simulator. The frequency resolution for his simulation was one-tenth of an octave from 125 to 6000 Hz, except at the resonant peaks, where the resolution was increased to one-fiftieth of an octave. He also compared the frequency response in a simulated 2-cm^3 coupler and noted the decrease in high-frequency response as compared to that in the modified Zwislocki ear simulator. Simulations were performed with the middle-ear impedance varied to reflect otosclerotic and disarticulated pathologic conditions.

Egolf (1978, 1980) compared the computer simulation of hearing-aid frequency responses to actual frequency responses obtained by measurement of hearing aid performance on an artificial ear using ear molds having no vent, a side-branch vent, and a parallel vent. His results show strikingly similar performance obtained between computer-simulated and measured conditions. One of the most difficult aspects of modeling a hearing aid fitting is to represent the transducers accurately, particularly the receiver of the hearing aid, in analogous electronic parameters.

Bade et al. (1984) predicted the magnitude and phase of the output sound-pressure level of a hearing-aid receiver-earhook and ear-mold system in a 2-cm^3 cavity on a Hewlett Packard 85 personal computer. The computer programs used were written in ENHANCED BASIC, which, in combination with the limited computing speed of the processor, resulted in very long computing times. Corrections were made to model the effects of tubing attached to the microphone within the hearing aid case. For each simulation made, a corresponding actual measurement was obtained in order to test the validity of the simulation. It was found that the predicted values of output sound-pressure level were within 5 dB of the actual measurements over the frequency range 100 to 6000 Hz.

A Hewlett Packard 85 personal computer has also been used by Karzon and Niemoeller (1983) to model a commercially available hearing aid for the purpose of predicting the output speech and noise-spectrum levels to be expected as input levels are varied. Unique to this model is simulation of the hearing aid being driven into saturation by speech and noise. The model was developed empirically from the input/output characteristics of a hearing aid fitting obtained with speech and with narrow bands of noise at 250, 500, 1000, 2000, and 4000 Hz. Parameters measured included the effects of adjusting gain control, tone control, and output-limiting potentiometers. Second-order polynomials were found that produced the best fit with the empirical data. Validity of the model was checked by comparing the simulation predictions with data obtained from actual measurements. The occluded ear simulator (Zwislocki) was used as the termination for the hearing aid. The resulting discrepancies were found to be less than 4 dB under any input or control-adjustment condition. The authors concluded that the modeling technique could be applied in the actual fitting of hearing aids only if (1) all hearing aids could be easily modeled, including those with automatic gain control, (2) individual ear, head, and torso diffraction could be accounted for, (3) one could predict the effect of speech and noise combined while the aid was in saturation, and (4) the output of the simulation was in a form that could be easily correlated to the output format of conventional hearing aid measurements.

MEASUREMENT OF ELECTROACOUSTIC PARAMETERS

The electroacoustic tests defined by the American National Standards Institute (ANSI) Standard S3.22-1976 to measure the performance of hearing aids for quality-control purposes became required labeling in 1977 at the instigation of the Food and Drug Administration. As a result, these tests have been implemented on several microprocessor-based hearing-aid analyzers. The use of computers for this application became a necessity because of the time-consuming averaging and subtraction required for manually calculating the reference-test gain-control setting.

Prior to the S3.22-1976 ANSI Standard, computers were used to a limited extent in hearing aid analyzers to control automatically the sequence of tests performed. In this function, the measurement data from the hearing aids were not converted to the digital domain, but remained in analog form. Thus, the computer was used only for process control, rather than for generating the stimuli and for operating directly on the data. However, in more recent hearing aid analyzers, the computer actually generates the sine-wave stimuli, and the data are converted to digital form by an analog-to-digital converter and stored in memory for future calculations and output (Feldman and Malacek, 1977). This enables the digital computer to perform calculations of such parameters as average gain, average SSPL90, equivalent input noise, and total harmonic distortion. Basic to the use of a digital computer for a hearing-aid analyzer application is the critical requirement that enough bits are used to provide adequate amplitude resolution over at least a 50- to 150-dB sound-pressure level and that enough frequencies are sampled to provide an accurate representation of frequency response. Deficiencies can result in loss of fine structure detail in frequency-response curves.

One of the most important functions performed by the computer in some hearing-aid analyzers is the equalization or leveling of the loudspeaker output across frequency in the test chamber. Such a calibration procedure is required, for example, to ensure that a 60-dB input sound-pressure level is maintained at the hearing aid microphone inlet at all frequencies while a frequency-response curve is being obtained.

IN SITU MEASUREMENTS

Computers can be used to equalize the sound field for manikin and real-ear measurements of hearing aid performance in situ much in the same way that they are used to level or equalize the sound field produced by a loudspeaker in a hearing aid-analyzer test chamber. The result is that the computer will control the level of the sound field at the location of the control microphone in the test booth during the leveling or equalizing calibration sequence. The location of the control microphone, and the resulting operations performed on the data acquired by the computer, for example, determine whether insertion gain or in situ gain is measured. In order to measure insertion gain, the unaided sound-pressure levels must be subtracted across frequency from the aided sound-pressure levels. The computer in a hearing-aid analyzer is ideal for this subtraction function.

COMPUTER-BASED HEARING AID DISPENSING SYSTEMS

Popelka and Engebretson (1983) have suggested a computer-based audiologic system that includes modification of a commercially available hearing aid analyzer to interface it to a central computer. Results of all patient tests, including hearing aid characteristics, would be stored in the computer to allow future comparison and correlation.

Similarly, a computer-based hearing aid fitting system was suggested by Preves (1982). This system would consist of a computer-based audiometer, a computerized fitting prescriptor, a wearable computer-based fitting simulator, and a computerized hearing aid tester. These devices would "talk" to each other when connected together on a communications bus. For example, the fitting prescriptor could automatically calculate the recommended electroacoustic characteristics as a starting point for the hearing aid fitting from the audiologic data transmitted to it from the audiometer. The fitting simulator would automatically set up its gain, SSPL, and frequency response to the coordinates transmitted to it by the fitting prescriptor. The performance of the fitting would be verified by the hearing aid analyzer with conventional 2-cm^3 coupler or ear-simulator measurements, or by obtaining real-ear measurements on the patient in situ. Any adjustments required would be automatically transmitted back via the prescription verifier to adjust the electroacoustic parameters produced by the fitting simulator.

REFERENCES

Agnew, J. The role of the small computer in hearing aid fittings. *Hear. Instr.* 34:7, 1983.

Bade, P., Engebretson, A., Heidbreder, A., and Nielmoeller, A. Use of a personal computer to model the electroacoustics of hearing aids. *J. Acoust. Soc. Am.* 75:617–620, 1984.

Berger, K. W., and Gans, D. P. *Hearing Aid Selection by Computer.* Kent State University: Speech and Hearing Clinic, 1984.

CID (Computer Software-Phase IV). St. Louis: Central Institute for the Deaf Publications, 1985.

Cole, W. A. Prospects for the applications of high technology to hearing aids. *Hear. Instr.* 3:1, 1983.

Craig, C. H., and Siegenthaler, B. M. Preliminary hearing aid selection by computer. *Hear. Aid J.* 34:2, 1981.

De Jonge, R. Computer simulation of hearing aid frequency responses. *Hear. J.*, 36:27–31, 1983.

Donnelly, K. G. Computer assisted hearing aid fitting. *Hear. Instr.* 33:7, 1982.

Egolf, D. Computer predictions of hearing aid sound spectra. *Hear. Aid J.* 31:6–8, 1978.

Egolf, D. P. Techniques for Modeling the Hearing Aid Receiver and Associated Tubing. In G. A. Studebaker and I. Hochberg (Eds.), *Acoustical Factors Affecting Hearing Aid Performance*. Baltimore: University Park Press, 1980.

Engebretson, A., and Miller, J. A computer program for fitting a master hearing aid to the residual hearing characteristics of individual patients. *J. Acoust. Soc. Am.* 72:426–430, 1982.

Engebretson, A., Morley, R., Popelka, G., Niemoeller, A., and Heidbreder, A. A digital hearing aid. Presented at the 18th International Congress of Audiology, Santa Barbara, Calif., 1984.

Feldman, S. What is Certifit? *Hear. Instr.* 33:7, 1982.

Feldman, S., and Malacek, R. Signal processing techniques in a computerized hearing aid test system. *J. Acoust. Soc. Am.* 62:1457–1462, 1977.

Gans, D. P., VerHoef, N., and Berger, K. W. Hearing aid selection by computer. *Hear. Instr.* 34:5, 1983.

Glascoe, G. *Hearing Aid Manager*. State College, Pa.: Parrot Software, 1984.

Glascoe, G. *Select a Hearing Aid*. State College, Pa.: Parrot Software, 1984.

Glascoe, G., and Johnson, R. Computer oriented management for the selection of hearing aides. Scientific display, Annual Convention of the American Speech, Language and Hearing Association, 1975.

Graupe, D., Beex, A., and Causey, D. ARMA filter and method for designing the same. U.S. Patent 4,188,667, 1982.

Karzon, R., and Nielmoeller, A. A model for predicting hearing aid performance. *Scand. Audiol.* 12:275–284, 1983.

Katz, K. Computers . . . every office needs one! *Hear. Instr.* 34:7, 1983.

Katz, K. *Hearing Aid Computer Simulation and Sales Program* (3rd ed.). Tucson: Katz Computer Software, 1984.

Lauridsen, O., and Nielsen, H. B. A new computerized method for hearing aid fitting based on measurements at the ear drum. *Scand. Audiol.* 10:109–113, 1981.

Levitt, H., Neuman, A., Mills, R., and Schwander, T. A digital master hearing aid. *J. Rehabil. Eng. Res. Dev.* Submitted.

Mangold, S., and Leijon, A. Programmable hearing aid with multichannel compression. *Scand. Audiol.* 8:121–126, 1979.

Mangold, S., and Leijon, A. Multichannel compression in a portable programmable hearing aid. *Hear. Aid J.* 34:6–10, 1981.

Moomaw, D. G. *Systematic Hearing Aid Prescription* (SHAP) User Guide. Youngstown, Ohio, 1984.

Nielsen, H. B. Evaluation of hearing aid evaluation by listening to the test signal at the eardrum. *Hear. Instr.* 35:1, 1984.

Nunley, J., Staab, W., Steadman, J., Wechsler, P., and Spencer, B. A wearable digital hearing aid. *Hear. Aid J.* 36:29–34, 1983.

Pascoe, D. P. An approach to hearing aid selection. *Hear. Instr.* 29:6, 1978.

Pascoe, D. P. Clinical implications of nonverbal methods of hearing aid selection and fitting. *Semin. Speech Lang. Hear.* 1:217–229, 1980.

Popelka, G., and Engebretson, A. M. A computer-based system for hearing aid assessment. *Hear. Instr.* 34:6, 1983.

Preves, D. The potential of computers and signal processing for hearing aids. *Hear. Instr.* 31:15–16, 1982.

Preves, D. *Computerized Fitting Analyzer (CFA) Software.* Minneapolis: Starkey Laboratories, 1984.

Rasmussen, S. B. How insertion gain measurements can take the guess work out of hearing aid fittings. *Hear. Instr.* 35:1, 1984.

Skinner, M. W., and Miller, J. D. Amplification bandwidth and intelligibility of speech in quiet and noise for listeners with sensorineural hearing loss. *Audiology* 22:253–279, 1983.

Skinner, M. W., Pascoe, D. P., Miller, J. P., and Popelka, G. R. Measurements to Determine the Optimal Placement of Speech Energy within the Listener's Auditory Area: A Basis for Selecting Amplification Characteristics. In G. A. Studebaker and F. H. Bess (Eds.), *The Vanderbilt Hearing Aid Report.* Monograph in Contemporary Audiology, 1982.

Stacey, J. St.G. *Hearing Aid Selection Procedure Using a Small Home Computer.* Sheffield, U.K.: Hearing Aid Tinnitus Services, 1984.

Stein, L. K., and Dempesey-Hart, D. Listener-assessed intelligibility of a hearing aid self-adaptive noise filter. *Ear Hear.* 5 (24): 199–204, 1984.

Voroba, B. Perspectives on the state of hearing aid fitting practices. *Audecibel* 31:12–16, 1982.

Voroba, B. A tool for the optimization of hearing aid fittings. *Hear. Instr.* 86:1, 1984.

Walden, B. E., Schwartz, D. M., Williams, D. L., Holum-Hardegen, L. L., and Crowley, J. M. Test of the assumptions underlying comparative hearing aid evaluations. *J. Speech Hear. Disord.* 48:264–273, 1983.

Walden, B. H. Validating Measures for Hearing Aid Success. In G. A. Studebaker and F. H. Bess (Eds.), *The Vanderbilt Hearing Aid Report.* Monographs in Contemporary Audiology, 1982.

14

Computers in Research Design and Analysis

James R. Murphy

"If we don't know where we are going, what does it matter how fast we get there?" If there is ever a contest for an official caveat of the computer age, the above sentence will be a definite contender. While the computer has given us new freedom from some of the drudgery of data collection and analysis, our responsibility to ensure that we know what we are doing has increased. Piles of meaningless printed output, as well as unexpected and inexplicable results need to be guarded against as much as conventional problems such as poor experimental design and arithmetic error.

Since the computer makes it easy to explore a data set, and since the probability structure for discovered results is different from the structure for a priori hypothesized results, the researcher must take care before requesting, and especially when interpreting, a myriad of computer output. This warning presupposes that the right data were collected, that the data were correctly entered into the computer, and that the data have been correctly stored over time.

MICROCOMPUTER SELECTION

The following advice is for those who have not yet purchased their computer. The computer is the used car of the twenty-first century. There are as many options, deals, and discounts in the computer market as there are on the used-car sales lot. There is even a developing market in used computers, and, because of the rapid advance of technology, there is built-in planned obsolescence. All of this means that the first-time buyer needs to arm himself or herself with a bit of knowledge before the purchase commitment is made.

The best armament is having a clear idea of exactly what you want your new system to do for you. Since computers are usually multipurpose machines, they can probably do more than you plan initially. However, if the computer does well the major thing that you planned for it, the rest is gravy. Moreover, if your system is doing what you planned for it to do in an efficient way, it does not matter quite so much that if you had just waited one more year to purchase it, it would have been faster, smarter, had more memory, etc.

Having a few well-planned projects in the back of your mind is a great help when dealing with salesmen. There is nothing that puts the damper on unintelligible sales jargon faster than asking for a demonstration of the computer's capabilities to perform a project of your choosing. This does not mean that you should not learn something about the function of a computer and the attendant terminology before you begin the serious effort involved to purchase one. Knowing a little bit of the jargon and how it relates to the function of the computer is very useful. This chapter will give you some ideas about what to look for in a computer that has as one of its main functions the handling of *research data*.

Some final observations for those who have not purchased their microcomputer include the following advice:

1. Make a checklist of what you want the microcomputer to do for you—today, next month, next year, and in 3 years.
2. Ask for a demonstration of the computer's ability to do the one or two major things that you want it to do (benchmarking).
3. Be aware that you may need to make some changes in your physical plant to provide a reduced-static, low-dust, moderate-temperature environment for the computer.
4. Find a group of people who are already using the type of microcomputer that you want to buy (a user group), and talk with them. Chances are that someone in the group has an application similar to yours and can tell you how that microcomputer works for that application.

DATA COLLECTION

To the computer, there are two types of data that can be collected: analog-signal data and digital data. Analog data is generated by changes in the flow of electrical current. Oscilloscopes, strip charts, and a particular type of computer that has been constructed to deal with changes in electrical current are examples of analog processors. Microcomputers are digital processors, which means that they deal with data as discrete packets of information and not as changes in a continuous flow of electricity. Analog data can be captured, stored, processed, transformed, and transferred on microcomputers, but the data is chopped up into discrete packets, and this requires some additional processing capability that does not come as standard equipment on most microcomputers. If your research application requires that you capture analog data, be prepared to spend some time and effort making this work correctly.

The major part of research data is captured as digital data. Even a straight or curved line can be stored as a very large number of individual Y-axis values that correspond to small incremental changes in the X axis. These data are entered into the computer from the keyboard or in some cases from an electronic drawing pad. The point of concern is that these data be entered correctly, stored correctly for varying lengths of time, and transferred correctly to output devices such as printers.

Correct data entry requires an interaction between the person entering the data and the computer. The human side of the equation requires an easy-to-read computer screen, a comfortable place to work while entering data for long periods of time, and a system that is easy to work with, as described in Chapter 2. The computer requires an environment that is free of dust and static with adequate cooling, and software that meets the user's needs.

Most research done on human subjects requires the collection of a variety of different types of data—age, sex, etc. This type of collection is best done using some type of data-base management system (see Chap. 4).

The system should be easy to learn and use, provide for checking to ensure that variables being entered are within specified ranges of correct values, provide an easy way to put together specified groups of variables, and create reports. Try reading the sections on data entry and report generation in the instruction manuals of any data-base management system that you intend to buy. This will give you some idea of how easy it will be to use the program.

Plan ahead because when the operator becomes competent in the use of the system, processes such as menus, which made the system easy to learn, will become cumbersome. You should look for a system that allows easy access and a great deal of assistance for the novice user, and a quicker way of performing the same tasks for the accomplished user. If the tasks in mind require many back-and-forth comparisons between different sections of text, it may be useful to look for a system that allows different "windows" into the file that can be displayed simultaneously.

All data should be backed up several times for microcomputer systems—that is, make several copies of data disks. It is also desirable to have as a part of the data-base management program, or as a separate program, an easy way of comparing the data on two disks. This allows the user periodically to check one of the backup disks against another to make sure that the data are maintaining their integrity during storage.

Data-base management programs are among the most complex software available for purchase for the microcomputer. The user must plan on spending 3 to 6 months in training to use the program to its full capacity. Check with the supplier or manufacturer of the data-base program to see if training is available; also check with the supplier or manufacturer to see whether they provide support if something goes wrong—for example, a hotline number you can call to get help while using the program. Database systems will use up much of the microcomputer memory. Be sure that enough memory space is available to run the project you have in mind before purchasing the data-base program.

The report-generating abilities of the data-base system are where all the tables are put together for presentation. The system should be capable of outputting data in such a way that the data can be tabled and incorporated into a written report in your word-processor program. The system should also be able to put together a data set that can be used by your statistical-analysis program and your graphics package. In short, merely collecting the data on your data base will not be useful unless it is easy to interface the data-base systems with other areas where the data can be used.

QUALITY CONTROL

The computer is an excellent resource for maintaining data quality. In addition to providing range-checking on input and comparison of data disks, the microcomputer provides an easy way to look at the data often and in a variety of configurations. Coupling some simple data analysis closely in time with the data-collection process during data entry often helps identify errors early while the errors are still relatively easy to correct.

Printing a frequency table for discrete data will reveal discrepancies that may have slipped past the data-entry routines. A word of caution is in order, however, because it is generally better to establish a specific value for missing data than to use blanks or zeros. Not all microcomputers handle blanks and zeros in the same way. Some computers cannot even distinguish the difference between a blank and a zero. Should a blank be used to indicate a missing value, you are never sure if the value is really missing, or if someone just forgot to ask the question.

Look at the data often and in a variety of ways. This is the best safeguard against errors. Do not drop the data in the "black hole" of the data-base manager and expect the data magically to produce error-free results 5 years later.

RESEARCH DESIGN

There are as yet no packaged programs available for microcomputers that provide a design scheme and sample-size calculations. Sample-size programs are easy to write if a statistics book is handy and someone is available who is reasonably well versed in a language that works for the microcomputer in use. However, the computer can be incorporated into the management of a particular research design. For example, if you are conducting a study that requires that data be collected at several different times, a date command can be activated on computers having an internal clock that will print a list of all data that needs to be collected on a given day. What might be done with a microcomputer to help manage the particular project depends on what the project is and the level of programming help available.

Table 14-1 contains a brief description of basic research designs. Included for each design is an indication of the statistics that are usually computed for that design and an indication of what a microcomputer might do to help manage that design. Since this chapter specifically concerns research, nonexperimental (observational) designs—those without a comparison or control group—are excluded. A control group is a comparison group that was defined before the experiment began so that it would contain a specific set of individuals. Inferences can then be made with respect to the specific characteristics of the control group. For example, selecting a control group of all women without breast cancer to compare with a group of women with breast cancer in order to determine the difference in the smoking habits of the two groups is better than selecting a comparison group of hospital patients (both men and women) who happen not to have breast cancer.

DATA ANALYSIS

Statistical-analysis programs for microcomputers do not have the same demand as spread-sheet or word-processing programs. Accordingly, there is only a limited variety of statistical-analysis programs available, and they tend to be mixed in their performance capabilities and quality of programming.

An important consideration for a statistical-analysis program is the ease of use. It is convenient to find a program that allows data entry on a case-by-case basis. The statistics program should be able to save, retrieve, and transform raw data as the need arises. It should also be able to take the output from one analysis for use as input in a second analysis. For ex-

*Table 14-1. Commonly used experimental designs.**

I. *Self-Comparison Designs*
This design (sometimes referred to as pretest–post-test, before and after, cross-over, or repeated-measures experiments) compares each subject to itself. These are most frequently analyzed with a cross-over or repeated-measures analysis of variance, or paired t-tests. Data-base management systems can be programmed so that interventions are given in the proper sequence, with appropriate washout periods observed and nonpaired data dropped out.

II. *Independent Comparison (Control) Group Designs*
Differences between a study or treated group and an untreated (comparison) group are examined. Typical statistical tests are the t-test for differences in means or the chi-square test for differences in proportions. The microcomputer can quickly provide the means and standard deviations of any variable in either group and select out the number of observations that fall in a given range while calculating proportions.

III. *Randomized Control-Group Designs*
To overcome possible selection bias of Designs I and II, subjects are randomly selected from some specified population to go into either a treated group or a control group. The statistical tests for these designs are similar to the tests in Design II, but the inference may be quite different. A computerized random-number generation program can select a truly random sample from the population.

* For further reading on research designs and their inherent problems, see Michael et al., *Biomedical Bestiary: An Epidemiologic Guide to Phantoms, Flaws, and Fallacies in the Medical Literature*, Boston: Little, Brown, 1984. Consult with a statistician before becoming too involved in a complex design, data collection, or analysis scheme.

ample, the statistics program might calculate the means of observations at 20 different points in time from the raw data, and then run a regression analysis on these means.

Another important consideration is the accuracy of the results produced by the analysis program. Accuracy is determined by the number of digits that are used for computation, by the rounding or truncation procedure used when the number of digits that can be carried is exceeded, and by the actual algorithms used to carry out the statistical computations. A simple check for the accuracy of calculations is to have the analysis package compute the mean and standard deviation first for the digits 1 through 9 and then for the numbers 1,000,001 through 1,000,009. In the first problem the mean should be 5 with a standard deviation of 2.73861279. In the second problem, the mean should be 1,000,005 with a standard deviation that is exactly the same as that found in the first problem—that is, 2.73861279. If you do not get the same number of significant digits for the standard deviation of 1 through 9, the computer may not be carrying enough digits in its computations to provide an accurate output. If a different value is noted for the standard deviation of 1,000,001 through 1,000,009, the algorithms being used for computations are not the best available. In either case, complex statistical operations and computations involving a large number of observations should not be done with such a limited system.

Other slightly more complicated checking can be done for procedures such as regression (Lachenbruch, 1983). Even if the analysis package and

Table 14-2. Commonly used statistics and statistical tests for normally distributed (continuous) and binomially distributed (discrete) data.

A. Single variable

Statistical Interest Measure	*Continuous*		*Discrete*	
	Descriptive	Inferential	Descriptive	Inferential
Central tendency	$\bar{x}$ (sample mean)	Z score, one sample test	p (sample proportion)	Chi-square binomial test
	Median mode			
Variance	s^2 (sample clearance)	One sample Chi-square	p q/n	
	s (sample standard deviation)			
	$s/s\sqrt{n}$ (sample standard error)			
	$s/\bar{x}$ (sample coefficient of variation)			
Distribution	Frequency histogram			
	Cumulative frequency histogram			
	Quantiles			
	Box plots			

B. Two variables

Statistical Interest Measure	*Continuous Inferential*	*Discrete Inferential*
Means	Paired observations	Paired observations
	Paired t-test	McNemar's test
	Independent observations	Independent observations
	T-test (equal variance)	Fisher's exact test
	T-test (unequal variance)	Binomial test
		Chi-square test
Variances	Two-sample F-test	
Distribution	Scatterplots (descriptive)	
Association	(r) (correlation)	
	Linear regression	
	Polynomial regression	

C. More than two variables

Statistical Interest Measure	*Continuous Inferential*
Means	Analysis of variance
Association	Multiple regression

computer system pass all the checks, it is a good idea to have a set of test data for which the statistical results are known. This test set should be run periodically on the microcomputer to check the output of the statistical packages.

A second set of test data that can be used when evaluating a statistical-analysis package is one with a number of known errors in it. Running this set of data will allow you to check the error diagnostics (error messages) embedded in the statistical package. Of course, the statistical package should be able to find all the errors that are placed in the data set.

Writing personal programs for data analysis is something to be considered. However, since errors in numeric output are often difficult to spot, be prepared to do a lot of checking of results with test-data sets. It is a good idea to set up a regular testing schedule, once a week, once a month, etc., to make sure that the personal program has not been accidently changed.

The following general rules apply when writing your own programs: (1) Back up personal programs—that is, make several copies. (2) Protect personal programs so that others cannot accidently write over or change your code. (3) Spend considerable time planning the program before beginning to write it. Consider the following questions: How many ways do you want to get the data into the program? What do you want to do with the data? How many people will be using the program? What kind of instructions and data labeling are needed? (4) Make each function of the program a separate unit or module so it will be easy to change parts of the program without changing the whole thing. (5) Determine if you have the best algorithm for what you want to do. There are many different ways to do statistical computations, and some are better for use on microcomputers than others. For additional suggestions on program writing see Ledin and Ledin (1979).

Table 14-2 contains some commonly used statistics that most microcomputer statistics programs should have. For more information on these statistics and their use, consult a general statistics test such as Snedecor and Cochran (1971).

DATA PRESENTATION

In addition to a word processor, a printer and possibly a graphics program may be needed to preserve the data in some permanent form. If a large number of reports must be printed out, the printer will become a bottleneck to an efficient operation. Printers print reports at rates from 10 to 300 characters per second. Microcomputers can send data at speeds up to 9600 characters per second. This difference in processing speed creates the printer bottleneck. Printer bottleneck is alleviated by the purchase of a printer buffer. This buffer is a piece of hardware that holds data sent by your microcomputer until the printer can process it, permitting the computer to continue processing data while the report is being printed. Unfortunately, there may still be a wait for the printer to finish printing a lengthy report.

A variety of printers are available for use including ink-jet, thermal, dot-matrix, and daisy-wheel printers. To decide on an appropriate type of printer take into consideration the initial cost, the quality of print desired, the cost of maintenance, and the speed at which printed output is produced. Take additional care that the printer can be connected to your microcomputer and that some reputable firm will take responsibility for service of both the microcomputer and the printer. Otherwise, you may wind up dealing with two groups of service people, each blaming the other for the malfunction of your computer-printer combination.

Make sure the printer will produce the graphic output you need. Almost all printers will produce graphics of some kind, but the pictures produced may not be sufficiently smooth (have a high enough resolution) to be of publishable quality. To get very good-quality graphics and the ability to produce charts, tables, pictures, etc., in multiple colors, a plotter may be necessary in addition to the printer. There are printer-plotters on the market, but consider carefully how much the plotting capability slows down the printing capability, whether the device can make plots in multiple colors, and how much manipulation is required (e.g., it might be necessary to change pens to achieve a particular plot).

If your microcomputer has a color monitor (television screen), consider taking photographs directly from the screen for slide presentations. A high-resolution monitor and graphics package is required for high-quality slides. A certain amount of practice with various camera lens openings and exposure times is necessary to produce good slides inexpensively.

Figures 14-1, 14-2, and 14-3 illustrate some standard graphic proce-

Fig. 14-1. Plot of the minimum, maximum, and mean and standard deviation of fevers for hospitalized patients in four different outcome groups. The means for the groups are connected by the jagged line. The standard deviations about the means are represented by the vertical lines with tic marks at each end, and the minimal and maximal fevers are at the ends of the vertical lines.

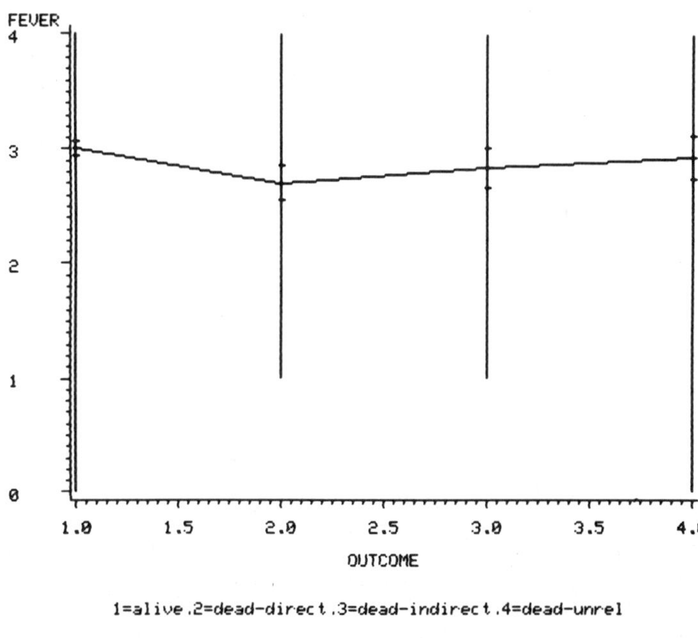

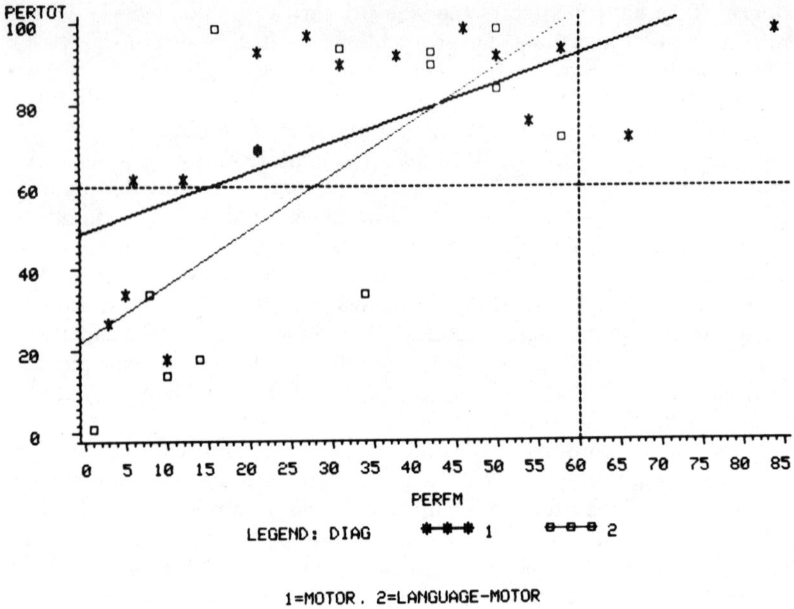

Fig. 14-2. Discrimination using performance versus fine motor. Scatterplot of two groups of subjects with linear regression lines with reference axes. The ability to plot data with different characters (and □) is useful. Overlaying the regression lines indicates a similar correlation between PERTOT and PERFM for both diagnostic (DIAG) groups. The reference axes make it clear that this is not a random scatter of points, i.e., most of the observations for both diagnostic groups fall above 60 for PERTOT and below 60 for PERFM.*

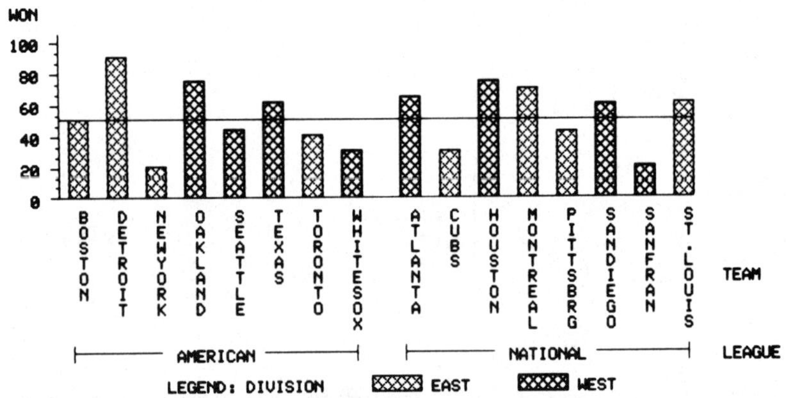

Fig. 14-3. Basic histogram showing the percentage of games won by each team (broken down by division). The horizontal line is at the 50% point. This graph illustrates a variety of type fonts and label options.

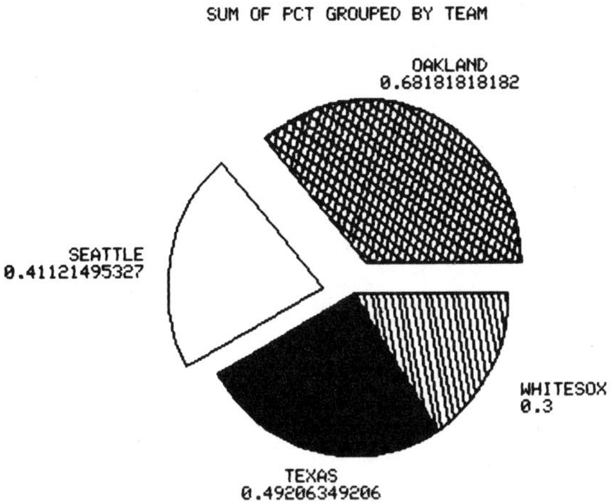

Fig. 14-4. Worst of the American League West. Pie chart in which the area of the circle allotted to each team represents the proportion of games won in relation to the other teams represented in the circle. For example, the total proportion of games won by all teams in the circle is 1.88. Oakland contributed a proportion of 0.68 to that total, so Oakland gets 0.68/1.88 = 0.36, 36%, or a little over one third of the area of the circle.

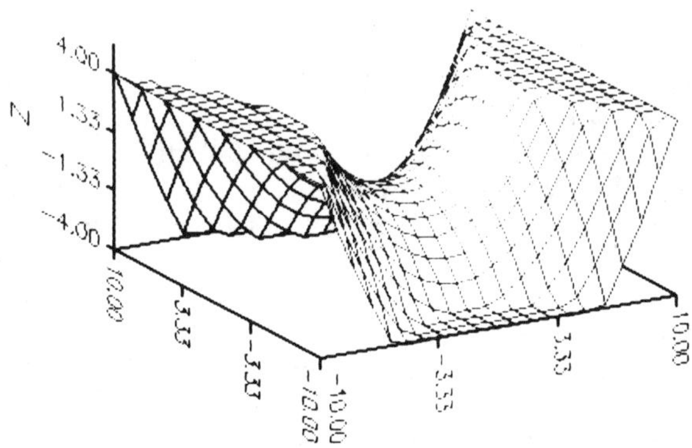

Fig. 14-5. Three-dimensional plot of a mathematical function. The ability to tilt and rotate such plots may be useful in certain research areas. Projected large axis labels and tic-mark labels are perpendicular to axes.

dures frequently used in research presentations. Figures 14-4 and 14-5 are optional graphics that may be useful for certain research projects. These graphics were done with the *SAS/GRAPH* program using a Tectronix 4165 terminal and a Tectronix 4695 printer.

Colored graphics allow you to put a great deal of information on a single plot. Also, having different type fonts for titles, axis labels, and footnotes helps make graphs more readable. It is also useful for a graphics software program to have default (prespecified) values. Default values allow the user to do a rough plot quickly, but later, as shown in Figure 14-1, it might be an improvement to go back and make changes. For Figure 14-1 the changes might involve removing the 1.5, 2.5, and 3.5 horizontal tic marks and moving the lines for outcome group 1 away from the vertical axis.

In addition, the ability to expand specified areas of a plot or drawing in order to achieve greater detail and the ability to animate certain figures may be useful graphic options in specific research areas. Adding these options makes the hardware and software more expensive, as you might expect.

OTHER CONSIDERATIONS

Because of the lack of good statistical-analysis programs on microcomputers, or for other reasons, it may be useful to connect the personal computer to a larger mainframe computer. Sending individual lines (strings) of data between machines is usually easy to accomplish over telephone lines using a modem, which changes electronic pulses into sound pulses. There are a few requirements that must be met to match up the microcomputer and the mainframe computer, so you will need to work with someone to determine the type of data coding used (ASCII or EBCIDIC), the type of transmitting protocol (asynchronous or synchronous), etc. In general, however, transmitting data strings between personal and mainframe computers is not a serious problem.

If a large amount of data is involved, however, the process can be speeded up by transferring a large number of strings (files) quickly. At this point, the transfer of information between micro- and mainframe computers becomes considerably more difficult. Each type of computer has special instructions that are placed in files to define such things as the beginning and ending of the file and the length of the data strings (now called records) in the file. Data-base files contain more characters to establish links between records, and word-processing files have still more characters. In addition, record and file sizes may be different between the microcomputer and the mainframe computer. Unless the special characters and file and record sizes are recognized in the same way by both computers, a special program is required in order to transfer large blocks of data such as files.

To enter text or data-base material through the microcomputer to the mainframe computer is far more difficult than simply sending a file of already collected data to the mainframe computer in order to use its statistical analysis capabilities. Check with the people in charge of running the larger mainframe computer about how this data transfer can be accomplished.

In order to take complete advantage of the capabilities of both the microcomputer and the mainframe computer while they are connected to one another, the microcomputer must act like (emulate) a terminal with which the mainframe computer is familiar. Terminal-emulator programs are not plentiful, and if you want to use your microcomputer in this manner, take particular care in its selection and purchase so that the microcomputer can actually work with the mainframe computer.

In addition to connecting the microcomputer to a larger mainframe computer, it may be useful to connect together more than one microcomputer. This can be accomplished with telephone modems by sharing disks. If the microcomputers are the same brand and model, there should be no problem. If the microcomputers are different brands or different models of the same brand, however, it is necessary to verify that they are able to communicate. Problems can be present, however, even when the microcomputers are the same brand and same model if, for example, the disk heads are not aligned the same way on both disk-drive mechanisms.

Connecting several microcomputers together so they can share memory or computing power (networking) may someday be a viable consideration in any facility, clinic, or research laboratory. At the time of this writing, problems in maintaining accurate communication, loss of processing speed, and problems with rapid memory transfer make networking a specialized area that most microcomputer users will find cumbersome.

Sharing information using electronic mail, or using large data repositories (information utilities) is certainly an enjoyable part of owning a microcomputer. Face it—it is fun to scan and print sections of the *New York Times* on your microcomputer! The research application of this capability may be limited, however. To retrieve abstracts, bibliographies, or articles from a data base, such as MEDLINE, requires training to learn the special indexing system. Sharing up-to-the-minute research information with colleagues is an intriguing idea, but it requires an always-available host computer so that telephoning is, in fact, probably less expensive.

For further reading in the area of research design and analysis, see the Selected Reading list at the back of the book.

15

Microcomputers in Office Management of Speech and Hearing Facilities

Larry L. Ball,
Charlie D. Anderson, and
Christopher Schweitzer

The addition of microcomputers to any environment really implies that the functions currently performed need to be speeded up or implemented in a different fashion to be more consistent with new requirements. In the implementation of this change, it may become clear that not everyone supports the change. The people who are going to be involved in the process or who are affected by the change must be educated and made aware of the possible problems along the way. The trick, of course, is to minimize the impact of new tools on the user's expectations of his or her job performance. Fear and lack of identification with new technology are nowhere more accentuated than in the office environment. In order to overcome the initial resistance that accompanies fear and lack of identification, the potential user must be made to feel comfortable with the mechanism of automation and its implementation. The rest of this chapter will deal with the objective issues, as opposed to the subjective issues, of office automation. The wise office manager must acknowledge that new hardware, software, and networking will not make the system work without the full cooperation of the essential ingredient—the human being.

TECHNICAL INGREDIENTS

Office automation means different things to different people. All the technologies of computer science, electronics, and mechanical engineering come together in the office environment of today to window what we can expect in the twenty-first century. In today's world, office automation means that we have at our fingertips the following technology:

1. Complete information retrieval on patient demographics, financial relationship to the practice, test results, clinical notes, and special analytical results—in other words, an *integrated data base*
2. Complete networking of workstations within the practice, should multiple functions and high-volume usage be required
3. Variability of printer output, such that drafts, graphs, and letter-quality documents can be generated from the same system
4. Graphics capability at the workstations and at suitable printers
5. Accessibility to outside information sources, such as bibliographic searches and electronic reimbursements
6. Full range of software products to support all office information needs and functions

These features usually come packaged in the form of a display medium, a keyboard, and other ancillary hardware. Some of these features are found in products sold in common business or computer stores. All of these features, however, are only found in special-purpose systems designed or programmed for practices in the hearing and speech sciences. The hardware features alluded to are seldom found in common computers, because such machines are usually inexpensive and therefore possess minimal capability. The software systems found in home computers also leave much to be desired, because sophisticated programs such as the ones required in this medical specialty cannot be accommodated on such limited workstations.

INTEGRATED DATA BASE

Office administration is integrally associated with clinical data and, in this regard, not only does a sophisticated data base have to be available to the office user, but also it has to be a data base that can access both types of information. For instance, patient demographic information—such as address, insurance carrier, date of birth, and identification number—is as important to the clinical application as it is to the administrative system. Figure 15-1 shows a complete demographic data set for a particular patient in a clinic as it might appear on a computer. The entry of such data requires the same effort (or less) as that required to enter the same data on typewritten cards. The significant difference, however, is that once entered into the system, the data can be used to support a variety of functions, such as data-base searching or automatic appending of information to insurance forms, none of which requires repetitious typing as it would in the manual environment. (It is here that word processing has changed the life of the person who has been introduced to it.)

This same information is also used in the clinical environment to associate records of some sort with the appropriate patient. In order for the office system to manage this environment adequately, a variety of information must be accommodated. This information comes in the form of clinical test results, clinical notes, schedules, account status reports, etc. This requires that the software system be able to accommodate a variety of formats and a large number of patient files as well. The formats for a typical clinical operation could vary considerably in number and style, an example of which (a patient history) is shown in Figure 15-2. An ideal program is one in which the format for each type of form can be designed on the screen by the user. All forms, whether they be patient histories, hearing-aid inventories, or anything else, should be capable of being recalled at the user's discretion. Finally, each form with patient information included should be able to be recalled instantly. The technology required to implement such a sophisticated feature is a large "hard-disk" permanent-storage medium and a software program to implement this electronic filing system.

Special analytical or test results derived from patient visits are an integral part of the office-management function because demographic data, scheduling, and (of course) billing functions support the patient visit. The analytical and test results become part of the system's data base by way of automated collection or by manual input. In the automated environment,

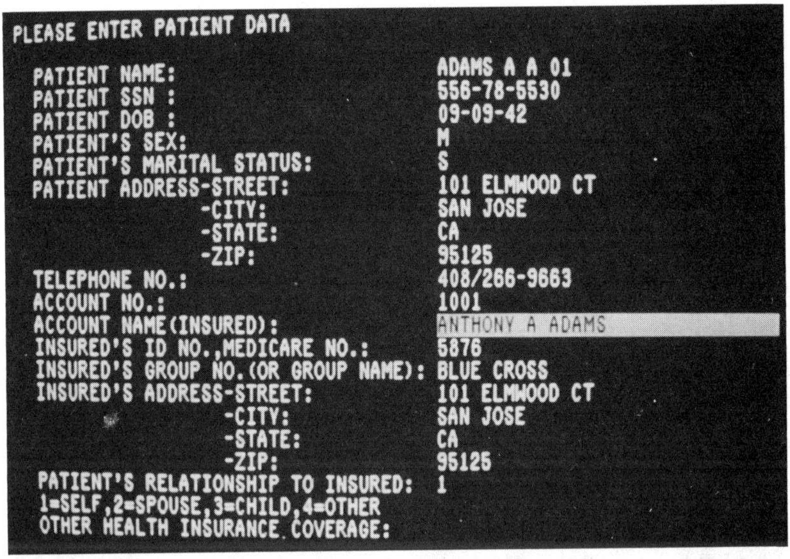

Fig. 15-1. Computer screen showing typical demographic data set for a patient.

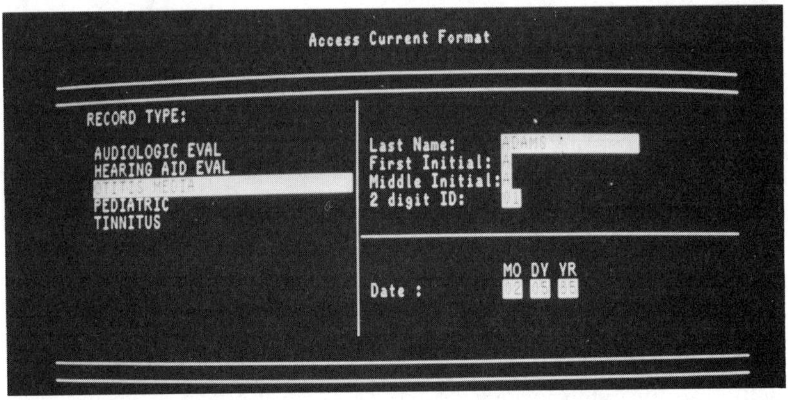

Fig. 15-2. Computer screen showing typical patient history information.

the examiner has minimal involvement with the data and can therefore devote his or her time to involvement with the patient. The data are automatically collected by some appropriately designed hardware unit, such as the one shown in Figure 15-3, which converts the signals to a form that can be read by the computer system. Administrative annotations, such as a patient's social security number or date of birth, are either added manually or appended automatically from a previously existing data base. This data base comes from the information already known about the

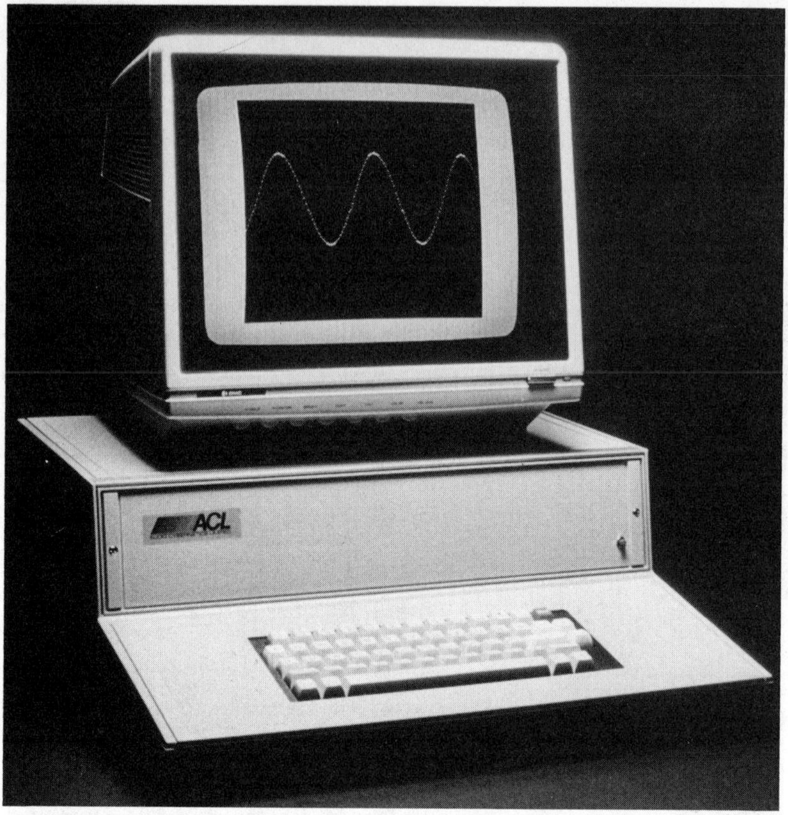

Fig. 15-3. ENG acquisition terminal.

patient as a result of his or her declarations to the office management function.

Patient scheduling is an office function that also fits well within the integrated scheme of things. It allows the clinician to schedule as well as track patient visits and past testing through the clinic environment. This facility is illustrated in Figure 15-4. This is just one small example of the additional functionality and capability of an integrated information environment.

The subject that receives the most attention these days is that of accounts receivable. The efficiency of a well-run office is probably best reflected in its patient-billing capabilities. This is truly the focal point of the operation, where all information on intake from patients, costing, traceability of various payments and charges, and test information come together. A recent innovation in this all-important function is that of electronic reimbursements. This feature allows the clinician to apply for insurance reimbursement through the Medicare and Medicaid systems and probably soon will support paybacks from private carriers, too. Bill-

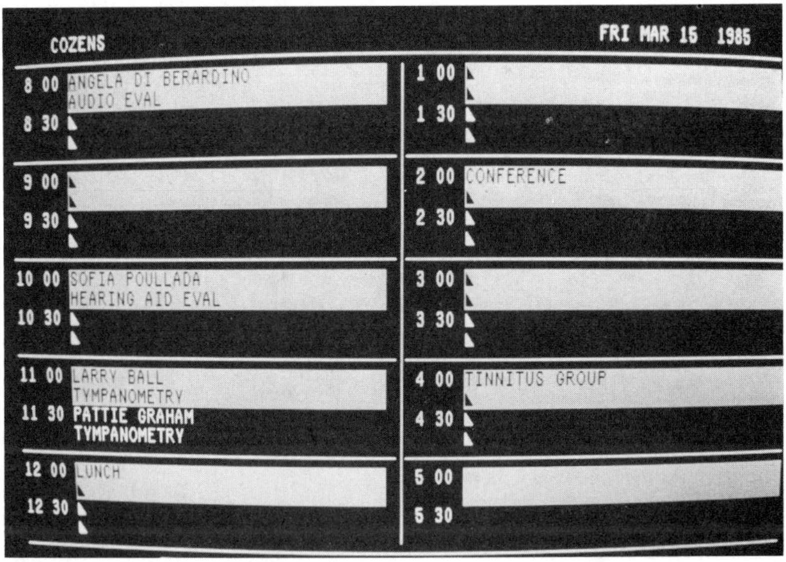

Fig. 15-4. Scheduling screen.

ing systems should be able to support a large variety of requirements. Some of these are inventory control, accounts payable, purchasing, payroll, and general ledger. A minimum of functions must be integral to the cost-recovery capability. These features include management of postings to several different clinicians, individual patient accounts with up-to-date totals of charges, payments, and aged-account information (Fig. 15-5). Printing of monthly statements and insurance forms for Medicare, Medicaid, and private insurance companies is necessary during the interim until replacement with electronic billing. Accounts should be aged on a monthly basis. A monthly billing-report capability should compile comprehensive, printed reports that categorize financial information. These should include a list of new and returning patients, revenue balances itemized by procedure or test, revenue balances itemized by clinician, payment totals itemized by reimbursement method, and delinquent accounts. These reports are updated and printed monthly.

NETWORKING WORKSTATIONS

All office functions are part of the major clinical scheme of things in which all functions are tied together by common data-recall capabilities, and in which all workstations are capable of "talking" to each other by some sort of networking scheme. It really makes no difference how cost-effective an integrated data-base system may be if all functions have to be performed at the same unit. The utility of the system is voided in cases in which the users cannot perform their own required functions simultaneously with others in the clinic. The clinical environment of today is one

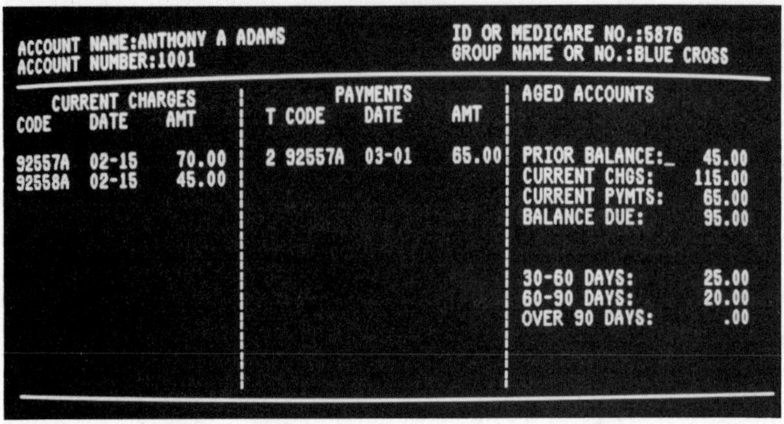

Fig. 15-5. Patient account screen.

in which the entire staff is accessing the same data base for both clinical and administrative needs and in which all information is available to the entire staff (within the realm of security). The adequate patient-information management system has the capability to provide all programs and data to anyone at any workstation. The basic scenario requires that each workstation in the network can run a different program simultaneously, and that all stations still have access to the patient-data files stored electronically within the system. High-volume operations are considerably enhanced by networks because simultaneous performance of the same function can be accommodated.

Each user needs to have his or her own password so that selective control of information can be maintained by the office manager. Such capabilities are not expensive, nor do they require that the clinic hire a computer expert. In some cases the clinical manager may want to protect receivables and reports pertaining to certain items by requiring the use of a password to access information in these areas.

PRINTED REPORTS

Two major types of printing are available today: letter quality and dot matrix. The letter-quality printing found in the office environment is identical to that generated by the conventional typewriter, where each stroke printed is generated by a preformed character on the typeball or typewheel. The dot-matrix form of printing is generated by a series of tiny ink dots that form the desired letters, numerals, or special characters. The dot-matrix printer is especially favored in those situations in which graphic representations are desired. This, of course, is required in much of the test-reporting in audiology. The letter-quality printer is favored in those more traditional situations in which communications are required, such as insurance reimbursements or referral reports. The point is that both types of printer should be accommodated in the typical office system. The user should also assure that the system can function with any letter-quality printer or dot-matrix printer, because it is never certain that the same printer will always be used. For instance, as the clinic grows, a faster printer may be required, and therefore new communications requirements may be necessitated that should be under software selection and control.

WORKSTATION PRESENTATIONS

The office system should be capable of displaying graphic presentations for the user. Patient-test results and analyses can be effectively shown only when they can be replicated on the computer at any time. The minimal system of one workstation must therefore be capable of graphics output, both on the display screen and on the dot-matrix printer. Because of the color scheme used in audiology, it is an advantage, but not necessary, to have color graphics. In those cases in which multiple workstations comprise the network, then at least one of the units must be a graphics station.

OUTSIDE SOURCES OF INFORMATION

The office environment may, from time to time, need to access outside information. This function can be supported only if the office system has communications capabilities with the outside world. Communications channels on a modem (a unit that conditions signals so that they can be handled over transmission lines) and telephone lines are necessary to do this. The modem usually operates in conjunction with a telephone receiver or has a dialing mechanism built into it. The only other requirements are that the user knows what he or she wants to tap into and has the appropriate passwords to enter the desired data base.

FULL RANGE OF SOFTWARE PRODUCTS

The clinical office supports many different functions as well as administrative tasks. This role requires that a wide range of software products be available to accommodate all such needs. It is entirely possible for anyone to develop his or her own software and hardware to meet individual needs. The question is, however, do you have time for such projects? Usually, the answer is *no*. It is much more advantageous for us to have a market to which we can go for our office automation needs, because our primary functions are in the clinic and not in the support of peripheral activities associated with the primary function.

It is much more advantageous for us to seek commercially developed software programs for our office automation needs and direct our professional energies toward patient-care activities. The commitment to develop new, specialized software for clinical-administrative computer automation is a long and expensive process, which often results in reinventing the wheel.

The potential for automating speech-hearing-language administrative responsibilities is easily at hand. Although incorporating automated, computer-managed functions into daily clinical routine is at first laborious and cumbersome, the end result is usually worth the initial effort. Integrated software will provide information that is useful to everyone on the staff and make the accountability of providing clinical speech and hearing services easier to evaluate.

Selected Reading

Carpenter, J., Deloria, D., and Morganstein, D. Statistical software for microcomputers. *Byte* 9:234–264, 1984.

Computers: should you take one into your home? *Consumer Reports* 48:461–488, 1983 (Part I); 48:531–551, 1983 (Part II).

Electric Industries Association. *How to Buy a Home Computer: A Guide for Consumers.* EIA Consumers Electronics Group. P.O. Box 19100, Washington, D.C. 20035, 1983.

Lachenbruch, P. A. Statistical programs for microcomputers. *Byte* 8:560–570, 1983.

Ledin, G., and Ledin, V. *The Programmer's Book of Rules.* Belmont, Calif.: Wadsworth, 1979.

McWilliams, P. *The Word Processing Book.* Los Angeles: Prelude, 1983.

McWilliams, P. *The Personal Computer Book.* Los Angeles: Prelude, 1983.

McWilliams, P. *The Personal Computer in Business Book.* Los Angeles, Prelude, 1983.

Michael, M., Boyce, W. T., and Wilcox, A. J. *Biomedical Bestiary: An Epidemiologic Guide to Flaws and Fallacies in the Medical Literature.* Boston: Little, Brown, 1984.

Snedcor, G. W., and Cochran, W. G. *Statistical Methods* (6th ed.) Ames, Iowa: University of Iowa, 1971.

The Carpenter and Lachenbruch articles contain useful information on selecting statistical packages. The articles in Consumer Reports *contain practical advice. Ledin and Ledin show how to make the program intelligible and helpful to the user. The books by McWilliams, a nontechnical series describing the use, misuse, frustration, frivolity, and ubiquitous nature of the microcomputer, are very readable introductions to various aspects of computer processing. Michael et al. has a wider scope than the title indicates and is a good introduction to several different research designs and their problems.*

GENERAL AND TECHNICAL MAGAZINES

There are a number of useful periodicals available to aid in the selection of microcomputer components and systems, including Byte, Creative Computing, Datamation, Family Computing, Personal Computing, *and* Popular Computing. Datamation *(business oriented) and* Byte *(hobbyist or engineering oriented) are especially useful in terms of keeping abreast of new products, projecting trends, and reviewing available software and hardware. In the field of speech synthesis devices for the handicapped,* Communication Outlook, *a quarterly from the International Society for*

Augmentative and Alternative Communication, is a good source for new product announcements, reviews of existing devices, local and regional interest groups, and upcoming conferences and workshops on nonoral modes of communication (c/o Artificial Language Laboratory, Computer Science Dept., Michigan State University, East Lansing, Mich. 48824) and PRC Current Expression, a quarterly from Frentke-Romisch Co., contains information on a wide variety of communication aids; the company also maintains an electronic bulletin board that can be accessed by users with telecommunications equipment (c/o Frentke-Romish Co., 8759, Twp. Road, Shreve, Ohio 44675 (216-567-2001).

USERS' GROUPS

An active users' group for speech-language—hearing professionals has been established under the leadership of James L. Fitch, Ph.D. Interested individuals are encouraged to join Computer Users in Speech and Hearing (CUSH) by writing to Dr. Fitch at the Communication Sciences Laboratory at the University of South Alabama, Mobile, Alabama 36688.

Index